THE   REHABILITATION   MEDICINE   SERVICES

The Rehabilitation Medicine Services

By

LAURENCE P. INCE, Ph.D.

Center for Learning Disabilities

Briarwood, New York

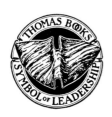

CHARLES C THOMAS • PUBLISHER

Springfield • *Illinois* • *U.S.A.*

Published and Distributed Throughout the World by
CHARLES C THOMAS • PUBLISHER
Bannerstone House
301-327 East Lawrence Avenue, Springfield, Illinois, U.S.A.

© *1974, by* CHARLES C THOMAS • PUBLISHER
ISBN 0-398-02852-4
Library of Congress Catalog Card Number: 73-4548

Printed in the United States of America

N-1

Library of Congress Cataloging in Publication Data
Ince, Laurence P.
    The Rehabilitation Medicine Services
    1. Physically handicapped—Rehabilitation.
I. Title.
[DNLM: 1. Physical therapy. 2. Rehabilitation.
HD 7255 136p 1973]
RD795.153   362.4   73-4548
ISBN 0-398-02852-4

This book is dedicated to my parents

and to my grandmother

PREFACE

Following World War II, the first comprehensive physical rehabilitation center in a general hospital was initiated at Bellevue Hospital in New York City under the direction of Howard A. Rusk. This early effort marked the true beginning of the field of rehabilitation medicine. Since that time well over 250 rehabilitation centers have been set up in hospitals and as separate institutions throughout the world.

Rehabilitation, broadly defined, is the restoration to as normal a life as possible of the person with a chronic physical disability. The objective of any rehabilitation program is to educate the man, woman or child with a residual handicap to function maximally within the limits imposed by that handicap. In rehabilitation, the emphasis is on the whole individual, encompassing his physical, psychological, educational, vocational and social needs. It is always the positive aspects of a patient's potential which are stressed. The attitude of those who work in the rehabilitation field is not that a patient cannot perform various life activities because of a particular disability, but instead, that there is a great deal which he can do despite the handicap. Rehabilitation then, is an endeavor requiring the skills of many trained professionals working together as a team toward a common goal, retraining a patient to live a satisfying, productive life despite a severe disability through making the fullest use of his remaining capacities following crippling disease or injury.

As greater numbers of our population become handicapped or disabled by injury and disease there is a growing need for multi-disciplinary facilities which combine many services. Among these services are physiatry, the medical specialty of rehabilitation medicine, physical therapy, occupational therapy, speech therapy, psychology, vocational counseling, social work, recreation therapy and nursing. This book, which has been more than three years in the writing, is about these services. It is designed to acquaint students planning on entering the rehabilitation field, new health workers in the field and rehabilitation professionals with the various disciplines which combine to form the rehabilitation team.

While the profession of physical rehabilitation has been rapidly growing, the literature has not kept equal pace with its growth. This book is an attempt to fill the void by describing, in detail, the rehabilitation services, their roles and functions. Conspicuously absent is a section on the role of the physician in rehabilitation. Such a section was omitted because a complete discussion of medicine is beyond the scope of the book and because there are many excellent texts available, such as the volume by Rusk, which provide thorough coverage of this material.

The first section of the book defines and describes the types of patient disabilities which are encountered in a rehabilitation setting. These chapters are not intended as a general medical text, but rather as a guide and orientation to the disorders which require physical rehabilitation. The remainder of the book is devoted to the various rehabilitation services and is intended to provide the reader with as complete a picture as possible of what the rehabilitation process encompasses.

I have gained pleasure and have learned much through my writing of this book. If the reader can also claim enjoyment and new knowledge through his reading of it I can ask no further reward.

New York, N.Y.   Laurence P. Ince

ACKNOWLEDGMENTS

No book, even if singly authored, such as this one is, is ever entirely the work of one individual. There are always others without whom the book either could not have been written or would not have been of the same quality or thoroughness. I would like to take the opportunity to mention those who have had a share in this work.

Grateful acknowledgment is given to the many people who have improved upon the quality of this book through their initial suggestions, their critical reading of various portions of the manuscript, their careful listening to my own readings and their patient answering of my many questions.

My heartfelt thanks go to Muraleedhara Menon, Alice Eason, Margaret Hundley, Yvette Coelho, Ann Goerdt, Dorothy Reiss, Lynn Singer, Matilda Lang and Leroy Carmichael.

I wish to express my appreciation to Arleen Mandia for her careful proofreading of the final manuscript.

All photographs other than those which were supplied by the manufacturers listed in the Permissions and Copyrights section were taken by Raoul Hurwitz.

I want to thank several people who, although they were not directly involved with the writing of this book, enabled me, through their teaching or kindness, to reach the stage in my career where I was able to engage in such work. They are Dwight Gardiner, G. M. Gilbert, Joel Greenspoon, Harold Cottingham and Joan Bardach.

To the many patients from whom I have learned much over the years goes my sincere gratitude.

And finally, since no author's work springs full-blown from his brow, but rather rests upon the efforts of those who have preceded him, I acknowledge my debt to the many authors cited at the end of each section of the book from whose labors I have profited.

L.P.I.

COPYRIGHTS AND PERMISSIONS

The following photographs are reprinted by permission of the Chattanooga Pharmacal Co., Chattanooga, Tenn.: the Hydrocollator® steam packs and Hydrocollator® master heating unit on p. 149; and the cold packs and Hydrocollator® master chilling units on p. 157.

The following photographs are reprinted by permission of the Ille Electric Corp., Williamsport, Pa.: the mobile paraffin bath on p. 150; the mobile hydrotherapeutic tank unit on p. 152; the Hubbard tank and therapeutic tank and pool on pp. 154 and 155.

The following photographs are reprinted by permission of the Burdick Corp., Milton, Wisc.: the infrared lamp on p. 159; the ultraviolet lamp on p. 162; the short wave diathermy unit on p. 167; the microwave diathermy unit on p. 170; and the combination electrical stimulator and ultrasound unit on p. 174.

The following photographs are reprinted by permission of Medco Products Co., Inc., Tulsa, Okla.: the ultrasound generator on p. 172.

The following photographs are reprinted by permission of the Florida Brace Corp., Winter Park, Fla.: the cervical collar on p. 181.

The following photographs are reprinted by permission of S. H. Camp and Co., Jackson, Mich.: the lumbosacral corset on p. 181; the back brace on p. 182; the axillary crutch on p. 186; the Lofstrand crutch on p. 188; the canes on p. 192; and the walkers on pp. 194 and 195.

The following photographs are reprinted by permission of Everest and Jennings, Inc., Los Angeles, Calif.: the Standard Universal wheelchair and the Hollywood wheelchair on p. 196; the Traveller wheelchair and tiny tot wheelchair on pp. 197 and 198; and the power drive wheelchair on p. 201.

The following photographs are reprinted by permission of L. Mulholland and Associates, Ventura, Calif.: the children's wheelchairs on pp. 198 and 200.

The following photographs are reprinted by permission of Institutional Industries, Cincinnati, Ohio: the reclining back wheelchair on p. 202; and the standard wheelchair on p. 204.

The following photographs are reprinted by permission of Rolls Equipment Inc., Division of Invacare Corp., Elyria, Ohio: the reclining wheelchair on p. 203; and the standard wheelchair on p. 204.

The following photographs are reprinted by permission of the Veterans' Administration Prosthetics Center, New York, N.Y. through the courtesy of Mr. Henry F. Gardiner: the lower extremity prostheses on pp. 208 and 210; the APRL voluntary closing hook on p. 277; the APRL hand on p. 278; the upper extremity prostheses on pp. 280 and 281; and the "Boston Arm" on p. 281.

The following photographs are reprinted by permission of Nilus Leclerc, Inc., L'Isletville, Que., Canada: the patient operating the foot-powered loom on p. 245; the weaving loom on p. 249; the weaving loom adapted for bed use on p. 251; the table loom on p. 255.

The following photographs are reprinted by permission of G. E. Miller, Inc., Yonkers, N.Y.: the "Deltoid-Aid" Brand® arm counterbalance on pp. 274 and 275.

The following photographs are reprinted by permission of Voiceprint Laboratories Corp., Somerville, N.J.: the sound spectrograph on p. 318.

The following photographs are reprinted by permission of Precision Acoustics Industries Inc., New York, N.Y.: the visible speech and articulation trainer on p. 320.

The following photographs are reprinted by permission of RIL Electronics, Inc.: the Echorder® training unit and the Echorder in use with a group of children on p. 334.

The following photographs are reprinted by permission of Tracor, Inc., Austin, Tex.: the two-channel clinical audiometer on p. 364; and the clinical Bekesy audiometer on p. 365.

The following photographs are reprinted by permission of the Beltone Electronics Corp., Chicago, Ill.: the two-channel pure tone and speech audiometer on p. 367; and the two-channel clinical research audiometer on p. 367.

The following photographs are reprinted by permission of Eckstein Brothers Inc., Hawthorne, Calif.: the binaural speech and auditory trainer on p. 374.

The following photographs are reprinted by permission of HC Electronics, Inc., Bellevedere-Tiburon, Mill Valley, Calif.: the Phonic Mirror® on p. 374.

The following photographs are reprinted by permission of Electronic Futures, Inc., North Haven, Conn.: the Audio Flashcard Reader® on p. 375.

The following photographs are reprinted by permission of Amsco Marketing, Erie, Pa., Division of American Sterilizer Co.: the floor loading steam sterilizer on p. 540.

The following photographs are reprinted by permission of the Castle Co., Division of Sybron Corporation, Rochester, N.Y.: the straightline steam sterilizer on p. 541; the table top steam sterilizer on p. 542; and the table top model autoclave on p. 543.

The following photographs are reprinted by permission of Vernitron Medical Products, Inc., Carlstadt, N.J.: the bulk sterilizer on p. 542.

The following photographs are reprinted by permission of Pharma-seal, Glendale, Calif.: the Foley catheter system on p. 557.

The following photographs are reprinted by permission of the Posey Co., Pasadena, Calif.: the foam heel protector on p. 558.

Contents

THE REHABILITATION MEDICINE SERVICES

THE DISORDERS AND DISABILITIES
OF REHABILITATION PATIENTS

Chapter 1

DISORDERS OF THE GENERAL ADULT PATIENT POPULATION

A s the life span of man continues to increase there is a corresponding rise in the incidence of chronic disability in the population. These are the patients for whom preventive and curative medicine and surgery have been employed to their utmost, but a residual physical disability remains. While these individuals constitute a minority of the general hospital patient population, they include within their group some of the most serious illnesses and severest injuries which are encountered within the health fields.

Rather than being acutely ill and requiring brief medical and paramedical therapeutics, the patients seen in a rehabilitation setting require either continuing, often lifelong medical treatment and therapeutic care, or a long, intensive period of general rehabilitation followed by occasional services. The former concerns the chronically ill whose constant need for care resembles that given to short-term patients. The latter are the persons who are chronically disabled as a consequence of acute disease or traumatic injury. Once they have received maximum benefit from therapy their needs for medical and paramedical services do not, with certain exceptions, differ greatly from the rest of the population.

Among the group of patients considered to be rehabilitation patients are those with spinal cord injuries, hemiplegia with or without aphasia, neurologic and neuromuscular disorders, muscular and musculoskeletal disabilities, metabolic diseases, pulmonary problems, cancer, cardiovascular diseases and geriatric disorders. With the exception of the last-named category these groupings can include children as well as adults, and it is, in fact, largely through efforts in the rehabilitation field that many children who were formerly destined to lead an unhappy, bedridden life can now look forward with optimism to a self-satisfying future.

SPINAL CORD INJURIES

Although spinal cord damage may be caused by either injury or disease, in the majority of patients undergoing rehabilitation it is a consequence of trauma. Direct traumatic insult to the spinal cord results in loss of bodily function, the return of which is quite limited. Such trauma encompasses concussion, compression, contusion, puncture, laceration, transection, vertebral dislocation and fracture-dislocation. Some of these injuries are a consequence of such behaviors as diving into shallow water and striking the head on the bottom of the enclosure, jumping from a height and landing on the feet so that the force of the impact is conducted upward with sudden violent flexion of the lower spine, or from athletic or automobile accidents, or from knife or gunshot wounds.

When the spinal cord is injured function is lost or impaired at the site of the injury and below. Loss is in both motor and sensory modalities and the degree of impairment is a consequence of both the level of the spinal cord at which the insult occurred and the extent of the damage produced by such insult. The resultant paralytic disability of spinal cord injury is termed either *quadriplegia,* when there is involvement of all four extremities, or *paraplegia,* when only the lower extremities are impaired, or *triplegia,* when three extremities are affected. Transections of the spinal cord typically produce motor and sensory paralysis or extreme weakness (hence, quadri-*paresis* or para*paresis*), loss of reflexes, loss of bowel and bladder control and generative function disorder. Medically, neurosurgery, urologic management and orthopedic surgery either in combination or as isolated procedures are required to reduce dislocations and compressions, muscle spasticity, intractable pain and bladder dysfunction. Nursing care is also highly important, particularly in the prevention of *decubiti,* or bedsores, which in the nonmobile patient can present serious problems.

The quadriplegic patient will always require some attendant care in the management of his person and his life. Attendant care for the paraplegic is dependent upon the level and extent of spinal cord injury, the paraplegic with damage in the cervical region of the cord being as limited in ambulation as the quadriplegic, but without sed-entary activity deficiencies.

The paraplegic patient with a high thoracic lesion has full upper extremity strength. He can transfer in and out of a wheelchair and is independent in self-care. Some ambulation with full bracing may be possible, but it is usually nonfunctional and he is primarily a wheelchair patient. A patient with a mid-thoracic lesion has good upper extremities and thoracic stabilization. Ambulation is possible on level surfaces. The paraplegic with a low thoracic lesion has, additionally, abdominal muscle strength. Thus, if adequately braced, he can climb stairs and curbs. The patient with a low lumbar or sacral lesion requires minimal bracing and is completely independent in all activities with only moderate deficiencies in ambulation and in some elevation activities.

HEMIPLEGIA

The term "hemiplegia" refers to a paralysis of the muscles of one side of the body which results from damage to parts of the brain on the side opposite, or contralateral to the muscular impairment. The brain areas most usually affected in hemiplegia are the cerebral cortex, the brain stem and the pyramidal tracts.

While this disability can be caused by tumor, cerebral anoxia, trauma or disease, the most frequent etiological factor seen among adult rehabilitation patients is a cerebrovascular accident (CVA) or *stroke*. Strokes may be due to a thrombosis, when a blood clot forms locally in an artery, an embolism, when a blood clot forms in the heart and travels to a cerebral artery, or when any body, such as an air bubble or piece of high-grade tumor lodges in an artery causing blockage or occlusion, collapse of a cerebral artery (spasm) or hemorrhage, as when a blood vessel bursts.

Thromboses and hemorrhages usually are found in arteriosclerotic vessels, hence in older individuals, with or without hypertension also being present. Cerebral emboli may occur following myocardial infarction or auricular fibrillation in arteriosclerotic cardiovascular disease, or following or during surgery, or during blood transfusions or intravenous procedures. When hemorrhage is the cause of the CVA the blood which has escaped from the vessel enters brain tissue and forms an expanding lesion with increasing symptoms.

Whatever the etiological determinant, the result of the CVA is a failure of circulation of oxygen-carrying blood to an area of the brain. The consequence of this is damage or death of the brain cells of the involved area. This is a *cerebral infarction* which is productive of hemiplegia.

Since hemiplegia is a functional deficit involving paralysis or paresis of one side of the body, ambulation and use of the upper extremity of the affected body side are prevented or largely restricted. The hemiplegia results from involvement of the corticobulbar and corticospinal tracts, and hence, there is, in addition to the paralysis or paresis of arm and leg, contralateral lower facial paresis and often, hemisensory deficit. Dependent upon which cerebral arteries are occluded a variety of clinical syndromes are seen. In addition to the above, when the internal carotid artery is affected blindness may occur on the side of the lesion if the ophthalmic artery is involved. If occlusion is in the distal branches of the anterior cerebral artery one lower extremity only will be affected and the patient will thus be *monoplegic.* Occlusion of the middle cerebral artery or the main posterior cerebral artery produces *homonymous hemianopsia,* or blindness for one half of the visual field of each eye. If the thalamus is involved the patient may experience pain, tremor, ataxia and involuntary choreoathetoid movements and emotional disturbances, the *thalamic syndrome.*

If the brain damage occurs to the dominant cerebral hemisphere the resulting language problems are generally grouped with the category of *aphasia.* Aphasia means, in fact, loss of language, and it refers to all aspects of language loss, including in addition to speech, writing, telling time, reading, arithmetic, spelling, typing, counting, recognizing objects and understanding what is being communicated. Since aphasia is most often a consequence of a CVA, the majority of patients who are aphasic are past the age of 50.

There are several possible disgnoses of aphasia. They are described only briefly and are covered more thoroughly in the section dealing with speech and language disorders.

Expressive aphasia is the inability to express oneself primarily through the mediums of verbal and written communication. It is a disorder of language output and the patient with expressive aphasia will experience difficulty in finding words, naming objects, using words in their proper order and context, counting, telling time, typing, spelling and writing. He often speaks in jargon without awareness that he is not communicating effectively or appropriately. *Receptive aphasia* is a disorder of language input. It is the inability to understand either spoken or written language. Such patients become confused when given instructions, or when watching television or reading, since these activities all require correct reception by the patient of the material being presented. When a patient has approximately equal difficulty in using and understanding language he is said to have *expressive-receptive,* or *mixed aphasia.* When the language impairment is so severe that there is complete or nearly complete loss of all language skills so that there is virtually no ability to communicate, the term *global aphasia* is used.

There are other communication disorders which occur frequently in hemiplegic patients. *Dysarthria* is an organic disorder in speech production. Impairment of the speech musculature, such as incoordination, paralysis or weakness produces impairments of respiration, phonation, resonance, articulation, volume, rate, voice quality and intonation. Motor aspects of speech production are the symptoms of dysarthric limitations of movement or weakness of the peripheral speech mechanisms. The most commonly manifested dysarthric speech symptom is slurred, disarticulated verbal production. When the symptoms are of sufficient severity to render speech unintelligible, the patient is termed *anarthric*.

Verbal apraxia is the inability to perform purposeful movements of the speech musculature although no neuromuscular paralysis exists. There is an inability to voluntarily move the tongue, lips and appropriate facial muscles. Verbally apractic patients typically demonstrate dysfunction of phoneme production. Apraxia is generally considered to be a subcategory of aphasia.

NEUROLOGIC AND NEUROMUSCULAR DISORDERS
Static Disorders of the Brain
Trauma

The term "brain damage" is frequently employed to describe a variety of symptoms. What is often not realized, however, is that the single phrase "brain damage" is not a very useful one either in diagnosis or prognosis of a patient's condition, and in fact, generally raises more questions than it answers. When one is speaking of a patient as being brain injured, one must be aware that the significance of such injury lies in its extent and anatomical locus and not merely in the fact that brain cells have been damaged or destroyed. Furthermore, many professionals when speaking of brain damage are generally referring to traumatic insult to the cortex, whereas the damage may be a consequence of either trauma or disease and need not be in the cortex at all.

Trauma is generally defined as a wound or injury inflicted usually more or less suddenly by some physical agent.

A lesion anywhere in the motor pathways of the cerebral cortex, internal capsule, corticospinal and pyramidal tracts will produce spastic paralysis of the affected muscles. This upper motor neuron lesion is commonly characterized by loss of voluntary movement, accentuated deep tendon reflexes, clonus and pathological reflexes, such as the Babinski sign. Lesions occurring above the point of origin of corticobulbar fibers to the cranial nerves (supranuclear) give rise to hemiplegia or quadriplegia. When the lesion occurs in the midbrain or below there is specific cranial nerve involvement or possible paralysis of cranial nerves on one side of the body and paralysis of the extremities on the other body side (*hemiplegia alternans*).

Damage to the cerebral cortex, internal capsule and brainstem may involve both motor and sensory pathways, resulting in a contralateral hemisensory deficit. Sensations of temperature, pain, touch and position may be affected to varying degrees.

The extrapyramidal system includes the basal ganglia and nuclei of the reticular formation. Trauma results in muscular rigidity and hence, difficulty with voluntary movement, loss of involuntary, automatic movements, disorders of muscle tone, choreiform and athetoid movements, and, on occasion, dystonic torsions are also observed.

Cerebellar injury typically produces incoordination of motor activities. The resultant disabilities are ataxia and atonia, or lack of normal tone or tension, causing muscle flaccidity.

Lesions in the brainstem give rise to spastic paralysis if corticospinal or pyramidal tracts are involved, contralateral hemisensory deficit if spinal thalamic tracts and the medical lemniscus are involved and specific cranial nerve palsies. Should there be damage to the reticular formation in the brainstem the ability to maintain an adequate state of wakefulness is impaired. Lesions characteristically produce apathy, lethargy and somnolence.

Injury involving the structures of the limbic system can result in a variety of problems which may affect rehabilitation. These are primarily emotional, as when the septum, amygdala, anterior thalamus or hypothalamus are involved, motivation and learning when the cingulate gyrus, septal region and amygdala are affected, and memory, when there is hippocampal damage.

Disease

Encephalitis is an infection of the brain which may be localized or diffused throughout the brain tissue. It may be an extension of *meningitis*, which is an inflammation of the meninges, or membranes which surround the brain and spinal cord. Etiological factors include bacteria, such as the tuberculosis bacillus, viruses, such as meningococcus, streptococcus and staphylococcus, parasites or fungi. If the infection has extended into the brain tissue encephalitis can result.

Patients who recover may have brain damage manifested in neurological, intellectual and emotional impairments. Transient paralysis as well as permanent plegic disabilities involving one or more extremities are one consequence of encephalitis. Concurrently, there may be cranial nerve deficits, blindness, aphasia and deafness.

Although patients may have meningitis without the extension of the infection into the brain itself, or may have bacterial infection leading to a brain abscess and possible residual hemiplegia, the patients seen most frequently in rehabilitation have residual effects of encephalitis.

Static Disorders of the Brain and Spinal Cord
Poliomyelitis

Acute anterior poliomyelitis is a viral infection of the spinal cord and brainstem. Lesions are localized primarily in the anterior horn cells, usually of the cervical and lumbar regions of the spinal cord, although the brainstem is often involved. In the group seen in rehabilitation, symptoms include manifestations of central nervous system involvement, plus the characteristic findings of weakness and paralysis of the trunk and extremities. This, then, is paralytic poliomyelitis. Paralysis is asymmetrical, with weakness of isolated muscles or individual limbs.

Spinal poliomyelitis is evidenced by trunk, pelvic, shoulder girdle, neck or extremity weakness. Diaphragm and chest muscles may be affected so that the patient requires artificial respiratory aids.

Bulbar poliomyelitis is marked by weakness and malfunction of muscles supplied by the lower cranial nerves, with impairment of facial movements, phonation and swallowing. Also seen are disturbances of medullary respiratory control resulting in shallow, incoordinated, irregular breathing, and deficits in vasomotor control with resulting hypertension and cardiac problems.

Bulbospinal poliomyelitis is characterized by loss of respiratory independence requiring breathing aids, and loss of protective cough and swallowing reflexes. Bowel and bladder problems and bone demineralization are also frequently present.

The residual paralysis in acute anterior poliomyelitis depends upon the distribution of motor cells which fail to recover from the viral infection. Paralyzed muscles are flaccid, and muscular atrophy begins to develop after several weeks. The muscles may eventually be replaced entirely by connective and adipose tissue. The severely paralyzed polio patient is also characterized by limb deformities. There are no concurrent sensory losses.

Although the patient with poliomyelitis presents some of the most difficult and complex problems for rehabilitation, both medically and psychologically, the recently developed Salk and Sabin vaccines have dramatically reduced its incidence of occurrence in the United States. Thus, while the problems of the individual patient are still great, the percentage of new patients in rehabilitation with poliomyelitis is far smaller than in the years preceding the use of the vaccines.

Guillain-Barré Syndrome

Upon initial examination, Guillain-Barré syndrome, or *ascending polyneuritis,* may be occasionally confused with poliomyelitis, since the presenting symptoms may be quite similar.

This disease is generally considered to be of viral origin, involving the peripheral nerves, spinal nerve roots and the spinal cord. Inflammation can be of one or more of these areas. The disease varies from mild temporary impairment of muscle strength to severe muscular weakness and/or flaccid paralysis. There is, concurrently, parasthesia of the extremities and absence of tendon reflexes.

Patients with Guillain-Barré syndrome often have sphincter involvement resulting in problems of bowel and bladder control. The course of the disease is typically characterized by progressive paralysis ascending from the lower limbs to the trunk, arms, and occasionally, the facial muscles. Once past the acute stage, the disease and disability may last for weeks or months, but the prognosis for recovery of motor and sensory function is favorable.

Transverse Myelitis

Also viral in origin, transverse myelitis is an inflammation involving the entire thickness of the spinal cord resulting in softening of the cord. It is manifested by acute onset of total paralysis of the areas of the body which are innervated by the cord segments at and below the level of infection. Bowel and bladder control are lost to the patient, with additional impairment of generative functions. Sensation is also abolished in the affected parts. The most frequent site of spinal cord involvement is in the mid-thoracic area. Prognosis for recovery of sensory and motor functions is poor.

Peripheral Neuropathy

Peripheral neuropathy is an inflammatory disease of the peripheral nerves resulting in a disturbance in sensory and motor functioning. It can involve a single nerve or many nerves (polyneuritis) in which case it is a more serious problem. There is partial destruction of various peripheral nerves which is frequently bilateral although nerves in scattered locations throughout the body may be involved. Manifestations of this disease are most clearly seen in the distal parts of the extremities.

Although the disability is primarily due to muscular paresis, complications arise from the resultant muscular atrophy and contractures. Sensory losses are also characteristic of peripheral neuropathy, often producing ataxic states due to the loss of function of proprioceptive fibers. Anesthetic skin is also prone to injury with delayed healing and decubiti as additional problems.

Peripheral neuropathy can result from several possible causes, the most frequent being metabolic disorders and deficiency states, such as diabetes mellitus and chronic alcoholism, and infectious conditions. It is a long-term and possibly a permanent disability.

Progressive Disorders of the Brain and Spinal Cord
Parkinsonism

Parkinson's disease is a slowly progressive condition resulting from lesions in the extrapyramidal system. Brain abnormalities include degeneration in the basal ganglia and substantia nigra. It can occur in younger persons as a consequence of encephalitis. In older individuals the cause may be arteriosclerosis involving this general region of the brain.

Characteristic signs of Parkinsonism include increasing rigidity of muscle tone, slowness and difficulty in initiating and executing voluntary movements and tremor, which is likely to be more severe during relaxation than during voluntary activity. Alternating flexions of the fingers produce the "pill-rolling" tremor commonly associated with the disease. The facial lines of the patient with Parkinson's disease are smooth and facial expression is fixed (masked face). Tongue muscles can also become involved and the patient may experience difficulty with chewing and swallowing. Speech may become slurred and soft.

The typical patient with Parkinsonism stands with head lowered and shoulders stooped. His gait consists, primarily, of short, slow, shuffling steps and his arms are held at his sides rather than exhibiting the rhythmic swing with the legs which is automatic in normal persons. There is difficulty in taking the first steps and often the patient stops in the middle of an ambulation pattern with difficulty in resuming ambulation movements ("freezing"). Frequently, once walking is initiated, the pace becomes increasingly rapid and the patient has difficulty stopping.

If a patient with this disease becomes ill, or for some reason has not received exercise for a period of time, his condition will deteriorate more rapidly. In advanced Parkinsonism there is progressive physical deterioration and losses in the psychological sphere which can lead to total incapacity.

Myasthenia Gravis

Myasthenia gravis is a functional disorder of neuromuscular transmission. It is a chronic disease involving, primarily, the muscles of the arms and legs, but including muscles of the trunk, eyes, face and swallowing. Various cranial nerves are impaired in function as well as the skeletal muscles. The disease is characterized by easy fatigability of the muscles after a few contractions due to a failure of neuromuscular conduction from the nerve endings to the muscles.

Since there is an impairment of transmission of nervous impulses to the muscles, they become weakened. Common symptoms of myasthenia gravis include ptosis, or drooping of the eyelids and diplopia, or double vision. As the muscles of the face are bilaterally weakened the face assumes a blank expression. When the soft palate is involved nasality of speech results. Due to weakness of the extremities ambulation and activities requiring functional use of the arms become limited. Although exercise is fatiguing to patients with this disorder, deformities rarely develop since they do not have abnormalities of muscle tone or true paralysis as in poliomyelitis or other plegic disabilities.

The course of myasthenia gravis is quite variable, with frequent daily fluctuations in the severity of the symptoms. Although it is progressive in nature it may remain static for long periods of time and with adequate treatment most patients can remain active for up to twenty years following its onset.

Friedrich's Ataxia

This form of ataxia represents a degeneration of the cerebellum and posterior spinal cord. It is hereditary in origin and may occur in several children of the same family.

The gait of a patient with Friedrich's ataxia is broad-based and staggering, resembling that of an intoxicated person. There is slow progressive deterioration of balance, cerebellar function and vision. The patient's feet exhibit a high arch, and as the disease progresses marked foot drop and inversion may occur. Visual defects associated with the disorder include nystagmus, diplopia and visual impairments resulting from optic atrophy. As the course of the disease continues the patient becomes necessarily confined to a wheelchair.

Multiple Sclerosis

Of unknown cause, multiple scerosis is one of the more frequent neurologic diseases seen in rehabilitation. It is highly variable in its course and symptomatology, and can be characterized by frequent remissions and exacerbations.

Multiple sclerosis is a demyelinating disease involving loss of the myelin sheaths of the tracts of white matter of the central nervous system. In the later stages nerve tissue may be replaced by scar formation. The gray matter of the brain and spinal cord is usually not affected.

Although remissions may occur with corresponding recovery of function which can last for several years, the course of the illness is inevitably progressive. With each improvement of the patient he generally does not attain the level of ability he was at previously. Some episodes of multiple sclerosis may be acute and terminate in the fatality of the patient. Usually several areas of the nervous system are involved rather than the disease being localized to one system or area of the body.

The first symptoms commonly are motor weakness and incoordination, intention tremor and visual disturbances, including double vision, blurred vision or impaired color perception, all of which show increasing impairment as the disease advances. In the early stages these signs may be transitory with complete remissions. In the later stages remissions are less striking and occur with reduced frequency.

Characteristic of the patient with multiple sclerosis is a spastic paresis of the lower extremities. Usually there is involvement of the arms as well. Intention tremor of upper and lower limbs increases with the progress of the disease. This tremor is noted during volitional movements and becomes more marked as the acts continue.

Speech becomes slurred, occasionally monotonic, and fluctuations in pitch frequently occur due to lack of control of vocal musculature leading to incoordination of the vocal cords and respiratory mechanisms. A more advanced disorder of speech is "scanning", in which words are spoken almost as if they were being spelled out.

Bladder dysfunction producing urinary incontinence or urgency is a common symptom.

As a consequence of numbness and parasthesia, decubiti can develop, particularly if the patient is forced to remain for long periods of time on affected body areas.

In the later stages, emotional symptoms such as euphoria and depression occur, with increasing intellectual deficits occasionally culminating in severe psychological impairment.

Multiple sclerosis progresses from the early symptoms discussed above to increasing disability, requiring the use of a wheelchair, to total disability.

Amyotrophic Lateral Sclerosis

This is a degenerative disease of unknown cause which progresses fairly rapidly, culminating in the death of the patient usually within five years of its onset. There is degeneration of the anterior horn cells of the spinal cord resulting in progressive muscular atrophy which produces a flaccid paralysis of the extremities.

The muscle weakness and wasting of the limbs usually begins in the small muscles of the hands and slowly extends to involvement of whole extremities. This condition alone is termed *primary spinal muscular atrophy*. Degeneration of the pyramidal tracts resulting in spastic paralysis of lower extremities is called *primary lateral sclerosis*. If there is degeneration of the motor nuclei in the brainstem giving rise to problems of swallowing, articulation, weakness of facial musculature and hoarseness of voice, the condition is known as *progressive bulbar palsy*. When these three conditions are present in a single individual, the diagnosis is one of amyotrophic lateral sclerosis. Although it may begin as one manifestation or form, the disease eventually progresses, without remissions, to include all three.

MUSCULAR AND MUSCULOSKELETAL DISORDERS

Although muscular dystrophy and amputations are among the disorders encountered in rehabilitation which belong in this general group, the former is a disease occurring primarily in children and the latter is often a geriatric problem and they will therefore be discussed in the appropriate sections below.

Chronic Back Pain

Back pain can result from a variety of causes, including trauma, excessive effort and cumulative stress and strain, or may develop without obvious cause. Etiologically, there may be pathology of the intervertebral discs in the spine, muscular weakness or imbalance, or psychological factors may play the largest role.

Strain of any of the muscles or groups of muscles attached to the spine will produce damage to the muscle or its tendon or point of insertion, producing local hemorrhage with a tendency to resultant scar tissue. The elasticity of the remaining muscles is reduced temporarily by protective spasm.

In the majority of patients who have suffered acute spasm or strain of a ligament, the pathology will be resolved as the local tissue damage heals. With some patients, however, the total elasticity of the posterior muscles becomes altered resulting in painful restrictions of the trunk muscles. When this persists for a prolonged period of time muscular fibrosis occurs. This causes back pain in patients who have been subject to prolonged postural defects. Sprains of ligaments in the lumbosacral area produce strain of the sacrospinalis muscles. Muscle tone then increases as a compensatory mechanism, but this causes, in time, changes within the joints and fibrosis of the muscles. When these are accompanied by already present osteoarthritic changes, the result is pain, restriction of motion, and loss of spinal elasticity leading to more pain.

Acute back pain resulting from externally imposed trauma can be easily treated by orthopedic procedures and generally shows spontaneous healing. It is when the tested methods of treatment fail and the pain persists for an undue period of time that the acute back case becomes a chronic back problem and orthopedic procedures yield to rehabilitation therapies. Despite medical, surgical and therapeutic intervention, symptoms may persist for years and a large number of patients do not return to their former occupations or levels of activity.

When medical examination reveals no physical lesions which would warrant the symptoms of the patient, or when the medical evidence is not sufficient to explain the disability, or when treatment methods which have been previously successful with like or similar cases fail, then a psychologic etiology must be suspected. The person with a chronic back pain may be receiving some secondary gain from his disability, such as attention from significant persons in his life. It may be preventing him from engaging in a perhaps necessary, but undesired activity. It is both interesting and important to note that the majority of patients with chronic back pain receive psychotherapy concurrent with their physical therapy. In a minority of patients, psychotherapy must be given prior to any other treatment and an approximately equal number of cases receive psychotherapy as the only form of treatment.

METABOLIC DISORDERS
Arthritis

The term *arthritis* refers to inflammation of a joint. The arthritides inflict one of the highest tolls in morbidity of all chronic diseases, while at the same time the mortality rate is low. Thus, the number of living persons disabled by arthritis is great.

Arthritis is a syndrome of varying etiology, and there are many possible causes. It may be a result of infection from a specific bacterium resulting, typically, in a single joint involvement, either acute or chronic, depending upon the nature of the infectious agent. Immediate medical attention is required to prevent tissue damage. These patients are not frequently seen in rehabilitation. There are, however, other forms of arthritis which are chronic and can be extremely disabling, and afflicted patients are given the rehabilitation therapies. Although there are several large classifications, certain forms of the disease are statistically more prevalent and receive the majority of treatment services. The two which are most frequently encountered are discussed herein.

Degenerative Joint Disease

In the process of aging there are certain degenerative changes which take place in articular structures. They appear initially in childhood in the articular cartilage and gradually increase in frequency and severity with time. Similar changes occur in adults of middle age, but in joint tissue other than cartilage. The degree of development of this senescent deterioration varies widely in individuals, microscopically or macroscopically, past the age of fifty. These changes are called degenerative joint disease, senescent arthritis, hypertrophic arthritis, or most commonly, *osteoarthritis,* each term actually emphasizing a different aspect of the disease.

The etiology of this disease is not fully understood, but it may be that the "microtraumas" inflicted by continual usage of a joint contribute directly to the degenerative changes. It is the often-accompanying synovitis and inflammation of the ligaments which gives the name of arthritis to this disease. When articular tissue changes, growing to macroscopic proportions, produce major defects in the articular surfaces, the result is a mechanical friction and irritation with consequent inflammation and pain as the irregular articular surfaces move against each other. The joint inflammation, or arthritis, is a result of friction upon use of a joint, produced by intra-articular changes.

Joints which have become previously damaged may become the sites of premature osteoarthritis. In non-injured joints, those most commonly affected are the weight-bearing joints and those subject to the most trauma, e.g. knees, hips and lumbar and cervical segments of the spine. Also commonly involved are the terminal interphalangeal joints of the fingers and the carpometacarpal joints of the thumbs, resulting in the knobby enlargements known as Heberden's nodes.

Degenerative joint disease is an uncomfortable, often painful, and occasionally limiting disease. It does not, however, produce the severe disability of rheumatoid arthritis. It occurs primarily in older people and is almost universal in persons past the age of fifty, yet only a small percentage of affected individuals present the symptoms of pain, stiffness of joints and limitations in range of motion and mobility. When it is found in younger persons, other factors such as congenital pathology, previous injuries and other disease must be considered.

Rheumatoid Arthritis

Rheumatoid arthritis is the most frequently occurring among the arthritides and is also the most severely disabling. It has a high potential for crippling among a relatively young population and once the disease is firmly established the duration of the symptoms is lifelong. Mortality rates are low and when death does come it is usually from a complicating disease and not from the arthritis itself.

Although the symptoms of rheumatoid arthritis may initially have their onset in infancy or old age, the average age at onset is between the middle of the second and the middle of the fifth decade of life. Several etiological factors have been suspected, such as hereditary or constitutional variables, body physique and endocrine imbalance, auto-immunity, environmental factors—e.g. temperature and humidity, nutrition, physical stress and emotional problems; but no one factor or combination of factors has been definitely established as productive of the disease.

On a pathological level, there is inflammation of connective tissue with fibrinoid degeneration. In the early stages of the disease proliferation of synovial cells with thickening of the synovial membrane occurs, in addition to effusion of the joint and swelling of the soft tissues which surround the joint. The proximal interphalangeal joints are frequently the first to become involved, with fusiform, or spindle-shaped swelling. As the disease progresses the inflammatory changes and proliferation of synovial cells increases. Inflammatory tissue overgrows eroded and possibly destroyed cartilage. Decalcification and destruction of bone adjacent to the affected joint takes place. These factors eventually lead to deformity commonly seen in advanced arthritic patients. If the disease continues to advance, fibrous or osseous fusion of the bones forming the joint may occur with consequent ankylosis, or fixation of the joint. Alternately, the affected joint and its adjacent bone may be destroyed entirely and reduced to scar tissue. In patients with severe rheumatoid arthritis every joint in the body may become involved.

Clinically, the joint manifestations of the disease typically are pain and heat, swelling, stiffness, wasting of the muscles, limitation of range of motion and deformity, which can be extreme. The general symptoms include fatigue, insomnia, depression, agitation, anorexia with subsequent weight loss, fever, chills and anemia, which can occur together in various combinations and with varying degrees of severity. It is possible for a patient to have involvement of only one joint, and remissions do occur which may last for many years.

A variant form of this disease is *rheumatoid spondylitis*, or *Marie-Strumpell's disease.* This is rheumatoid arthritis of the spine which, in its severe form, progresses until there is total fusion of the patient's spine. The patient with spondylitis tends to develop a kyphosis of the spine which may involve only the lumbar region or it can include the entire spine, depending upon the nature and extent of the disease. Development of a kyphotic deformity produces a loss of erect stature and a decrease in respiratory excursion due to forward compression of the thoracic cage. Hips and shoulders are affected in approximately fifty per cent of all cases and other joints show less frequent involvement.

Rheumatoid arthritis is extremely variable in its forms. It can advance rapidly resulting in death within one year of onset. It may progress swiftly for a period of time and then slow down, progressing at a slow rate for several years. A well established case will steadily continue its advance over the years at an intermittent, but sure, gradual pace. On the other hand, it can be a very mild disease with only slight involvement of the joints of the fingers.

Since the cause is unknown there are no specific treatments. Physical therapy has no curative effect and does not alter the disease's course of progression.

PULMONARY PROBLEMS

Emphysema

Obstructive pulmonary emphysema is an irreversible condition resulting from tissue destruction which is characterized by an abnormal inflation of the lungs and obstruction of air flow. It is a disease of the alveoli, or air cells, in the lungs in which these sacs become over-distended. The patient is able to inhale but has difficulty exhaling due to a loss of the elasticity of the lungs. This leads to a failure to expel air in the normal manner. Since only a small amount of air in the alveoli can be expelled, there is a limitation placed upon the amount which can be inhaled in the next breath.

This slowly and inexorably progressing disorder leads to respiratory insufficiency and, occasionally, heart failure. There are several possible predisposing conditions, including chronic bronchitis and bronchial asthma.

Although progressive, obstructive pulmonary emphysema is characterized by a course of remissions and exacerbations. During exacerbation periods several clinical symptoms are present. Dyspnea, or shortness of breath, may be noted initially only during moderate or severe exertion. As the illness continues, the dyspnea appears even upon only mild exertion, such as walking one block at a slow pace. Cold weather increases the dyspneic symptoms. Coughing is commonly associated with emphysema, as is abundant expectoration. These symptoms are more marked upon arising in the morning than during the night. A patient's efforts to expel sputum may be so great as to result in fainting, or syncope. Fatigue is also a typical finding among emphysema patients, particularly affecting the limbs in the early morning hours. Concurrent with the respiratory problems and consequent limitations in ambulation is a tendency towards ready irritability. This is probably due to the frustration felt by the patient as he encounters difficulties in performing activities which previously presented no problems to him.

The emphysema patient typically exhibits forward bending of the upper trunk with raised shoulders and a "barrel" chest. This kyphotic posture is commonly and habitually assumed in order to permit easier breathing. However, this requires additional muscular effort, adding an increase to the already high expenditure of energy thus requiring an increased oxygen supply. In addition, the abdominal muscles tend to lose their tonicity and become flabby and atrophied. Consequently, they lack the power to move the viscera up to assist the diaphragm in normal breathing.

Persons with emphysema are highly prone to respiratory infections, such as influenza or pneumonia, which are dangerous for them to the extent of being potentially fatal. Recurring upper or lower respiratory infections can produce irreversible damage to the tracheobronchial tree. Each such episode is frequently followed by reduced function. The disease generally progresses until death occurs, generally in the sixth or seventh decade of life. The patient's demise is usually due to severe insufficiency in ventilation or to heart failure.

CANCER

Over the past several decades as the health and longevity of our population has been steadily improving, cancer has become an increasingly significant problem. Of all diseases, a diagnosis of cancer is perhaps the most terrifying one which a physician can communicate to a patient. This fear is partly justified since cancer is the second-ranking cause of death in the United States, being exceeded in mortality rate only by cardiovascular diseases. The magnitude of the problem can be seen when it is realized that over half a million new cases of cancer are diagnosed each year and that approximately fifty per cent of these occur during the most productive years of life, between the ages of twenty-five and sixty-five.

Cancer is currently considered to be a group of diseases having a similar developmental course and pathological effects on the patient, yet also having separate, unique characteristics which can result in varied prognoses for affected persons.

Many different types of cancer are described today, each having varying degrees of severity for the host. Some types are localized lesions which are largely curable, while other forms are metastatic in nature and are difficult or impossible to eradicate. As a general term, cancer may be defined as a variety of malignant neoplasms, or new growths, due to largely unknown and probably multiple causes. It can arise in all tissues of the body which are composed of potentially dividing cells, and results in adverse effects on the host organism through invasive growth and metastases.

Cells which make up particular tissues have the property of division called mitosis which is ordered and disciplined growth needed to maintain tissue bulk. In cancer these cells do not conform to the orderly growth process and become capable of independent growth not susceptible to normal regulatory and inhibitory "laws." This type of autonomous growth, which may occur at sites away from the tissue of origin is known as *metastasis*. Such uninhibited and generally rapid growth of cancerous cells in multiple organs and tissues of the body produce extensive damage which may eventually result in the death of the host.

There are several theories regarding the causes of cancer. One position holds that in some forms of cancer chronic irritation of an area is the cause, citing as an example the incidence of lip cancer in pipe smokers. Another view maintains that trauma is a possible causal factor. However, a traumatic event, when linked to cancer, is usually linked in a correlational way and not in a cause-and-effect relationship. The trauma frequently serves to bring to attention a pre-existing cancer condition. Repeated trauma to a particular area, such as cuts and abrasions of the lips or burns on the skin may play a role in cancer development in these areas.

A theory of hereditary transmission is supported by evidence from animal studies, but in humans the relationship is unclear. Certain forms of cancer have strong hereditary factors while others, in fact the most prevalent forms, do not show this. In general, genetic variables probably do play a part, but the extent and method by which they do is not well known at this time. A current theory presents an argument for a viral origin of cancer, and modern detection devices, such as the electron microscope, are providing supporting evidence. In laboratory animals viruses produce a variety of malignant neoplasms, yet no case of human cancer has been definitely linked to a viral cause.

Carcinogenic factors in the environment have been receiving increasing attention as cancer-producing agents. Among these can be included arsenic, tar, oil, radioactive chemicals, the rays of the sun, and recently, "smog" and soot. It remains for future research to determine which of the current theories, if not all, are valid and to what extent, or to find possible causes not accounted for by present viewpoints.

Tumors can be either benign or malignant and, technically, the term cancer reflects the malignant type only. A benign tumor is an abnormal growth of cells which can occur anywhere in the body. Generally, these are circumscribed lesions, and even when multiple can be clearly differentiated from surrounding tissue. Aside from certain exceptional instances they are not fatal.

A malignant neoplasm tends to invade adjoining tissue so that the separation between the tumor and adjacent structures is lost. They can metastasize, or grow autonomously in tissues distant from their origin. A metastatic malignancy is often fatal, depending upon the extent of its invasion of various body organs. Not all malignant tumors metastasize, but rather produce disorders and disability at the site of local growth until the disease is very far advanced.

Patients seen in rehabilitation are those who have undergone successful medical or surgical treatment for benign tumors, yet have some residual disability, or who have had surgical removal of certain organs with malignant tumors and require retraining in the associated activity. The following section describes those forms of tumors most frequently associated with rehabilitation patients.

Tumors of the Central Nervous System

Brain Tumors

ASTROCYTOMA. This is a neoplasm of the brain in which the predominant cell is the astrocyte, a neuroglia cell. It is a slow-growing, well demarcated tumor occurring most often in the cerebellar lobes of children and in the temporal or frontal lobes of adults. Symptoms begin with recurrent, increased intracranial pressure manifested as headache, vomiting and papilledema. These may extend over six months to nine months before cerebellar, frontal or temporal signs appear with their concomitant losses of function.

MENINGIOMATA. Most meningiomas are extracerebral, as they do not infiltrate the brain, but slowly replace brain tissue. They rarely occur in youth, but are seen most frequently in patients between the ages of thirty and fifty. Their rate of growth is slow and they most commonly occur at the folds of the dura adjacent to dural sinuses, or over the cerebral cortex, or at the base of the skull. Meningiomata are usually not malignant.

The symptoms of meningiomata depend upon which area of the

brain is involved. Tumors originating along the longitudinal sinus often begin with Jacksonian seizures, followed by hemiparesis and sensory disturbances involving the lower extremity to a greater extent than the upper one. Those tumors crossing the falx can produce bilateral spasticity and sensory signs. Meningiomata in the occipital lobe or posterior fossa result in hemianopsia or cerebellar signs.

CEREBELLOPONTILE TUMORS. Cerebellopontile, or acoustic, tumors arise from the vestibular portion of the eighth cranial nerve and are situated between the cerebellum and the pons. They occur most frequently in mid-adult life and grow at a very slow rate.

Early symptoms begin with tinnitus which may last for years and progress to unilateral deafness and reduced vestibular function. Other symptoms include unilateral facial parasthesis of a transient nature, diminished corneal reflex and, occasionally, highly painful trigeminal nerve irritation. When the tumor encroaches upon the cerebellum and pons the resultant signs are periodic staggering gait, hand incoordination, ataxia, nystagmus, thickened speech and contralateral hemiparesis. If the tumor is entirely removed by surgical means, complete facial paralysis may result.

Spinal Cord Tumors

A spinal cord tumor is any new growth occurring within the vertebral canal. Such neoplasms can develop at any age but are usually found past the age of ten. Approximately fifty per cent of all spinal cord tumors arise in the thoracic region. About thirty per cent occur in the cervical area and twenty per cent are found in the lumbar region. Approximately sixty-five per cent of spinal neoplasms arise dorsal or dorsolateral to the cord but they can be located ventrally or in intermediate areas. Spinal cord tumors may lie above or below one or more spinal nerve roots, producing tension on them and, in fact, may be attached to or involved with the nerve root or adjacent membrane. The symptoms of spinal cord growths are due, primarily, to irritation and compression of nerve roots, compression and dislocation of the cord itself, or obstruction of vascular flow.

There are certain general signs of spinal cord neoplasms. Typically found is back pain due to irritation or compression of the cord and nerves. The pain becomes increasingly severe, often made worse by activity. Supination, which stretches the spinal cord, may increase the pain and force the patient to sleep in a sitting position. Another symptom may be sensory impairment, either due to compression from a malignancy or to hemorrhage within a benign growth.

Deficits in sensation of pain, temperature and touch may precede losses in vibration and position sense. The sensory impairment can progress to complete anesthesia. Concurrent with sensory losses is motor weakness, incoordination and spasticity. Increasing loss of control over sphincter functions may begin with urinary retention and incontinence. A late symptom is lack of rectal sphincter control.

In addition to the general symptoms of spinal neoplasms certain neurological signs occur depending upon the region of the spinal cord which is involved. Tumors in the cervical area produce pain in the back of the neck, particularly with neck movements. Weakness, clumsiness and muscle spasticity begin in one upper extremity and gradually spread to the other limbs. Atrophy of shoulder girdle muscles, upper extremities and intrinsic hand muscles may occur. Sphincter involvement may be late or absent. Tumors of the thoracic region produce hyperasthesia just above the site of the sensation impairment. Also occurring are spastic pareses of the lower limbs and sphincter disturbances. Tumors of the conus and filium terminals begin with severe low back pain radiating down one leg at first and then down the other. Weakness may begin with foot drop in one lower extremity, spreading to involvement of the entire leg, and finally, to the other lower extremity. Early signs include sphincter disturbances and impairment of sexual function.

It is encouraging to note that more than eight-five per cent of primary spinal cord neoplasms are benign and can be removed completely through surgical procedures. Following laminectomy, over ninety per cent of these patients make a complete recovery. Recovery may be very slow, requiring the efforts of a rehabilitation team, but these patients finally become able to resume their normal premorbid activities.

Cancer of the Lung

While the causes of lung cancer have yet to be firmly established, most physicians feel that cigarette smoking is a primary agent. Other factors, such as radioactive ores, nickel and chromates are also capable of producing lung malignancies, but lung tumors among non-smokers are far less common than among smokers.

Symptoms of lung cancer include coughing, chest pain, loss of weight and hoarseness of voice, the latter three signs occurring in advanced stages of the disease.

The disability which results from treatment for lung cancer (surgery or radiation therapy) is manifested as pulmonary insufficiency producing shortness of breath. The extent of this depends upon how much of the lung tissue was damaged or excised. If a lobe of a lung is removed the pulmonary insufficiency will be minor. If, on the other hand, an entire lung is removed, the patient will experience varying degrees of shortness of breath during work or exercise. Minor recurring upper respiratory infections will further impair functioning. Rehabilitation consists of training the patient to plan his activities and work within the capability of the remaining lung.

Cancer of the Larynx

The larynx, or "voice box," is intimately concerned with three important functions. These are phonation, or the utterance of sounds, deglutination, or swallowing, and respiration. Thus, cancerous growths in this body area present complex problems in rehabilitation.

Some tumors, particularly those occurring superficially on one of the vocal cords, can be removed through radiation therapy with satisfactory return of voice. In some laryngeal areas, however, the preferred or required treatment is surgery. Where the cancerous neoplasm in the larynx is extensive, or where radiation therapy cannot be performed, a total laryngectomy must be performed.

The chief disability resulting from removal of the larynx is loss of voice, since the patient can no longer phonate. Rehabilitation consists of retraining the patient to speak in a new way, such as teaching him to develop an "esophageal voice." When this is not feasible or the technique cannot be mastered by the patient, an artificial larynx may be prescribed.

CARDIOVASCULAR DISEASES

Heart Disease

Heart disease is one of the most important problems facing the nation today. In terms of human lives it has the highest mortality rate of any illness in the United States, causing nearly one million deaths each year. Over fifty per cent of all deaths in this country occur from cardiovascular diseases. From an economic viewpoint the toll is great. More than four billion dollars are spent annually on heart disease and over four billion dollars of gross income are lost to industry every year as a result of more than fifty million working days being lost by individuals with cardiac conditions. These data, of course, do not take into account the losses in happiness, comfort and security suffered by patients with heart disease and by the members of their families. The needs, therefore, of the patient with heart disease for rehabilitation and future life planning are great.

Not all patients with heart disease come to the attention of a physician. There are those who have no obvious symptoms or are not aware of a cardiac condition. These individuals are not limited in their activities and are not disabled by the disease. On the other hand, those patients with symptoms are conscious of the fact that they have an illness and both they and their physicians recognize the need for treatment and regulation of activities.

There are several types of heart disease which are important to classify since each type presupposes variations in treatment and planning for future employment and recreation. There are, however, certain symptoms which occur to some extent in virtually all forms of heart disease.

One common symptom is heart failure. In order to meet the body's demands the heart must pump adequately. When it fails to do so the patient may experience feelings of weakness, most noticeably upon effort, and fatigue in activities which formerly were non-tiring. Ready fatigability is a typical sign of heart failure. As the disease progresses, the fatigability signs occur even during activities which do not require much exertion. Also, during exertion dyspnea, or rapid, distressed breathing occurs. When the patient becomes dyspneic while at rest, the indication is of advanced heart failure. In the case of left heart failure, a typical symptom is orthopnea, a discomfort in breathing while in any but an erect or sitting position. Orthopnea is produced by fluid entering the lungs. Thus, when the patient is in a reclining position, gravity tends to bring the fluid into the lungs resulting in shortness of breath. As the disease becomes more severe the patient must lie in an increasingly erect position to sleep.

Syncope may occur during exercise as a result of a disproportion between the needs of the muscles for blood and the amount of blood which the heart can pump out, or an inability of the heart to increase in rate.

Some patients with right heart failure also have abdominal pain due to congestion of the abdominal organs with blood which has backed up from the right atrium, or upper chamber of the heart.

A second general symptom of heart disease is chest pain. The pain which clearly indicates cardiac distress is known as *angina pectoris*. This term describes a constricting pain in the center of the chest below the sternum. The pain may not be very sharp and the "squeezing" or pressing sensation may go relatively unnoticed. However, the sign means the same thing even when not occurring as severe pain. *Anginal distress* refers to a severe chest pain, often radiating to the left shoulder and down the arm to the fingers.

Symptomatic dysrhythmias are also typical of heart disease. When a rhythm abnormality has been present for a long period of time and has not been called to the attention of the patient by a physician, the patient is usually not aware of its presence. But when there is an acute onset of a rapid or irregular heart rhythm the patient becomes suddenly conscious of palpitations in the chest. Although such rhythm irregularities usually occur during effortful activity, they also occur during rest when a patient is seriously ill. Two kinds of rhythmic abnormalities occurring in heart disease are *tachycardia,* or heart rate in excess of one hundred beats per minute, and *bradycardia,* which is a heart rate of less than fifty beats per minute.

An important initial step in rehabilitation planning for the cardiac patient is a functional and therapeutic classification of heart disease.

A functional classification is an estimate of what a patient's heart will permit him to do. There are four classes of patients which may be so grouped. *Class I* includes cardiac patients who have no limitations in physical activity. Their normal activity does not produce symptoms of heart disease, such as fatigue, dysrhythmias, dyspnea or angina pectoris. *Class II* patients have slight limitations in activity and are comfortable at rest. Ordinary physical activity results in fatigue, palpitation, dyspnea or anginal pain. *Class III* patients have marked limitation of physical activity and are most comfortable while resting. Even slight effort produces the symptoms of their disease. *Class IV* patients cannot carry on any physical activity without discomfort. Even while at rest they may suffer cardiac insufficiency or angina pectoris.

A therapeutic classification of heart disease acts as a guide to the management of a patient's activities, primarily in terms of daily routine physical actions. The categorization is as follows: *Class A* patients have cardiac disease but their activity need not be restricted in any way; *Class B* patients need not restrict their ordinary physical efforts but are advised against strenuous or competitive activity; *Class C* includes cardiac patients whose ordinary activities should be limited in moderation and who should discontinue strenuous exertions; *Class D* patients must markedly limit their ordinary physical activity; *Class E* comprises the group of heart-diseased patients who should be at complete rest, confined to a bed or wheelchair.

Diseases of the Heart

ARTERIOSCLEROTIC HEART DISEASE. Arteriosclerotic, or coronary heart disease, is a consequence of the narrowing of the coronary arteries by atherosclerosis. This is an infiltration of the intima, the inner lining of a blood vessel, such as an artery, by lipids with a consequent reduction in the vessel's lumen and thus, in the blood supply to the organ served by the vessel. In addition to restricting vascular flow, this condition predisposes the vessel to the presence of clots which can precipitate acute cardiac distress.

Acute coronary heart disease is manifested by acute myocardial infarction, usually produced by the presence of a thrombus, or new clot, in one of the larger coronary arteries. Often there is no actual clot, but an extreme narrowing of the vessel. This leads to necrosis, tissue death in one or more zones of the heart, generally accompanied by anginal pain and frequently also by congestive heart failure, dysrhythmia and shock. If the patient survives, the heart heals in a relatively brief period of time by the formation of scar tissue. Chronic coronary heart disease, however, may cause small scars in various heart regions and larger scars due to one or more myocardial infarctions. In time, such hearts tend to dilate and hypertrophy and to become insufficient.

RHEUMATIC HEART DISEASE. Rheumatic heart disease is primarily a disorder of the younger population and, as such, will be discussed in Chapter Three (see p. 52).

Peripheral Vascular Disease

The generic term "peripheral vascular disease" refers to disease of any of the peripheral vessels, that is, those which are distant from the heart and excluding the brain. Disease is caused either by injury, such as inflammation, or by impairment of the circulation within the vessels.

There are five major etiological factors which are productive of peripheral vascular diseases. They are as follows: stenosis, or narrowing of a vessel resulting in impaired circulation below the point of stenosis; obstruction of a vessel producing interruption of circulation below the point of closure which is generally a result of slow growths of clots within a vessel or of pressure on the vessel emanating externally; inflammation, which may result from physical trauma or infection; aneurysm formation caused by chronic dilation of a segment of a vessel because of weakening of its walls by disease; and arteriovenous fistula, an abnormal connection between an artery and a vein.

The disability which is produced by peripheral vascular disorders arises either from the symptoms or from indirect complications of the disease, such as a limb amputation which may be necessary in certain cases.

When there is interference with circulation one resulting symptom is pain which, in acute cases, is always present until relieved, and in chronic cases occurs on effort. Pain can also be caused by inflammation of a vessel. When there is tissue injury, or inflammation, or blockage of venous or lymphatic drainage in a body part— notably an extremity— edema, or swelling, occurs from an increase of fluid in the tissues. With impaired circulation the skin becomes predisposed to infection and ulceration of the skin of the affected areas may occur. As a consequence of pain, edema, skin breakdowns and weakness in involved body parts, ambulation becomes impaired, often to a marked degree.

In a large percentage of patients with peripheral vascular disease, rehabilitation techniques can be of great value in the restoration of function.

Chapter 2

GERIATRIC CONDITIONS

O NE CONSEQUENCE of the greater longevity of mankind has been an increase in the number of elderly patients seen in rehabilitation. The philosophy of rehabilitation remains the same for the aged as for their younger contemporaries. Old age is not a disease in itself although persons in the geriatric population do tend to have more than a proportionate share of disabling diseases and chronic illnesses. The current thinking in the rehabilitation field is that the elderly should not be excluded from any of the restorative processes unless there are serious contraindications, such as cardiac or respiratory disease, which place limitations on applying certain therapies with these patients.

There are few illnesses which are confined to the old age group. Most of the diseases and disabilities occurring in younger individuals are also found in the geriatric population and, conversely, the majority of the problems of the elderly confront youth. There are, however, certain disabilities which occur with a significantly greater frequency in the aged and these will be discussed in this chapter.

HIP FRACTURES

Fractures of the hip and connected bones have been on the increase in the elderly and hence, have been causing greater problems for the population than ever before.

With advancing age the entire skeleton becomes more brittle and, as a result, even minor trauma can result in fractures. The most common fracture sustained by the aged which requires rehabilitation is that occurring to the femur, particularly the femoral neck. While such fractures may be a consequence of direct traumatic insult, such as an automobile accident, they are very often the result of a fall in which the elderly person could not react quickly enough to check the fall by extending an arm.

There are two main groups into which femoral fractures can be divided. An *intracapsular fracture* is one at the articular end of a bone, such as the femur, within the line of insertion of the capsular ligament of the joint. Included within this category are subcapital fractures which occur just below the head of the femur, transcervical fractures occurring across the neck of the femur, and fractures at the base of the femoral neck. An *extracapsular fracture* is a fracture of the articular extremity of a bone but outside the line of attachment of the capsular ligament of the joint. The extracapsular heading subsumes all fractures occurring in the trochanteric region (pertrochanteric, intertrochanteric and subtrochanteric) which is the area lying between the greater and lesser trochanters, the bony processes at the upper end of the femoral shaft.

Treatment for intracapsular fractures involves either surgical replacement of the head of the femur with a metal prosthesis or fixation by a nail and plate. In the case of an extracapsular fracture conservative treatment is often successful since the break readily unites, but in the elderly the enforced bedrest can lead to complications. This makes surgery the treatment of choice in most cases. With early care followed by intensive rehabilitation the majority of patients with hip fractures can be restored to functional living.

AMPUTATIONS

Amputations may be necessary in any age group, yet over seventy-five per cent of those currently performed are carried out on individuals past the age of sixty. In this elderly group amputations usually are not isolated mechanical problems as they might be in traumatic cases, but rather, are additional complications superimposed upon patients who have vascular problems or other chronic diseases.

Amputations are unique in that the disability is a result of a form of treatment which has eliminated a pathology rather than from the pathology itself. It is possible that the limitations imposed by a remaining diseased extremity can be greater than those of an amputated limb with a prosthesis.

An amputation may be of an upper or a lower extremity, but in rehabilitation the most frequently encountered patients are those with lower extremity amputations.

The Causes of Lower Extremity Amputations

Vascular insufficiency associated with artericsclerosis or diabetes mellitus is a frequent cause of leg amputations in the elderly. As a result of impaired vascular flow death of tissue occurs, necessitating the surgery.

When a patient with diabetes mellitus which is not medically controlled sustains a wound to an extremity, and medical attention is not given to the injury, infection leading to gangrene can occur. Amputation is then a required treatment.

Necrotic tissue resulting from peripheral vasospastic conditions, such as Buerger's disease (*thromboangiitis obliterans*), is often a cause of amputation.

Emergency amputation is carried out when there has been sufficient injury resulting from accidental violence to affect the blood and nerve supply of a limb, rendering it nonfunctional.

Malignant tumors require high proximal amputation as a life-saving measure.

Any acute infection which cannot be brought quickly under control and becomes chronic is extremely destructive to functioning tissues. If conservative treatment or surgery cannot restore function, amputation may be required.

Thermal injuries, such as excessive burns with contractures causing loss of function in an extremity, and extreme cold and frostbite in the presence of vascular insufficiency are often reasons for performing an amputation.

Levels of Amputation

There are standard levels of amputation for both upper and lower extremities. In this section the concern is with the latter.

In the lower extremity the most proximal amputation is the hemipelvectomy. In this operation half of the sacrum and the entire ilium, ischium and pubis are unilaterally removed. Although a prosthesis can be successfully fitted, a satisfactory gait is difficult to achieve for patients who have undergone this procedure. However, fair function can be restored and many patients who have had a hemipelvectomy are able to return to their daily routines.

Amputations below this level are referred to as disarticulation at the hip, and the surgery is performed between the knee and the hip.

Knee disarticulation takes place through the knee joint without cutting of any bone.

Below-knee amputations are carried out between the ankle and the knee, or, in the case of the partial foot amputation, on the foot alone.

When amputation is performed in cases of vascular disease, the level at which the surgeon operates is often determined by the adequacy of collateral circulation.

Rehabilitation, in the case of the amputee, is most often a matter of prosthetic prescription and training. Many factors are considered in evaluating a patient for a prosthesis. Age is important. Persons over the age of sixty will be slow in adapting to an artificial limb and take longer to achieve their highest potential than do younger amputees.

Physique, general physical condition, weight and coordination are also considered. The obese patient with a cardiac disease will experience far more difficulty in using a prosthetic limb than will the strong, slim and healthy person.

Sex plays an important role in deciding for a prosthesis, and a female patient may be rehabilitated for a homemaking career while a prosthesis may be less feasible for a working man.

The type of occupation which the amputee is engaged in often determines the type of prosthesis prescribed. A man engaged in manual labor requires a different device from the executive with a desk position.

A patient's desire for a prosthesis and his motivation to succeed with one are two highly important variables. The individual must be aware of the full nature of his disability, must have a good acceptance of it, must be willing to cooperate completely on a rehabilitation program and must be highly motivated to make the fullest use of any artificial limb given to him. Prescription of a prosthesis requires that the patient be realistic in his expectations of the device.

Finally, economic factors are considered. A prosthetic limb may not be feasible for the indigent person living alone, in a building with no elevator, who does not have the aid of a wheelchair and cannot afford an attendant.

The Functional Classification of Amputees for Prostheses

For purposes of establishing the functional objectives of the prosthesis, amputees are divided into several categories. This is a key step in the prescription process since it helps to determine the type of prosthesis given to a patient. Prostheses vary depending upon whether they will be put to a great deal of functional use, or whether they will be needed for the stability and protection of the wearer, or whether they will be worn for cosmetic reasons only. There are six functional classes.

Class 1—Full Restoration

Patients in this class are quite functional, having been restored fully to a function which is the equivalent of normal. They have a handicap but not a disability, and can perform at their former work and recreation activities with no restrictions. Few amputees attain this level.

Class 2—Partial Restoration

An individual in this group will be completely functional with an artificial limb. He will be able to work, although slight changes on his job may be necessary. Athletics may have to be eliminated, but activities such as walking and dancing may be continued, though curtailed.

Class 3—Self-Care Plus

Being placed in this group means that the patient is able to care for himself, personally, and do even more. He may require a cane or a crutch, but can work at a job which does not demand a great deal of walking or standing. Hiking, dancing and the like must be eliminated, but the patient is a functioning individual who can responsibly care for himself and his family.

Class 4—Self-Care Minus

Individuals so classified require assistance from others in their self-care. The amount of help needed varies. Stairs are unmanageable alone, as is going out from the home alone, because these amputees are not safe ambulators. If they have a desk-type job and can be transported to and from work by automobile, return to their former occupation may be quite possible. Such patients can live at home with their families, but not alone.

Class 5—Cosmetic-Plus

As the name of this class implies, the artificial limb is prescribed primarily for the sake of appearance. Persons included in this category fall short of being able to care for themselves and require considerable assistance from others. They can move about the home with the aid of crutches, but outdoor activity is largely excluded. Functionally, the prosthesis does not give them a much greater advantage over their handicap without a prosthesis.

Class 6—Not Feasible

The amputee in this group does not have a prosthetic limb prescribed for him. Instead, he is trained in self-care activities from a wheelchair.

OSTEOPOROSIS

Skeletal complaints, particularly of low back pain, in the aged are frequently attributable to osteoporosis. This is a condition in which bone mass become quantitatively reduced while the bone itself remains qualitatively identical to normal bone. The decrease in bone may result from two possible causes, an absolute or relative decrease in rate of bone matrix production, or an absolute or relative increase in rate of bone removal. Currently, the former explanation is preferred, although the evidence which supports it is clinical and not experimental.

While generalized osteoporosis may occur in any decade of life, its incidence increases with age and, in the elderly, is often referred to as *senile osteoporosis*. In women the balance of antianabolic and anabolic hormones is suddenly shifted with the menopause and the diminution of anabolic estrogens leaves a preponderance of antianabolic hormones. In men the decrease in anabolic hormones is more gradual and the shift to preponderantly antianabolic hormones occurs later and is less marked. Other factors which are associated with osteoporosis in the aged are immobilization and disuse of an area following a fracture, in which osteoporotic changes take place in the immobilized area, and diabetes mellitus.

Although senile osteoporosis is a generalized metabolic disease of the skeleton, symptoms most commonly involve the vertebral column. There is a predominance of back pain, especially of the lower back, which is due to gross structural changes occurring more often in the vertebrae than in other bones. The pain may be due to alterations within the bone itself, or the pressure of the altered bone on surrounding ligaments, muscles and nerves. The area of pain below the lesion may be extensive, often involving, in addition to the back, the hips and lower extremities.

Patients typically present a history of years of mild to moderate low back pain with a sudden increase in pain, often following mild trauma. In addition to the pain, osteoporosis can be responsible for fractures and vertebral compression because of the general fragility of the skeletal structure.

Concurrent with hormone administration and dietary regulation, energetic mobilization is important for osteoporotic patients to aid osteoblast formation. Physical inactivity or prolonged bed rest is to be avoided.

GERIATRIC GAIT PATTERNS (SENILE GAIT)

In the elderly, it is not uncommon to find anomalous gait patterns which can become incapacitating. A pathological gait creates problems in ambulation and can result in accidents.

While there are specific causes for various senile gait patterns, motor ability in the aged is generally considerably poorer than in younger persons. The gradual deterioration of accuracy and speed in motor performance of the elderly is due, primarily, to physiological aging and brain damage in the form of arteriosclerosis.

One etiological variable in an abnormal gait pattern is general locomotor disuse. This is the case where a disease has forced the patient to discontinue ambulation for a long period of time and, following remission of the illness, normal activity was not resumed. Rehabilitation can be very successful in restoring such cases to normal ambulation patterns.

Single muscle group disuse in the elderly also produces a form of senile gait. A patient with osteoarthritis of the knee, for example, who, because of some short-term intercurrent illness, remains quiescent for a period of time, will experience pain on attempting to ambulate following termination of the illness. The bed or chair rest produced disuse atrophy of quadriceps muscles, and when ambulation is initiated the inadequately protected knee joint accumulates minor trauma with resultant pain and swelling. Should the patient then rest to relieve the painful knee, the quadriceps weakness may become worse, leading to further pain. This cycle of pain and disuse atrophy may result in permanent discontinuation of ambulation if not treated by the appropriate medical and rehabilitation procedures.

A characteristic of advanced osteoarthritis of the hip is painful muscle spasm around the joint, predominantly in the hip adductor muscles. When this is combined with changes in the bony structure of the hip it can produce varying degrees of coxa vara, or curvature of the neck of the femur. This causes adduction of the thigh and shortening of the limb as the head of the femur is drawn nearer the shaft. Coxa vara can take place bilaterally, resulting in a "scissor" gait, and may greatly limit a patient's ambulation activities so that walking is achieved only with the aid of crutches.

Types of Senile Gait

Petren's Gait

Petren's gait is a consequence of neurological impairment and resembles, in some features, the gait of the patient with Parkinson's disease. There is a gradual disintegration of the patient's ability to initiate motor activities, especially walking.

In the initial phase, only episodes of Petren's gait occur, but in the advanced stage, the patient's feet appear to be glued to the floor. Gail consists of sliding the feet along the floor in very short steps. After every few steps the patient stops and then resumes ambulation for another series of small steps. Unlike Parkinson's disease, there is no rigidity of the major muscles and almost no coordination loss between the trunk and the lower extremities.

Intermittent Double Step Gait

Patients with hemiplegia, hip fractures and locomotor disorders frequently exhibit this gait pattern. The name describes the patient's stopping after every two steps, which is done to enable him to regain his uncertain balance.

Other causes of senile gait include disuse osteoporosis, pain or changes in the alignment of the long bones of the leg, ununited hip fractures, peripheral nerve involvements, motor system disease, tabes dorsalis, spinal cord diseases, arthritis and the myopathies. In a large percentage of cases rehabilitation can be of significant value to the elderly patient with a gait problem.

Chapter 3

DISABILITIES OF CHILDHOOD

M<small>ANY OF THE DISORDERS</small> found in adults are also met with in children, and conversely, a large number of primarily childhood diseases and disabilities are seen in the adult population. One reason for this general nonselectivity of disorders is simply that a particular disease may initially strike adults and children alike and is not restricted in its effects to any single age group. Another reason is that the greatest number of childhood diseases, with their resultant disabilities are not fatal and hence, are carried with the individual into adulthood. Thus, for example, the adult with cerebral palsy initially acquired the disorder at birth or shortly thereafter, and the older person with a deformed limb may have a congenital defect.

To distinguish disorders of children from those of adults, this chapter will discuss diseases and disabilities which occur initially in childhood, or primarily in childhood, or occur only in, and run their entire course during, the childhood years. Poliomyelitis, formerly the largest diagnostic group requiring rehabilitation, will not be dealt with herein. Due to the advent of the development and widespread use of the Salk and Sabin vaccines the prevalence of this disease has been markedly reduced and now has a relatively low frequency of occurrence in children in this country. The largest number of polio patients seen in rehabilitation today are adults with residual disabilities from childhood infection. Poliomyelitis was discussed in Chapter One (See p. 11).

OBJECTIVES OF CHILD REHABILITATION

Any rehabilitation program involving children must be based upon the belief that the patient with a disability is first and foremost a child. This means that not only the particular handicap is treated, but *the whole child* and his needs, desires and total behavior repertoire receive full consideration. Most children with a disability have a lifetime before them which does not differ appreciably in length from that of non-disabled children. It is the job of the rehabilitation team to help them to achieve their highest potential as a family member, as members of society, and most important, as individuals.

The objectives of rehabilitation with children must include aiding them towards the maximum physical, behavioral, social, educational and vocational possibilities within the limits imposed upon them by their disabilities.

Furthermore, the child with a fatal prognosis should not be denied rehabilitation services because his life span is relatively limited. Rather, all efforts should be expended to help him make the most effective use of his remaining time and to enable him to live as full a life as possible. The incurable disease of today may be cured or prevented tomorrow, as the recent advances in poliomyelitis illustrate. All children requiring rehabilitation have the right to receive it regardless of their diagnosis or prognosis. As is true for adults, the philosophy must not be that a child's disability will prevent him from doing many things, but instead, that his remaining abilities can be utilized for a happier life.

It is true that despite the best efforts of a rehabilitation team the majority of children on a therapeutic program will have a permanent physical disability. The objectives then, of such a program, are not "cure," in the general or traditional sense of the word, or habilitation to completely normal functioning, but rather, prevention and correction of deformities and the building up of muscle strength and endurance so that the child can be taught to perform all of the activities of daily living of which he is capable. Rehabilitation focuses on self-care in the bed and the wheelchair, maximum use of the hands, ambulation and elevation activities, speech and hearing, and the appearance of being normal, which becomes increasingly important as the child grows older.

There are many conditions which produce disabilities in children, but not all of them come to the attention of rehabilitation services as the term is used in this book. Of those which do, the most frequently seen are orthopedic disabilities which are primarily on neuromuscular, skeletal and musculoskeletal, and central nervous system bases, and cardiac disorders. A large number of children are multi-handicapped, as for example, the child with cerebral palsy who may have speech and hearing losses, visual defects and intellectual retardation in addition to neuromotor dysfunction.

Children with orthopedic disabilities often have their rehabilitation complicated by secondary deformities produced by contractures, and sensory and perceptual deficits. Despite the complexities of the problems of these children, much can be accomplished through an intensive rehabilitation program.

PROGRESSIVE MUSCULAR DYSTROPHY

Progressive muscular dystrophy is one of the more common primary diseases of muscle. It is characterized by weakness and atrophy of the skeletal muscles resulting in increasing disability and deformity as the disease progresses, frequently involving degeneration of cardiac muscles. There are several types of progressive muscular dystrophy but all forms show the muscular atrophy.

The etiology of the disease is unknown, yet all of the dystrophies have significant hereditary factors involved. Genetic patterns may be of a sex-linked simple recessive or dominant type. When the disease has been transmitted through a sex-linked or simple recessive factor, the symptoms tend to become manifest in early life. When a dominant mode of inheritance is involved, the onset occurs later in life. The disease is three times as prevalent in males as in females, and is also more severe and more rapidly progressive in males. It may be that different biochemical deficits are responsible for the various forms of the disorder.

All of the clinical forms of muscular dystrophy may be considered variations of a single disease, differing only in age of onset, affected muscle groups and rate of progression, although some authorities feel that the term "progressive muscular dystrophy" comprises a number of different diseases with similar characteristics.

Although classical nomenclature lists several distinct types, it is possible for an individual patient to exhibit the characteristics of more than one form of the disease.

Pseudohypertrophic Form

This is the most common and also the most serious type. Also called Duchenne type, childhood type or severe generalized type, it has its onset between the ages of two and ten years, most often prior to age five. It is transmitted by a sex-linked recessive gene and is rare in females.

The disease begins in the muscles of the lower back, trunk, hips and lower extremities, and progresses cephalically. Occasionally, the first signs become noticeable in infancy when the child experiences difficulty in standing or in learning to walk. It is more often the case that the child is observed to have gradually increasing weakness of the legs with a waddling gait and frequent falls. Eventually, the disorder progresses so that riding a tricycle, climbing stairs or even raising the arms above the head to comb hair become impossible. The child becomes unable to rise from the floor without a typical pattern of movements considered pathognomonic of muscular dystrophy. Once the child is standing, the abdomen is thrust forward, and there is severe lordosis, or anteroposterior curvature of the spine.

The muscles of the body are usually symmetrically involved. As the illness advances, more and more muscles become atrophied until late in the disease all muscles of the legs, spine, pelvis and shoulder girdle are atrophic. In some cases, large subcutaneous deposits of fat preserve body contours, while in others, contractures and skeletal deformities occur. Most children with this form of muscular dystrophy succumb to respiratory infection or from cardiac failure once the heart muscle becomes involved in the dystrophic process. Death usually occurs before the age of twenty.

Facioscapulohumeral Form

This type of progressive muscular dystrophy, also known as Landouzy-Déjerine, or mild-restrictive type, has its initial onset in both sexes between the ages of six and twenty, and most frequently between age ten and age eighteen. It is transmitted through a dominant mode of inheritance.

The muscles which are first affected are those of the face and shoulder girdle. The initial disability which is frequently observed is an inability of the child to raise his arms overhead. The face takes on an expressionless appearance and the patient is unable to close his eyelids, raise his eyebrows or wrinkle his forehead. The disease advances slowly to include muscles of the pelvis and lower extremities. The rate of progression is so slow that longevity is not significantly altered, although, in later life, severe disability does occur.

Limb-Girdle Form

This form of dystrophy is less severe than the pseudohypertrophic type and is more serious than the facioscapulohumeral form. The onset varies between the first and fourth decades of life. The disease may first attack either the pectobrachial or pelviformal muscle groups. It then spreads to the opposite girdle within two to fifteen years. It is transmitted hereditarily without sex linkage.

Juvenile Muscular Atrophy

Juvenile muscular atrophy (Erb's type) usually has its onset in adolescence or early adulthood. The shoulder girdle muscles are involved initially, with resultant winging of the scapulae. The child has difficulty in raising his arms above his head. This type of the disease is slowly progressive and the patient's status may remain unchanged for years.

Other forms of muscular dystrophy include *myotonic dystrophy,* which is characterized by initial involvement of the upper extremities, cortical cataracts, frontal baldness and gonadal atrophy, and *ophthalmophegic dystrophy,* in which muscle degeneration is largely confined to the extrinsic eye muscles.

ARTHROGRYPOSIS

This is a relatively rare disease. The term "arthrogryposis" means congenital contractures of joints in flexion or extension.

The etiology of the disorder is in doubt, some believing it to be a connective tissue disease, some claiming it is a consequence of myoblastic failure of development, and still others presenting evidence for a neurogenic origin. While it is generally not considered hereditary, cases have been described of autosomal dominant transmission for several generations of a family. The disorder may occur alone or in conjunction with other disabilities, such as arachnodactyly, abnormal length of the extremities, or premature synostosis, or fusion of the bones of the skull.

In arthrogryposis, the arms are rotated inward while the thighs are rotated outward. The elbows and knees are commonly ankylosed, or stiffly fixed in extension, although fixation of the knees in flexion also occurs. Fingers and wrists are flexed, and clubbed feet are a typical finding.

One form of the disorder is *arthrogryposis multiplex congenita* (multiple congenital articular rigidities), which shows additional symptoms. Commonly found are congenital stiffness of one or more joints, dislocation of the hips and other joints, palate and vertebrae malformations, and absence of sacrum and fibula.

Treatment consists of physical therapy, orthotic training and orthopedic surgery.

OSTEOGENESIS IMPERFECTA

Osteogenesis imperfecta is a familial disorder characterized by increased fragility of the bones so that they are easily fractured, even by mild trauma. Affected children usually have blue scleras and flaccid ligaments, and occasionally become deaf in later life.

Osteogenesis Imperfecta Congenita

In this form of the disorder fractures may occur *in utero* and the infant is born with deformed extremities due to the bones healing in abnormal positions. Fractures can occur during delivery.

The affected child has prominent eyes with blue scleras, dental changes, a short neck and, in severe cases, deformed chest and spine.

Many children with the severe congenital form do not survive long after birth. Children who do not succumb often suffer fractures of the extremities from slight trauma, the legs usually being the most frequently involved extremities. Marked deformities often result from such fractures.

Osteogenesis Imperfecta Tarda

This other form of the disorder, also termed *osteopsathyrosis,* has a milder course. The child appears normal at birth and fractures do not occur until after the first year of life. On occasion, this type is severe and resembles the congenital form, but usually only a moderate number of fractures occur and the tendency to easy breakage of bones ceases after puberty.

The bones of the extremities of affected children are long and slender, and heal rapidly, although deformities may develop. Flaccidity of ligaments and muscles may result in repeated dislocations. Frequently, with orthopedic treatment, these patients are able to live relatively normal lives.

CONGENITAL LIMB DEFICIENCIES

Amputations in children can be the result of either trauma or disease, or they can be congenital.

With the exception of the results known to have been produced by the drug thalidomide, the etiology of congenital limb deficiencies is not well known. The factors to be considered include the child's month and year of birth, the mother's age at the time of delivery, the presence of associated skeletal or other anomalies, complications during pregnancy, and familial abnormalities, including cancer.

Experimentally, known etiological agents are hereditary factors, diet, irradiation, hormones, chemicals and trauma. In humans, these agents have not been fully evaluated. The only teratogenic agent known to consistently result in congenital limb amputations and deformities is thalidomide, which is the active ingredient of a tranquilizing drug formerly widely used in Western Europe. Among limb deficiencies not related to thalidomide, the amputation is usually unilateral and most frequently involves the left upper extremity. Thalidomide-produced deformities generally involve both upper extremities with similar deformities, sometimes affecting all four limbs.

There are two types of skeletal imperfections to be considered in this section.

Terminal deficiencies may be likened to an axe cutting across the laminations of the extremity somites at any level from the trunk to the tips of the digits. If the "severation" is completely through the extremity, a terminal amputation exists at that site. If the "axe" cut through only the pre- or post-axial somites, then those areas fail to develop distal to the site of injury. The remainder of the limb develops paraxially, or parallel to the axis.

Intercalary deficiencies can be depicted as an animal bite in the extremity. Areas which are proximal and distal to the "bitten out" area survive and continue to grow. If the "bite" transects the limb entirely, the terminal portion survives in a foreshortened form. Should the metaphorical bite remove only a segment of the pre- or post-axial laminations, the somites survive distally and proximally and continue to develop, resulting in a paraxial intercalary deficiency.

The two types of congenital amputations which are most frequently encountered on a children's rehabilitation service are amelia and phocomelia.

Amelia refers to a complete absence of an extremity. Included within this classification are the following: *acheiria*, absence of the hand; *apodia,* absence of the foot; and *adactylia,* absence of digits.

Phocomelia describes extremities which are foreshortened as are the flippers of a seal.

In all cases, the desired rehabilitation goal is to enable the child to function as normally as possible with prosthetic devices.

SPINA BIFIDA

Spina bifida is a disability in which some of the child's vertebrae do not develop fully during gestation. In one form of the disorder, *spina bifida occulta,* although some of the vertebrae are incompletely developed, the spinal cord itself is normal. This condition occurs on approximately ten per cent of all births and generally does not present complex problems. The form of the disability which requires rehabilitation services is known as *spina bifida manifesta.* Here, the spinal cord fails to form properly and rather than developing in a tube-like shape forms as a flat plate (*myelomeningocele*) which protrudes from the surface of the back. It is not protected by vertebrae as is the normal cord, but is covered by the meninges alone.

The causes of spina bifida are, as yet, unknown, Experimentally, a number of compounds can be administered to pregnant animals of several species which will result in the condition. There is no evidence with humans, however, that any drug ingested during pregnancy causes it. Having had one child with spina bifida appears to increase the chances of having a second child with the same disorder, although the risk is small.

There are several problems associated with spina bifida manifesta. As a consequence of failure of the spinal cord to sufficiently innervate the muscles and skin, children with this disability usually are paraplegic or paraparetic and have accompanying sensory losses. The neural deficiency which causes the muscular weakness and sensory deficit also results in bowel and bladder incontinence. The child is unable to detect when his bowel or bladder is full, nor can he void normally since the muscles required for this act lack the strength to expel feces or urine because of an inadequate nerve supply. Thus, the kidneys continue to pass urine into the bladder until the pressure causes it to overflow without the child's volition or awareness.

An additional difficulty occurring in most patients with spina bifida manifesta is hydrocephalus, an abnormally rapid and excessive enlargement of the head. This is due to interference with circulation and absorption of cerebrospinal fluid in the ventricular and subarachnoid spaces of the brain. The fluid pressure in the brain rapidly increases, enlarging the skull. If the condition is permitted to continue without surgical intervention severe intellectual retardation can result.

Rehabilitation of children with spina bifida manifesta consists of surgery, bowel and bladder management and training, physical therapy and teaching the activities and daily living. Some affected children learn to ambulate without assistance of any kind while others always require the use of a wheelchair. In all cases, considerable independence can be achieved through prompt medical and therapeutic treatment.

AMYOTONIA CONGENITA

There are two main forms of this syndrome.

Werdnig-Hoffman disease is an inherited lower motor neuron disorder transmitted either as a dominant with low penetrance or as a recessive. It is a progressive muscular atrophy whose symptoms appear in the later half of the first year of life. The paralysis rapidly spreads from the trunk to the shoulder girdle and then to the muscles of the extremities. Most children with Werdnig-Hoffman disease do not live past the age of twelve.

Oppenheim's disease is characterized by general muscle weakness, hypotonia and hypermobility of joints. It is a disease of lower motor neuron degeneration and, presumably, has its onset prior to birth. Despite data which indicate that many affected children succumb within the first decade of life, the impression in the medical field is that Oppenheim's disease is a relatively benign condition with a good prognosis for recovery.

DYSTONIA MUSCULORUM DEFORMANS

Dystonia musculorum deformans is a disease involving the loss of cells, most notably the larger cells, in the basal ganglia. While relatively rare in the United States, it occurs more commonly in Eastern European Jewish families. There is no sex predilection.

The chief symptom of this disease is maintained torsion of the limbs and trunk. Signs are first noted before puberty and generally within the first decade of life. The initial symptom is a fixed position of one leg, with the foot extended and held *in pes cavus* with the toes flexed. Shortly after this symptom appears, the thigh flexes and adducts, the knee bends and the other leg becomes involved. Extreme lumbar lordosis appears early. After some years, the arms rotate internally, adduct, extend at the elbows and flex at the wrists. Finally, strong, involuntary torsion movements appear which involve the legs, arms and trunk.

Walking results in extreme writhing of affected parts. These movements are absent during sleep and made worse by emotional distress, although psychotherapy is of no help. Dystonia musculorum deformans has a long course ultimately resulting in the confinement of the patient.

CEREBRAL PALSY

Cerebral palsy is a nonprogressive brain disorder resulting from malfunction of the motor centers and pathways of the brain occurring during gestation, parturition or the neonatal period. It is characterized by paralysis, weakness and incoordination of motor function with resultant abnormality of movement and/or posture. This disorder is one of the leading cripplers of children, and is multi-handicapping, presenting problems in neurologic, orthopedic, speech, auditory, visual, intellectual and behavioral areas of function.

Cerebral palsy is termed *congenital* when the initial effect of the etiologic factor occurs prenatally or within the first two weeks of neonatal life. It is called *acquired* when the onset takes place after this period.

There are several possible causes of cerebral palsy and hence, it is considered by many to be a group of disorders rather than a single entity, with the common factor of brain dysfunction occurring in the prenatal or natal period. The single largest causative variable is infection of the central nervous system, such as encephalitis. Other etiologic factors include trauma, as in a blow to the head, cerebrovascular accident, neoplasms, post-seizure complications, surgical complications, developmental defects of the brain in regard to its biochemical maturation, hypoxia, hemorrhage, toxins and poisons, genetic defects and isoimmunization reactions. Regardless of the cause, cerebral palsy is a static condition which is nonfatal and noncurable.

Classifications

The classifying of children with cerebral palsy may be done on the basis of the type of neuromotor deficit and also on the topographic distribution of the neuromotor involvement.

Neuromotor Impairment

Spastic. This type is characterized by a pathologically exaggerated stretch reflex, increased deep tendon reflexes in the affected parts, "scissoring" and contractures affecting the anti-gravity muscles. *Clonus,* which is rapidly successive contractions and relaxations of affected muscles, is typical of the spastic type. It gives the child the spasmodic, uncontrollable movements of the trunk and extremities which are characteristic of this form of cerebral palsy.

Athetotic. Athetosis is marked by involuntary and incoordinate movement of the affected parts with varying degrees of muscle tension. Initially, the clinical sign may be hypotonia, and only during the second year of life will the athetotic symptoms become manifest. The main characteristics of this type are the slow, writhing, involuntary, unpredictable and random motions of the trunk and limbs while the child is at rest.

Ataxic. Ataxia is manifested as lack of coordination, balance and equilibrium due to disturbances of the kinesthetic and balance senses. Ambulation of the affected person resembles the reeling gait of one who is intoxicated. Hypotonia may be associated with the ataxia.

Rigidity. The primary clinical sign of the rigid patient is muscular hypertonicity which, in some children, is so extreme that no motion is present. It is due to continual resistance in agonist and antagonist muscles when the affected part is moved.

Tremor. Tremors are primarily involuntary and uncontrollable. They are reciprocal and occur in a regular rhythmic pattern.

Atonia or Hypotonia. This form is characterized by soft muscles and increased deep tendon reflexes. It is frequently a precursor of other types of involvement.

Mixed. Approximately one per cent of all children with cerebral palsy exhibit more than one type, but usually one form predominates.

Topographic Involvement

PARAPLEGIA. Involvement of the lower extremities. These patients are almost always of the spastic type.

HEMIPLEGIA. Involvement of upper and lower extremities on the same side of the body. Patients who are hemiplegic are most often spastic, but athetotic patients with hemiplegia are occasionally observed.

TRIPLEGIA. Involvement of three extremities. Generally, this refers to both lower extremities and one arm. Again, the disability is usually of the spastic type.

QUADRIPLEGIA. Involvement of all four extremities. Almost all patients with athetosis are quadriplegic. When the term "diplegia" is used it indicates greater involvement of the legs than the arms.

There are three main categories of severity of neuromotor involvement.

Mild

Such patients require no treatment. This means that there are no speech problems, ambulation is performed without the aid of devices or appliances, and the child is able to care for his daily needs.

Moderate

These children are in need of treatment. They are inadequate in speech, ambulation and self-care activities. They require braces and self-help appliances in order to function.

Severe

The severely involved patient is here referred to, and the degree of impairment is so great that prognosis for adequate speech, ambulation and ability to care for himself is poor.

In addition to the problems of impaired movement and posture, the child with cerebral palsy is likely to have one or more associated defects.

Seizures occur in approximately one-third of these children, either only once, or a few times, or with recurring regularity. The incidence of seizures in spastic cerebral palsy is three times greater than in the athetotic type. If seizures occur frequently, learning is interfered with. Furthermore, the possibility of falling becomes an ever-present danger, and additional brain damage may occur as a result of increased intracranial vascular pressure.

There is considerable variation in the reported incidence of hearing deficits among the cerebral palsied, ranging from five to eighty per cent. The affected children are primarily those with kernicterus, or jaundice of brain areas due to isoimmunization factors. With such patients there is probably a high incidence of hearing loss for sounds in the upper frequency range.

More than half of the children with cerebral palsy can be expected to have visual impairments. These deficits range from total and partial blindness to various forms of strabismus. Some affected children exhibit homonymous hemianopsia.

Sensory losses are common in cerebral palsy. Losses occur for light touch, stereognosis, two-point discrimination, position, vibration, pain and temperature. Patients with post-natal onset of spastic hemiplegia have nearly twice the frequency of loss of touch sense as do patients with prenatal or natal onset. Approximately twice as many spastic cerebral palsied children as athetotic children have losses in the sensory sphere.

Speech defects occur in about two-thirds of the patients. The severity of the impairment varies from minor handicaps which present no significant problems to unintelligible or completely absent speech. There is generally a direct positive correlation between the degree of motor handicap and the extent of speech loss. The incidence of speech absence is greatest in the spastic type and dysarthria is most typical of the athetotic type. In the ataxic type, although the frequency of speech problems is high, intelligibility is usually good. Dysarthria is more common in quadriplegic and diplegic children than in hemiplegics. Reports of aphasia have been noted, but children so diagnosed do not resemble adult aphasics and perhaps the term is a misnomer when applied in these cases.

Approximately one-half of the patients are intellectually retarded and test out to an IQ of below seventy, about one-fourth of these scoring below an IQ of fifty. The incidence of retardation is related to the frequency of seizures, speech impairments, emotional problems, perceptual deficits and learning disabilities. The degree of retardation is greater is spastic children than in those with athetosis.

Learning difficulties are common even among the nonretarded children. These patients are deficient in reading, arithmetic and other school subjects, generally being one or more grades below their age level. Children of the spastic type are, as a group, considerably lower than athetotic children in their educational functioning.

Although the brain lesion in cerebral palsy is static in nature, the neurological deficit is not unchanging. A small percentage of infants do improve with time and may, upon subsequent examination, appear normal. On the other hand, some children develop signs of neurologic impairment as they grow older, although late developing signs are usually mild. All children with the disorder can benefit to some extent from rehabilitation. While many will never be able to ambulate independently, independence in activities of daily living can be achieved with the great majority of affected children.

JUVENILE RHEUMATOID ARTHRITIS

Juvenile rheumatoid arthritis, or *Still's disease,* is a protean systemic disease with a wide spectrum of manifestations and joint involvement.

The disease is of unknown etiology, although a variety of factors influence its expression. There is a relatively high familial incidence. The frequency of occurrence is higher in temperate climates and in the spring months. It occurs more often in females under the age of six. Psychological stress appears to be linked to the onset and to exacerbations. It may be that the disease is a response to as yet unrecognized exogenous stimuli and is manifested by the interaction of several secondary variables.

Still's disease occurs twice as commonly in females as it does in males. The median age for its initial onset is about five years of age, with the mode being between two and three years. It can occur suddenly or insidiously with almost imperceptible development of stiffness in the joints, swelling, pain and eventual limitation of motion. This limitation may be localized to a single joint for months or even years, but eventually almost all joints become involved.

The affected child may sit characteristically in bed, guarding his joints against movement or contact. Pain results in reduced motion and swelling in the joints produces fusiform changes in the fingers. Limitation of motion can result in flexion contractures causing residual deformities.

In addition to the arthritic changes, carditis occurs in ten per cent or more of the cases and when this is associated with anemia the condition becomes quite serious. Ocular changes can also occur which lead to blindness.

The course of Still's disease is characterized by remissions and exacerbations. Generally, each exacerbation is less severe than the preceding one. The disease tends to become gradually quiescent, usually prior to puberty. During the acute phase, cardiac failure and toxicity may endanger the life of the patient but when these threats pass, the prognosis for life is good. The eventual prognosis depends upon the extent of residual deformity. Over one-half of affected children have complete functional recovery and over three-fourths can lead adequately functional lives.

RHEUMATIC HEART DISEASE

Rheumatic fever is due to a reaction to components of certain streptococci which initially result in an upper respiratory infection. While many children who contact rheumatic fever escape cardiac involvement, those who have had a difficult course during the acute stage of the illness will likely develop a heart valve abnormality.

Acute rheumatic fever usually occurs between the ages of eight and fifteen. The great majority of children survive, requiring prolonged bed rest followed by limitation of physical activity.

Chronic rheumatic heart disease develops as a result of scarring and distortion of the heart valves from the initial rheumatic inflammation. Many of the lesions are amenable to surgery or palliation although complications can arise, such as arrhythmias or heart failure requiring specific treatment.

Rheumatic Endocarditis

The term "endocarditis" describes an inflammation of the endocardium, the membrane lining the heart. The inflammation may involve only the membrane covering the valves (valvular endocarditis), or it may involve the general lining of the chambers of the heart (mural endocarditis).

Rheumatic involvement of the endocardium is the most common type of endocarditis affecting children. The mitral valve is affected most frequently, the aortic valve next most often, and the tricuspid and pulmonary valves less commonly.

As the infection subsides scars remain. Each repeated infection leaves more small lesions near the previous ones, involving the mural endocardium and the tendinous strands running from the papillary muscles to the mitral and tricuspid valves *(chordae tendinae).*

Mitral Insufficiency

Mitral insufficiency prevents normal closure of the mitral valve. It is most frequently rheumatic in origin.

Important signs include left atrial and ventricular enlargement, and an apical systolic murmur.

During convalescence, children with mild cardiac disease often make great improvement while those with advanced disease suffer from the effects of rapid growth of the involved parts. If there are further rheumatic infections the valvular condition becomes progressively worse.

Organic Mitral Stenosis

Nearly always of rheumatic origin, this disease results from sclerosis of the mitral ring and the base of the valve leaflets. It may take two or more years to become fully established, and it is frequently associated with mitral insufficiency.

Attacks of dyspnea are caused by left atrial failure. Other symptoms include: hemoptysis, or spitting of blood due to ruptured bronchial veins or pulmonary infarction; varying degrees of cardiac enlargement; apical murmurs; and a bluish and purplish tinge on the cheeks.

There are several complications of mitral stenosis, such as congestive heart failure, systemic emboli, subacute bacterial endocarditis, atrial fibrillation and functional tricuspid inefficiency.

The course and prognosis of the disease are quite variable. Some patients succumb during the adolescent years while others attain old age.

Rheumatic Pericarditis

Pericarditis is an inflammation of the pericardium, the fibroserous membrane covering the heart and beginning of the great vessels. It is usually a consequence of rheumatic fever.

The affected child becomes acutely ill with fever, dyspnea and pericardial pain. A common symptom, and one which is considered to be pathognomonic, is a friction rub, a leathery, "scratchy" sound in the heart.

If the child only suffers from pericarditis, serious after effects generally do not occur. However, there is usually extensive carditis making the prognosis a potentially poor one.

THE CHILD AND HIS PARENTS

In the rehabilitation of children, knowing the child is as important as knowing his disability. The patient's motivation is a key factor in determining the extent to which a rehabilitation program will be successful.

Parents must be made fully aware of their child's potential and their expectations of him must be geared to it. Unnecessary pressures placed upon a child's performance may retard progress rather than accelerate it. It is also highly important to keep the parents aware of the fact that the more independent a child becomes, within the expected performance range for his age, the more he will be able to benefit from educational, social and vocational experiences. Thus, while parents are urged not to push a child beyond his capacity, they are also cautioned against overprotecting him and shielding him from the necessary experiences of life.

Rehabilitation has been demonstrated to be possible and rewarding. With the team approach, including the parents, the future holds even more promise of satisfaction in making the youngest members of our society happier, more useful citizens.

———————————

Section I
References

1. Adams, J. C.: *Outline of Fractures, Including Joint Injuries,* 4th ed. Baltimore, Williams and Wilkins, 1964.
2. Blakeslee, B. (Ed): *The Limb-Deficient Child.* Berkeley, University of California Press, 1963.
3. Cecil, R. L. and Loeb, R. F.: *A Textbook of Medicine,* 10th ed. Philadelphia, Saunders, 1959.
4. Dacso, M. M. (Ed): *Restorative Medicine in Geriatrics.* Springfield, Thomas, 1963.
5. *Dorland's Illustrated Medical Dictionary,* 24th ed. Philadelphia, Saunders, 1965.
6. Gardner, E.: *Fundamentals of Neurology,* 3rd ed. Philadelphia, Saunders, 1959.
7. Gatz, A. J.: *Manter's Essentials of Clinical Neuroanatomy and Neurophysiology,* 3rd ed. Philadelphia, Davis, 1966.
8. Krusen, F. H., Kottke, F. J. and Ellwood, P. M. (Eds): *Handbook of Physical Medicine and Rehabilitation.* Philadelphia, Saunders, 1965.
9. Lee, P. R., Groch, S., Untereker, J., Silson, J., Dacso, M. M., Feldman, D. J., Monohan, K. and Rusk, H. A.: *Rehabilitation Monograph XV. An Evaluation of Patients with Hemiparesis or Hemiplegia Due to Cerebral Vascular Disease.* New York, Institute of Rehabilitation Medicine, 1958.
10. Long, C. and Lawton, E. B.: Functional significance of spinal cord lesion level. *Arch Phys Med, 36*: 249, 1955.
11. McCleary, R. A. and Moore, R. Y.: *Subcortical Mechanisms of Behavior.* New York, Basic Books, 1965.
12. Myers, J. S. (Ed): *An Orientation to Chronic Disease and Disability.* New York, Macmillan, 1965.
13. Nelson, W. E. (Ed): *Textbook of Pediatrics,* 8th ed. Philadelphia, Saunders, 1964.
14. Netter, F. H.: *The CIBA Collection of Medical Illustrations. I. Nervous System.* Summit, CIBA, 1962.
15. New York Heart Association: *Diseases of the Heart and Blood Vessels—Nomenclature and Criteria for Diagnosis,* 6th ed. Boston, Little, Brown, 1964.
16. Rusk, H. A.: *Rehabilitation Medicine. A Textbook of Physical Medicine and Rehabilitation,* 2nd ed. St. Louis, Mosby, 1964.
17. Shimkin, M. B.: Epidemiology of cancer. *Mod. Med, 28*: 81, 1960.
18. *Stedman's Medical Dictionary,* 20th ed. Baltimore, Williams and Wilkins, 1961.
19. Swinyard, C. A.: *The Child With Spina Bifida.* New York Assoc. for the Aid of Crippled Children, 1966.
20. Swinyard, C. A.: Progressive muscular dystrophy and atrophy and related conditions. In *The Pediatric Clinics of North America.* Philadelphia, Saunders, 1960, vol. 7, pp. 703–732.
21. Taylor, Martha L.: *Understanding Aphasia. A Guide for Family and Friends.* New York, Institute of Rehabilitation Medicine, 1958.
22. Wechsler, I. S.: *Clinical Neurology,* 9th ed. Philadelphia, Saunders, 1963.

SECTION II

THE PHYSICAL THERAPY SERVICE

Chapter 4

EVALUATION PROCEDURES—PART 1

PHYSICAL THERAPY lies at the very heart of the rehabilitation process. The majority of patients and many professional members of the rehabilitation team consider it to be the single most important aspect of training. In fact, many patients equate rehabilitation with physical therapy, and while they may occasionally be lax in their attendance at other classes, they will generally attend physical therapy sessions unfailingly. At evaluation and re-evaluation conferences following the medical report, it is the report of the physical therapist which is presented first, and when conditions such as a job "freeze" exist in hospital systems, physical therapy is most often unaffected. The primary consideration in deciding upon a patient's readiness for discharge from a rehabilitation institution usually is his status as determined in physical therapy.

Physical therapy, as the discipline is termed in the United States, or physiotherapy, as it is called in England and Canada, may be defined as the application of physical agents and forces to reduce pain and to improve or maintain function. This includes the use of physical and other effective properties of light, heat, cold, water, electricity, radiation and mechanical agents. Also included are the therapeutic principles of *kinesiology,* that part of the physiology of motion which describes and analyzes locomotor events or bodily motion as a reflection of mechanics or the action of mechanical forces.

Physical therapy is a part of almost every rehabilitation patient's regimen and, in fact, it is primarily the need for physical therapy which results in hospitalization in a rehabilitation center.

THE INITIAL PHYSICAL THERAPY EVALUATION

The initial evaluation of a patient's function, as conducted by a physical therapist, is designed both to assess the patient as a candidate for active rehabilitation and to point up strengths and weaknesses which should be considered in the planning of a therapy program.

The evaluation consists of several types, or classes, of procedures, including the testing of muscle strength by means of manual and electrical techniques, the assessment of active and passive range of motion in the joints, the examination of the patient's ability to stand, maintain balance and tolerate a standing position, the analysis of gait, the checking of orthopedic appliances, prostheses and orthoses, and the noting of special conditions which may be present, such as scoliosis—a lateral deviation of the spinal column—shortening of a leg, blindness or cardiac disease, to name but a few examples.

MUSCLE TESTING

While it is true that the physical therapist tests muscles in both upper and lower extremities as well as those of the trunk and neck, many of these muscles are also tested by the occupational therapist. Thus, there is some overlap of function between these two services. Since occupational therapy is primarily concerned with upper extremity function this will be discussed in the next section of this book, while the present section will focus on rehabilitation of the lower extremities. The reader will bear in mind, however, that these are not necessarily mutually exclusive categories, primarily because the rehabilitation services must all be concerned with the patient as a whole, a functioning, integrated individual.

Muscle testing is an integral part of physical diagnosis and is a key variable in the treatment and prognosis of muscular disorders. It is important for purposes of differential diagnosis and provides the therapist and the physician with information which cannot be obtained in other ways. The distinguishing feature of many neuromuscular disorders is a characteristic muscle weakness. Some conditions are typified by a lack of a specific pattern of weakness, some by the symmetry of the weakness, and others by the definite pattern which the muscle involvement takes. Muscle testing is also useful in determining the site of peripheral nerve lesions, since only those muscles which derive their innervation from the nerve branches distal to the lesion will exhibit weakness.

By recording the rate and degree of return of muscle power through comparing repeated testings with the findings obtained during the patient's initial evaluation, an index is provided for the prescription and alteration of treatment and for determining the prognosis of a pathological condition.

Basic Factors in Muscle Movement

Muscle testing requires a thorough knowledge of muscle anatomy and physiology. This includes an understanding of the origin and insertion of muscles, their anatomic, synergistic and antagonistic actions, and their role in fixation. It also requires the ability to locate the main segments of a muscle, to distinguish between normal and atrophied contour, and to recognize position abnormalities and the general appearance of a part. (Note: While muscles act cooperatively in a movement pattern, a single muscle can only relax or contract between the two points of its attachment. The word "origin" refers to the proximal anchoring, or immobile muscle attachment, and the term "insertion" refers to the distal, movable attachment of a muscle which moves the part. A muscle exerts equal tension at its origin and its insertion. Its regular or "reverse" action depends upon the stabilizing or opposing actions of other muscles.)

In the movement of an extremity there are three important factors involved. They are the power, or amount of force present in the muscles of the extremity, the coordination of muscular contraction required to bring about the desired movement, and the range of motion in the joints. In determining the ability of muscles to function normally, it is common to employ tests of strength. These are probably the most valuable single indicators of muscle function, but if a complete picture of a muscle or muscle group's capacity and ability is to be obtained, tests for strength must be supplemented by tests of endurance and coordination.

Strength is measured as the absolute force which the muscle is able to exert in a single contraction. Almost all of the tests involve the muscle acting as a prime mover, although in normal function a muscle can act as either a prime mover, an antagonist or a synergist. (Note: A muscle acts as a prime mover in a given movement when its action is such that it produces that movement. A muscle is an antagonist to a prime mover when its action opposes the prime movement. A muscle is synergistic to a prime mover when its action prevents some action of a prime mover which is not part of the prime movement considered. A synergistic muscle, therefore, is a partial antagonist to the muscle of prime movement.)

Strength is of limited use if the muscle has no endurance, and endurance is not necessarily equally affected by either disease or exercise. Endurance is the ability of a muscle or muscle group to maintain a given state of contraction over a period of time or to make repeated contractions through a given range at a given rate over a period of time.

The normal functioning of a muscle is also dependent upon coordination. This may be defined as the ease with which contractions can be made with speed and accuracy.

Each of these factors—strength, endurance and coordination—is considered separately in the evaluation of muscle function.

Purposes of Muscle Testing

First of all, muscle testing is necessary for purposes of differential diagnosis. It is important for diagnosing the variety of neuromuscular diseases encountered in a rehabilitation hospital.

Children who come to the hospital with problems of easy fatigability, minor limping at the end of the day, and gait and postural deviations have often been found, upon examination, to have a muscular weakness of a "spotty" nature which is distributed in one or more segments leading to a diagnosis of poliomyelitis which had previously gone unrecognized. There is often tightening of the heel cords, back, iliotibial bands, which extend between the ilium and the tibia, shortening of one extremity, or beginning scoliosis. These findings lead to the clinical impression that many patients with "idiopathic" scoliosis, back tightness and succeeding growth deformity, have suffered a bout of poliomyelitis. They will, upon careful muscle testing, frequently demonstrate a weakness in the extremities which is not secondary to the scoliosis *per se.* Following physical therapy most such children improve, many to normal gait, strength and endurance.

An early diagnosis of muscular dystrophy frequently rests upon adequate muscle testing. There are often signs, such as easy fatigability and minor gait disturbances, which can lead to detection. Muscle testing will reveal characteristic proximal weakness which can be confirmed by muscle biopsy and/or electromyography. An early diagnosis is important for the control of hip and plantar flexion contractures which are found in the disease. In addition, muscle strength may be maintained at a maximal level with therapy, thus prolonging functional independence.

The level of the lesion in peripheral nerve trauma can be ascertained through muscle testing. Muscles which receive their innervation below the lesion will be involved, either partially or completely, depending upon the extent of the lesion. Diagnosis is aided primarily by muscle tests. In peripheral nerve regeneration sensory return is often preceded by increased muscle strength and permits a better treatment of physical therapy.

Muscle testing is a diagnostic aid in milder cases of cerebral palsy where the spasticity was undiagnosed in the patient's earlier years. One symptom may be increasing difficulty in ambulation as a consequence of the development of heel cord contractures secondary to weak dorsiflexor muscles of the foot or spasticity of the plantar flexors. Testing which includes tests of muscle strength and range of joint motion may uncover the problems.

Post-fracture patients, particularly with fractures of the lower extremities, frequently experience a lengthy convalescence, poor functional recovery, continued joint pain due to muscle weakness and restricted motion of adjacent joints. The patient may be instructed to initiate ambulation before an appropriate assessment is made of muscle strength. Such action can result in the patient splinting the part and developing inefficient or disruptive patterns of muscle and joint activity. Normal strength may not return and secondary contractures can progress unless adequate strength and range of motion tests are conducted. When therapy is directed toward the weakened muscles and joint contractures, the patient will often rapidly return to full activity.

It is highly important to do a muscle test to determine weakness associated with other diseases. Weakness may be consequence of disuse of poor utilization resulting from incorrect or disrupted patterns of motion, particularly following painful or immobilizing states, such as arthritis, amputation or low back pain. Patients with arthritis are often encouraged to walk when their knee strength is not sufficient to provide stabilization. The knees are held stiffly during ambulation because of relative muscle weakness or pain. Reversal of this weakness with proper utilization of muscle strength in ambulation will frequently provide significant relief. Patients with chronic, painful conditions, such as osteoarthritis, find that when muscle weakness is reversed through physical therapy much of their pain is eliminated.

A second purpose of muscle testing is to guide a treatment program. A complete and accurate assessment of muscle strength patterns originally serves as a guide to the physician in prescribing physical therapy and to the therapist in planning a program of exercises and activities. As muscle strength patterns change during the course of treatment, therapy tasks are modified accordingly. Thus, periodic re-evaluative muscle testing is necessary.

The frequency of repeated testing is determined by the medical condition. In slowly recovering diseases, such as poliomyelitis, Guillain-Barré syndrome and nerve regrowth following severance and suturing, muscles may be retested every six to eight weeks. In conditions such as osteoarthritis and post-fracture states, muscle tests are performed weekly to avoid prolongation of treatment which may be unnecessary.

The third indication for muscle testing is as an assist in the prognosis of certain diseases. Based upon results of muscle tests a patient's future can be discussed more realistically with him and his family, and unnecessarily prolonged hospitalization can be avoided. If, for example, muscle testing reveals that all muscles of one extremity have not returned to good strength while all other body segments are at or near normal strength, the patient may be advised to wear a brace and to ambulate within a short time, since further return in the affected extremity is unlikely. Another patient who has only moderate involvement of the same extremity but a better prognosis for return of strength with continued therapy, may be kept nonambulatory or non-weight-bearing on that extremity for several months, depending upon the rate and extent of recovery demonstrated by serial muscle testing. Serial muscle testing in diseases such as muscular dystrophy, multiple sclerosis, Parkinson's disease and amyotrophic later sclerosis enables the rehabilitation team to more accurately predict the future course of the disability as well as the need for assistive devices.

Muscle testing is performed for a fourth reason, to assess the need for functional and assistive devices. Since appliances are designed for the individual patient's needs, it is essential that a careful muscle test be performed prior to the prescription of such apparatus. A child with no power in his quadriceps muscle and functional hamstring muscles will forcefully hyperextend his knee during ambulation. A brace will be required to correct this. Growth deformities due to unequal muscle stresses can similarly be corrected. Devices for ambulation or other activities of daily living also depend, for their prescription, upon an evaluation of muscle strength and endurance factors.

A fifth purpose of muscle testing is as a prerequisite to surgery. One form of surgery in which it is particularly valuable is the transplantation of muscle tendon. A tendon transplant implies some loss of strength in the transplanted muscle. Thus, the surgeon must be certain that the muscle to be used as a motor has sufficient strength to be of value in its new position. Otherwise, surgery is pointless. Satisfactory functioning of single or multiple muscle transfers is dependent upon the power of the muscles to be used as a motor. A good muscle test will determine this.

Following trauma to peripheral nerves, if reinnervation does not take place within the estimated growth period, surgical reunion of the nerve may be indicated. In various neurosurgical procedures, such as an anterior rhizotomy, where division is performed of the anterior, or motor spinal nerve roots, or in peripheral denervation procedures, as might be performed on patients with hemiplegia, paraplegia, multiple sclerosis or cerebral palsy, it is essential to know the strength of the surrounding muscles and segments.

The Measurement of Muscle Strength

Prior to about 1910 most methods of assessing muscle strength and range of joint motion were subjective in nature. Many of these methods are still in use but are now often supplemented by objective techniques. In the early subjective evaluation procedure the degree of muscle contraction, as estimated manually, was graded as being either normal, partly paralyzed or totally paralyzed. Later, this grading system became refined and is discussed in the next section of this chapter. The main disadvantage of the subjective technique is that it is crude. That is, it does not enable fine discriminations to be made between different levels of muscular activity, and it is dependent upon the personal impressions of an observer. Its foremost advantages are speed of testing, lack of requirement of special apparatus, and applicability to any muscle or joint in individuals of any age.

Objective methods of muscle strength evaluation have the advantages of reliability and accuracy. In addition, even small changes in muscle strength or amplitude of movement can be assessed. Some of the disadvantages of this kind of procedure are that it is time consuming, requires relatively expensive equipment and provides findings which require comparison with a standard. Furthermore, if an instrument is employed over a prolonged period of time, training or fatigue factors can confound the results of the test.

The general trend in muscle testing has been from relatively simple, subjective procedures to more complex, but more accurate, objective techniques.

There are four main classes of objective testing methods.

Spring-Balance Methods record the amount of resistance necessary to prevent a movement. The patient resists a pull instead of exerting strength in active effort.

Pressure Systems comprise a group of instruments which are designed to objectively measure muscle strength by means of a system in which pressure changes occur. An example of this is Newman's myometer, which consists of a pressure gauge and measures the resistance offered by a muscle in isometric contraction. The gauge's reading is proportional to the force required to overcome the isometric contraction of the muscle under test. The gauge is in a small cylinder which has a short shaft and a pressure transmitting button extending from one end. A hydraulic pressure converter which is built into the device transmits the linear force exerted on the button to the pressure gauge.

Weight-Lifting Techniques have been employed to assess muscle strength. In theory, the strength of muscles too weak to raise even the weight of the extremity against gravity, can be gauged by determining the minimum weight required to assist the muscle and permit movement to occur. In actual practice, however, it is very difficult to restrict the muscle to a purely passive role.

Strain-Gauge Methods are among the more recent developments in objective muscle evaluation. With the electrical strain gauge the applied muscle force is allowed to deform metal bars or rings to which the gauges are attached. The deformation produces a change in the electrical resistance of the gauges which can be recorded on a galvanometer or an oscillograph following amplification, or by pens. Electrical strain gauges are probably the most accurate measuring instruments of those just described.

The Measurement of Muscle Endurance and Coordination

The most common test of muscle endurance is of the ergographic type in which the patient repeatedly lifts a given weight load at a standard rate until a predetermined end-point is reached. The rate at which contractions should be made will be determined, in part, by the particular movement under study and whether or not the involved muscles are normal, and, in part, by the weight load.

The most frequently employed time intervals are one, two or three seconds. The end-point is determined as the point of exhaustion or as a given decrement in the distance which the weight is moved. It has been found that consistent results can be obtained only when ergographic loads induce exhaustion within a relatively short time, such as two minutes.

These tests typically involve graphic representation of the repeated exertions against a resistance provided either by springs or weights. Rather than providing only a single value of muscle strength, the record indicates the rate of onset of fatigue with a weight load that may initially be maximal or submaximal. In this way endurance is evaluated, and it is possible to calculate the total amount of work performed during a specified time period.

Another type of endurance test measures the length of time a contraction can be maintained at or above a given level. This test is comparatively simple to perform but it is so fatiguing that only a single reading can be obtained during any one session.

Muscle coordination can be crudely measured as the speed at which a given movement can be executed. Those tests which assess the accuracy of movements involve factors other than muscle coordination alone.

Grading of Muscle Strength

The first test of muscle strength was based upon factors of gravity and resistance, and muscle strength was graded on these variables. This was the test developed by Lovett in 1912. Since that date there have been revisions by Lovett and developments and modifications by several other investigators. Testing in the United States has been based primarily upon the principles of the Lovett method. While additions and changes in muscle testing have been made, and different systems of grading have been introduced, the use of gravity and resistance as key variables still remains the basis for manual muscle testing.

Systems for muscle grading were devised by Lowman, Legg and Merrill, Kendall and Kendall, Brunnstrom and Dennen, Kenny and Plastridge, and the National Foundation for Infantile Paralysis, Inc. which span the years from 1922 to 1946. Today, the most frequently employed systems date from the 1916 Lovett system, the 1932 Legg and Merrill revision of the Lovett system, the 1942 Medical Research Council of Great Britain system, the 1946 National Foundation for Infantile Paralysis system, the 1949 Kendall and Kendall system, the 1958 Mayo Clinic system, and the Warm Springs of Georgia system. These are described below.

The 1916 Lovett System

Zero	No contraction felt or seen.
Trace	Muscle can be felt to tighten but cannot produce movement.
Poor	Muscle produces movement with gravity eliminated, but cannot function against gravity.
Fair	Muscle can raise the part against gravity.
Good	Muscle can raise the part against gravity and against outside resistance.
Normal	Muscle can overcome a greater amount of resistance than a *Good* muscle.

The 1932 Legg and Merrill Revision

Gone	No contraction felt.

Other grades are the same as the 1916 Lovett system.

The 1942 Medical Research Council of Great Britain System

0	No evidence of contractility.
1	The muscle can be felt to tighten but cannot produce movement.
2	Movement with gravity eliminated.
3	Movement against gravity.
4	Movement against gravity and some resistance.
5	Normal, full strength. Movement against gravity and a greater resistance.

The 1946 National Foundation for Infantile Paralysis System

C or CC	Contracture or severe contracture.
S or SS	Spasm or severe spasm.
0% 00 Zero	No evidence of contractility.
10% 1 Trace	Evidence of slight contraction, no joint motion.
25% 2 P Poor	Complete range of motion with gravity eliminated.
50% 3 F Fair	Complete range of motion against gravity.
75% 4 G Good	Complete range of motion against gravity with some resistance.
100% 5 N Normal	Complete range of motion against gravity with full resistance.

The 1949 Kendall and Kendall System

Based upon Class II muscles of the wrist, elbow, shoulder, ankle, knee, hip and neck.

0	No evidence of contraction felt in muscle. No movement of the part.
5% and 10%	In muscle that can be seen or palpated a feeble contraction may be felt, or the tendon may become prominent during contraction. No apparent movement of the part.

20% and 30%	A twenty per cent muscle requires moderate assistance by the examiner in motion through a visible arc. A thirty per cent muscle requires slight assistance by the examiner.
40%	When the muscle attempts to hold the test position against gravity, there is a very gradual release showing inability to hold the anti-gravity position. Quadriceps muscles, hip rotators and deltoid muscles in the sitting position, and triceps and arm rotators in the prone position may be graded forty per cent if the muscle moves the part through the anti-gravity arc of motion almost to complete motion.
50%	The muscle holds the anti-gravity test position or the muscle moves the part through the anti-gravity arc of motion to completion.
60% and 70%	The muscle holds the anti-gravity test position against minimum pressure, or the muscle moves the part through the anti-gravity arc of motion and holds the completed position against minimum pressure.
80% and 90%	Same as above against medium pressure.
100%	Same as above against maximum pressure.

The 1958 Mayo Clinic System

4	No evidence of contraction.
3 plus Trace	Palpable contraction or visible tendon motion without limb motion.
3 Poor	Movement through available range with gravity eliminated.
2 Fair	Movement through available range against gravity alone.
1 Good	Movement through available range against gravity and resistance.
0	Normal.

The Warm Springs Foundation of Georgia System

0	No palpable or visible contraction; no motion of the part.
Trace	Palpable contraction.
Poor minus	Incomplete range of motion; gravity eliminated.
Poor	Complete range of motion, gravity eliminated—up to eighty per cent of range of motion.
Poor plus	Beginning motion against gravity—fifty per cent of range of motion or less.
Fair minus	Motion against gravity, though not full range—fifty to ninety per cent of range of motion.
Fair	Motion against gravity once—complete range of motion.
Fair plus	Motion against gravity several times, or once with mild resistance.
Good	Complete range of active motion with good resistance.
Good plus	Moderate weakness.
Normal minus	Slight weakness.
Normal	Considered normal for size, age, and sex of patient.

Procedures of Manual Muscle Testing

Muscles of the Trunk

TRUNK FLEXION AND ROTATION AND ABDOMINAL RETRACTION. The muscles involved in flexion and rotation of the trunk and in abdominal retraction are these: the *rectus abdominus,* which shortens the distance between the sternum and the pubis by either forward flexion of the thorax on the pelvis or flexion of the pelvis on the thorax; the *external oblique,* which acts to compress the portion of the rib cage to which it is attached, assists in initiation of flexion of the thorax on the pelvis, carries the thorax forward over the pelvis and helps to tilt the pelvis back, flattening the lumbar spine; the *internal oblique,* which rotates the thorax backward on the pelvis producing kyphosis of the dorsal spine; and the *transverse abdominus,* which compresses the abdominal viscera and, in expiration, helps to decrease the angle of the ribs.

To test these muscles the patient is placed in a supine, or face upward position on a plinth, a padded examining table, with his hands folded behind his head. The therapist stabilizes the patient's legs.

The patient is asked to raise himself to a sitting position by first raising his head, then his shoulders, and then his entire trunk. Flexion of the trunk is completed when the region of the seventh cervical vertebra is about eight inches from the plinth. At this point the hip flexor muscles complete the act of trunk raising.

For a functional grade of *fair* and above, resistance may be applied by pressure of the therapist's hand on the anterior upper sternum. Below this grade, and particularly below *poor plus,* palpation becomes more important in grading. The therapist may supply assistance in flexion by placing one arm around the patient's shoulders while palpating the rectus and oblique muscles to assist in grading.

During performance of this test, the patient's pelvis is observed by the therapist. With weak hip flexors the anterior superior spines will tend to move upward toward the patient's lower rib cage, with ineffective action of the abdominal muscles during trunk flexion. When this occurs, the examiner can achieve additional pelvic stabilization by pulling caudally over the anterior superior pelvic brim, the upper boundary of the pelvis cavity.

The therapist also notes whether the patient flexes straight upward from the plinth or rotates the shoulders to either side. Shoulder rotation to the patient's right indicates weakness in the rectus and probably also in the right external and left internal oblique muscles, and in this position the patient uses the left external and right internal obliques in attempting to flex his trunk.

In patients with lower motor neuron lesions, the upper abdominal muscles will be strong and the lower ones weakened. The therapist observes deviations of the umbilicus, the cicatrix marking the site of previous umbilical cord attachment, to detect this since the umbilicus will tend to deviate upward toward the strong muscles. Palpation of the upper and lower muscles will discover the areas of weakness and/or atrophy.

The oblique abdominal muscles, which rotate the vertebral column and compress the abdominal viscera, are tested by having the patient rotate the trunk as he flexes it, first to one side and then to the other.

In addition to the external and internal obliques, the muscles involved in trunk rotation are the following: the *latissimus dorsi,* the broadest muscle of the back and lateral thoracic region; the *semi-*

spinalis, consisting of muscle fibers that arise from transverse processes and run upward and medially to attach to the sinous processes; the *mulifidus,* which extends the thoracic and lumbar spine, and resembles the semispinalis, but has shorter fascicles, or bundles of muscle fibers, and is more obliquely placed in relation to the vertebral column; the *rotatores,* a series of small muscles deep in the groove between the spinous and transverse processes of the vertebrae; and the *rectus abdominus* (see above), which flexes the lumbar vertebrae and supports the abdomen.

With trunk rotation to the right, flexion of the left external and right internal oblique muscles will act in unison, producing diagonal flexion. In this test, the inferior angle of the right scapula, the flat, triangular bone behind the shoulder, should elevate one to two inches from the plinth when examination is for a functional grade. Elevation of the left scapula should be much higher.

Resistance is given against the forward-rotating shoulder while the patient's legs are stabilized as in the straight flexion test. Assistance may be given in trunk rotation by the therapist placing one arm behind the patient's neck and shoulders while palpating the external oblique with the other hand.

The patient will also be requested to approximate the left anterior rib cage to the umbilicus. In examining the right internal oblique muscle the therapist will cradle the patient's right leg in her right arm, directing the patient to approximate the right anterior iliac crest to the umbilicus, while she palpates the muscle with her left hand. In order to obtain further isolation of the muscle, the therapist can stroke, or point out to the patient the area to be tightened.

The right external and left internal oblique muscles are tested in the same way, namely by left trunk rotation and flexion.

When the patient is required to raise his trunk sideways from a side-lying position an imbalance may be revealed in the oblique muscles. This test is performed with the upper trunk, pelvis and legs in a straight line and the abdomen in retraction. The top arm is extended down the side of the body with the fingers closed so that the patient will not hold on to his pelvis and attempt to pull himself up with his arm. The underarm is forward across the chest with the hand holding the upper shoulder to exclude possible assistance by pushing up with the shoulder. The therapist holds the patient's leg firmly on the plinth and asks him to raise his under-shoulder from the examining table by raising his trunk.

If the legs and pelvis are held steady and not permitted to twist forward or backward from the direct side-lying position, the thorax is frequently rotated forward or backward as the trunk is flexed laterally. A forward twist indicates a stronger pull by the external oblique muscle, while a backward twist denotes a stronger pull by the internal oblique. If the back hyperextends as the patient raises himself, the quadratus lumborum, which fixes the twelfth rib and assists in unilateral pelvic elevation, and the latissimus dorsi are pulling strongly, and the direct anterior abdominal fixation is not sufficient to maintain the trunk in a straight line with the pelvis.

Testing of the lower abdominal muscles (trunk raising being a test of the upper abdominals) is performed by having the patient raise both lower extremities, simultaneously, from the supine position. When the abdominal muscles are weak and hip flexor muscles, which do the actual raising, are strong, the patient cannot hold his back flat as the legs are raised. The external oblique muscles and the rectus abdominus muscle flatten the lumbar spine on the plinth by pulling the pelvis into a position of backward tilt and holding it there. Attention, therefore, must be focused on the position of the pelvis during leg raising and not on the activity itself.

Movements of the arm can also be used in assessing abdominal strength. The arm must act against resistance or be held against pressure since unrestricted arm movements do not require action of muscles of the trunk for fixation. When there is weakness of the abdominal muscles, fixation for the downward push or pull of an arm can be provided by the back muscles alone. For diagonal movements of the upper extremity if abdominal muscles are unimpaired, the external oblique muscle on the ipsalateral side and the internal oblique muscle on the contralateral side contract to fix the thorax on the pelvis. If there is cross-sectional weakness in that line of pull, the opposite oblique muscles may act to provide the fixation.

Abdominal retraction is tested by assessing the functional ability of the transverse abdominal muscle. In a side-lying or standing position, the patient draws in his abdomen so as to reduce the size of his waist. All of the abdominal muscles assist in this action. Weakness will allow a bulging of the anterior abdominal wall without direct effect on the tilt or rotation of the pelvis or thorax.

Defects of Structure and Function Resulting from Abnormality of Major Trunk and Abdominal Muscles

Weakness of the rectus abdominus permits a separation of the pubis and sternum resulting in lordosis, an abnormally concave curvature of the lumbar spine. In the supine position, weakness results in decreased ability to flex the pelvis on the thorax or the thorax on the pelvis. Shortness of this muscle produces a dorso-lumbar kyphosis, or abnormally convex spinal curvature, with limitation of spine extension.

Bilateral weakness of the internal oblique muscle results in an inability to flex the thorax on the pelvis from a supine position. Unilateral weakness permits a forward rotation of the thorax on the weakened side. Bilateral shortness of the muscle depresses the thorax anteriorly, tending to pull the upper trunk into kyphosis. Unilateral shortness rotates the thorax backward on the side of shortness.

When there is bilateral weakness of the external oblique muscle, the result is either an anterior pelvic tilt accompanied by lordosis or an anterior pelvic displacement. Unilateral weakness permits the thorax to rotate backward on the weak side. Bilateral shortness of this muscle results in a posterior pelvic tilt. Unilateral shortness produces rotation of the thorax forward on the shortened side.

Weakness of the latissimus dorsi results in diminution of strength in lateral trunk flexion. Since this muscle is an accessory muscle of respiration, weakness interferes to some extent with forced expiration, as in coughing. Unilateral shortenss depresses the shoulder and displaces the thorax forward and toward the opposite side. Bilateral shortness depresses the shoulders downward and forward by the action of the muscle on the humerus, the bone which extends from the elbow to the shoulder.

Weakness of the middle and lower *trapezius* produces a kyphosis of the dorsal spine. The scapulae are abducted and elevated in a forward, round-shouldered position. (Note: The trapezius muscle normally rotates the scapula to raise the shoulder in abduction of the arm, and draws the scapula backward.)

Muscles of the Back

TRUNK EXTENSION. The muscles which are involved in extension of the trunk are as follows: the *erector spinae,* or *sacrospinalis* (intrinsic or deep back muscles) , which are the fibers of the more superficial of the deep back muscles originating from the sacrum and spines of the lumbar and eleventh and twelfth thoracic vertebrae and iliac crest. They split, and emerge as three vertical columns, the *iliocostalis,* the *longissimus* and the *spinalis* muscles; the *multifedus,* which extends and rotates the vertebral column; the *semispinalis,* which extends obliquely from the transverse processes of the vertebrae to the spines; and the *rotatores.*

The muscles of trunk extension are examined by having the patient lie prone, or face downward, on a plinth, with his hands at his sides or folded behind his head. The therapist stabilizes the patient's thighs and pelvis, and directs the patient to extend his spine, raising his shoulders and head from the examining table. The therapist applies resistance to the lower thoracic area of the spine.

Functional strength will elevate the body weight against gravity. Grading above *fair* depends upon the patient's ability to overcome increasing resistance. A grade of *poor plus* will enable the patient to begin extension but not to complete the range of motion. To estimate the passive range the therapist can assist the patient in completion of the full range of motion. Grades below the level of *poor plus* are determined, primarily, by palpation of the muscles.

Elevation of the Pelvis. The muscles of pelvic elevation are: the *quadratus lumborum,* which laterally flexes the lumbar vertebrae, fixes the twelfth rib and assists in unilateral elevation of the pelvis, and is commonly referred to as the "hip hiker"; the lateral fibers of the *external and internal oblique muscles;* the *latissimus dorsi;* and the *hip abductor muscles.*

The patient being tested lies in pronation (occasionally in supination) with the lumbar spine in moderate extension. He grasps the side edge of the plinth to stabilize the thorax and draws his pelvis up toward the thorax on one side. The therapist provides resistance above the ankles.

For patients with *fair* muscle strength the test is conducted with the patient is a standing position. The therapist stabilizes the thorax and the patient is asked to raise his pelvis toward the thorax on alternate sides. For patients with muscle strength graded below *poor minus,* the test is conducted on a plinth, and as the patient attempts to draw the pelvis upward contraction of the quadratus lumborum can be determined by deep palpation in the lumbar area under the lateral edge of the sacrospinalis.

Thoracic Muscles. The *diaphragma* (diaphragm) increases the length of the chest cavity decreasing intrapleural pressure and causing the lungs to expand on inspiration.

The patient is tested in a supine position. He is directed to keep his thorax fixed and to take a deep breath. With good diaphragm action the abdominal wall will protrude. Action of the diaphragm can be palpated by placing the fingers of both hands beneath the lower ribs, anteriorly on each side. On inspiration, the fingers will be pushed downward and outward. Severe weakness of the diaphragm results in rapid respiratory fatigue or distress if the thorax is fixed.

The *intercostal muscles* which draw the ribs together in respiration and expulsion stabilize the intercostal spaces, or spaces between the ribs which allows rib motion and chest expansion to occur without loss of stability of the costal (rib) cage. Laxity of these muscles affects the intrapleural pressure adversely during breathing.

No adequate test of the intercostals can be performed. If, however, the patient is of a thin build, the stability of the intercostal spaces can be observed and sometimes palpated, implying intercostal action.

Other thoracic muscles include the *levatores costarum,* which elevates the ribs and stabilizes the intercostal spaces, the *serratus posterior superior,* which elevates and rotates the ribs, and the *serratus posterior inferior,* which depresses or stabilizes the lower ribs in expiration.

While it is not possible to test these muscles individually, their action may be inferred. An estimate of function can be obtained by observation of rib rotation and elevation in the absence of the other accessory muscles of breathing.

Muscles of Hip Motion

FLEXION OF THE HIP. Hip flexion is provided by the *iliopsoas muscle,* which is divided into the *psoas major* and the *iliacus.* The psoas major muscle both flexes the trunk and flexes and medially rotates the thigh. The iliacus flexes the thigh and the trunk on the extremity. These are the prime movers of hip flexion.

Accessory muscles of hip flexion include the following: the *rectus femoris,* which extends the leg and flexes the thigh; the *sartorius,* which flexes the thigh and leg; the *pectineus,* which flexes and adducts the thigh; the *adductor brevis,* which adducts, rotates and flexes the thigh; the *adductor longus,* which adducts, rotates and flexes the thigh; the *tensor fasciae latae,* which flexes and adducts the thigh; and the oblique fibers of the *adductor magnus,* which adducts and extends the thigh.

Testing of patients with a functional grade and above is performed with the patient sitting on a plinth with his knees flexed over the edge of the table. This position reduces the action of the accessory muscles which assist the prime movers of hip flexion. The therapist stabilizes the patient's pelvis by pushing against it in a posterior direction. The patient is requested to flex his hip through the range of motion. He is permitted to stabilize his trunk by placing his hands on the edge of the table. The therapist applies resistance to the top of the distal thigh in a downward direction.

Patients graded *poor* or below are tested in a sidelying-position. The therapist stabilizes the pelvis and supports the weight of the lower extremity being tested to eliminate the effects of gravity. The patient is asked to flex his hip through the range of motion. Patients with *trace* or *zero* muscle strength are examined in supination with the lower extremity supported by the therapist. It may be possible, in such cases, to detect contraction in the psoas major muscle.

Defects of Structure and Function Resulting from Abnormality of Major Hip Flexor Muscles

Hip flexor weakness results in marked disability in stair climbing or in walking up an incline. It causes difficulty in rising from a reclining position. It makes ambulation a problem because it necessitates substitution of pelvic action for normal hip flexion action. In a standing position it tends to permit an anterior pelvic displacement.

Contracture of hip flexors produces hip flexion deformity with increased lumbar lordosis.

Shortness of the hip flexors results in an anterior tilt of the pelvis with lumbar lordosis.

In addition, unilateral weakness of the psoas major muscle is a causative factor in lumbar scoliosis, while bilateral weakness permits a lumbar kyphosis to occur.

ABDUCTION OF THE HIP. The muscles of hip abduction are as follows: the *gluteous medius,* which produces hip abduction with the hip extended and assists internal rotation with the hip flexed; the *gluteus maximus,* which extends, abducts and rotates the thigh outward; the *gluteus minimus,* responsible for abduction of the femur, internal rotation with the hip extended and stronger internal rotation with the hip flexed; and the *tensor fasciae latae,* which provides hip flexion and abduction.

Testing of the gluteus medius and gluteus minimus requires that the patient with muscle grades of *fair* or better lie on his side on the examination table. He abducts his thigh against gravity with hip and knee in extension. The therapist stabilizes the pelvis and applies resistance over the lower femur. Patients with muscle grades below *fair* are tested in supination. The weight of the lower extremity is eliminated by the therapist placing her hands under the thigh and leg. Abduction is graded according to the amount of active motion.

The gluteus maximus muscle is tested with the patient in pronation. He must extend his hip with the knee flexed to ninety degrees or more. Pressure is applied by the therapist in a downward direction against the lower part of the posterior thigh.

In patients with functional muscle power, testing of the tensor fasciae latae is conducted with the subject in a side-lying position. He is requested to abduct the thigh forward and with some internal rotation. Resistance is applied at the lower femur in an opposing direction, with the patient's trunk stabilized. For patients with muscle strength below functional grade levels, the test position is one of supination with hip and knee extended. The patient rotates his hip internally and the muscle is palpated at the outer edge of the anterior superior iliac spine, which is a blunt, bony projection on the anterior border of the ilium, the expansive superior portion of the hip bone.

Defects of Structure and Function Resulting from Abnormality of Major Hip Abductor Muscles

Weakness of the gluteus minimus reduces the strength of internal rotation and abduction of the hip. Bilateral weakness of the gluteus maximus makes ambulation very difficult, necessitating the use of crutches. Marked weakness of the gluteus medius produces a limp during ambulation. Slight weakness results in a postural deviation characterized by a raised pelvis on the affected side.

Contracture of the gluteus minimus and the gluteus medius produces an abduction deformity, seen upon standing as a low pelvis on the involved side with some lower extremity abduction. Shortness of these muscles produces leg abduction, if the pelvis is level, or a low pelvis, if the lower extremities are both in a position of midline adduction in relation to the trunk.

ADDUCTION OF THE HIP. The prime mover muscles involved in hip adduction are these: the *adductor longus,* which provides strong thigh adduction and assists in hip flexion and external rotation; the *adductor magnus,* which also serves to strongly adduct the thigh and, in addition, assists in extension of the hip and in external rotation with the hip in extension; the *pectineus,* providing adduction and assistance in hip flexion and external rotation; the *gracilis,* which adducts the thigh and aids in flexion of the hip; and the *adductor brevis.*

For patients with functional grades of muscle strength the test position is one of side-lying. The upper leg is supported by the therapist in abduction of from twenty-five to forty degrees. The patient is instructed to adduct, or raise the lower leg until it touches or approaches the supported leg. Resistance is applied over the lower femur of this extremity in a downward direction.

Patients with muscle strength graded *poor* or below are examined in supination. The lower extremities are abducted from thirty to forty-five degrees. Gravity is eliminated by the therapist supporting the leg being tested under the knee and ankle. The pelvis is held stabile. The patient adducts the supported extremity through the range of motion without rotating the hip. The amount of active motion determines the grade. For the lowest grades palpation of the adductors can be performed medially just below the pubis and on the medial thigh.

Defects of Structure Resulting from Abnormality of Major Hip Adductor Muscles

Contracture results in a hip adduction deformity. In standing, the pelvis tilts high to the side of the contracture.

EXTENSION OF THE HIP. Hip extension involves the following muscles: the *gluteus maximus,* responsible for hip extension and external rotation; and the *semitendinosis,* the *semimembranosis* and the *biceps femoris,* which flex and extend the thigh.

Muscle examination of patients with hip extensors graded as *fair* or above is conducted with the patient lying in pronation, knee flexed to ninety degrees and hip extended. The therapist stabilizes the lumbar spine with her hand and provided resistance by giving downward pressure over the lower posterior femur. The patient extends his hip through the range of motion.

Patients with muscle strength graded *poor* or below are tested in a side-lying position with the therapist supporting the upper leg to eliminate the pull of gravity. Extension of the hip is graded according to the amount of active motion present. The lowest grades are arrived at by palpation of the gluteal muscle.

Structure and function defects resulting from abnormality of the gluteus maximus, the primary muscle of hip extension, are described in a previous section.

EXTERNAL ROTATION OF THE HIP. There are six muscles which play a role in hip external rotation. The *obturatorius externus* and *obturatorius internus* rotate the thigh laterally. The *quadratus femoris* adducts and laterally rotates the thigh. The *periformis* rotates the thigh outward. The *gemellus superior* and the *gemellus inferior* rotate the thigh laterally.

For testing, the patient lies supinely on the plinth with the leg on the side being tested flexed over the end of the table. The extremity not under examination is flexed so that the heel of the foot rests on the table, thus providing adequate space for rotation. The therapist stabilizes the lower femur by supporting it so as to permit rotation only.

Her other hand holds the patient's ankle. The patient is requested to externally rotate his thigh. The therapist provides resistance by moving the patient's ankle in the opposite direction.

Patients with muscle grades in the *poor* range are tested in one of two ways. If the patient is able to stand, the extremity being tested is cleared of the floor. His pelvis is stabilized by the therapist's hand and he is asked to externally rotate his thigh through its range of motion. If the patient is unable to stand, he is tested in supination and is directed to externally rotate his thigh while the therapist stabilizes his pelvis. In patients with muscle grades below *poor,* the presence of contraction in the external rotators is determined by deep palpation behind the greater trochanter, the broad, flat process at the upper end of the lateral surface of the femur.

Defects of Structure Resulting from Abnormality of Major Hip External Rotator Muscles

Weakness in these muscles can produce internal rotation and adduction of the thigh resulting in a knock-kneed condition and external rotation of the lower limb in weight-bearing. It also results in a tendency toward an anterior pelvic tilt with lumbar lordosis.

Contraction of hip external rotators produces an external rotation of the thigh, usually in abduction.

Unilateral shortness of the involved muscles results in an external rotation of the femur, abduction of the hip joint in relation to the pelvis, or a rotation of the pelvis. If the shortening is bilateral, there is a tendency toward a flattening of the lumbar spine by posterior pelvic tilt.

INTERNAL ROTATION OF THE HIP. The hip internal rotators are the *gluteus minimus,* the *tensor fasciae latae,* the anterior fibers of the *gluteus medius,* the *semitendinosis* and the *semimembranosis,* the functions of which are described in previous sections.

The positions for testing these hip muscles are the same as those used in testing hip external rotators. The test consists of the patient internally rotating his thigh. Resistance is given by the therapist moving the patient's foot in an opposing, medial, direction. For patients with *trace* or *zero* muscle grades, the tensor fasciae latae may be palpated near its origin, posterior and distal to the anterior superior spine of the ilium.

Defects of Structure and Function Resulting from Abnormality of Major Hip Internal Rotator Muscles

Weakness will result in an external rotation of the lower extremity during standing and ambulation.

Contracture produces an internal hip rotation and a tendency toward a knock-knee if the patient has been weight-bearing.

Shortness results in an inability to fully rotate the thigh externally and to sit cross-legged.

Hip Flexion, Abduction and Internal Rotation with Knee Flexion. The prime mover is the *sartorius muscle,* which flexes the thigh and leg. Accessory muscles include the *hip flexors, knee flexors, hip external rotators* and *hip abductors.*

With patients whose muscle strength is graded above *fair,* the sortorius is tested in a sitting position with the legs flexed over the side of the plinth. The patient flexes, abducts and externally rotates his hip and flexes his knee. The therapist gives resistance to hip flexion and abduction with one hand placed above the knee joint. Resistance to hip external rotation and knee flexion is given with the other hand above the ankle joint.

Patients with *fair* muscle strength sit on the edge of the plinth with the heel of the leg being tested placed in front of the contralateral ankle. The therapist stabilizes the pelvis. The patient must raise his heel to the opposite knee with flexion, abduction and external rotation of the hip and knee flexion. The sartorius muscle is palpated near its origin at the anterior superior spine of the ilium.

If the patient's strength is in the *poor* range, the test is administered in supination. The therapist stabilizes the patient's pelvis and instructs him to slide the heel of the involved extremity to the heel of the contralateral extremity with flexion, abduction and external rotation and knee flexion being noted. The sartorius is palpated near its origin.

Defects of Structure and Function Resulting from Abnormality of the Sartorius Muscle

Weakness contributes to antero-medial instability at the knee.

Contracture results in flexion, abduction and external rotation deformities of the hip with flexion of the knee.

Hip Abduction from Flexed Position. The primary muscle involved in this action is the *tensor fasciae latae.* Additionally involved are the *gluteus medius* and the *gluteus minimus.*

For grades of *normal* and *good* the patient is tested in a side-lying position with the lower knee slightly flexed for balance and the leg being tested flexed to an angle of forty-five degrees at the hip joint. The pelvis is stabilized by the therapist and the patient is directed to abduct the leg through a range of motion of approximately thirty degrees. Resistance is applied above the knee joint.

For muscle grades of *fair* the test is the same but resistance is omitted.

A *poor* muscle is graded with the patient sitting on the plinth, knees extended. The trunk is kept at a forty-five degree angle to the table and is supported by the patient's arms. The therapist stabilizes his pelvis. The patient abducts his leg through a range of motion of approximately thirty degrees.

The test position for *trace* and *zero* muscles is the same. The therapist determines the presence of contraction in the tensor fasciae latae by observation and palpation below the origin of the muscle at the iliac crest and at the fascial insertion on the lateral side of the knee joint.

Testing for *poor, trace* or *zero* grades may be conducted with the patient in a supine position with his legs on a board which is tilted at an angle of forty-five degrees.

Defects of Structure Resulting from Abnormality of the Tensor Fasciae Latae Muscle

Weakness results in a thrust in the direction of a bow-legged position upon standing and a tendency of the extremity to rotate outward from the hip.

Bilateral shortness results in an anterior pelvic tilt and, occasionally, bilateral knock-knee. Unilateral shortness can lead to a pelvic tilt, knock-knee and internal rotation of the femur depending upon the involvement of other muscles.

Contracture produces flexion of the hip and a knock-kneed position.

Muscles of Knee Motion

FLEXION OF THE KNEE. The muscles which provide for knee flexion are as follows: the *biceps femoris;* the *semitendinosis;* the *semimembranosis;* the *sartorius;* the *gracilis,* which adducts the thigh and flexes the knee; the *popliteus,* which assists in knee flexion and medially rotates the tibia; and the *gastrocnemius,* which flexes the knee joint.

The tendons of the gracilis, sartorius and two other muscles are termed, together, the *inner hamstring muscles,* while the tendon of the biceps femoris is referred to as the *outer hamstring.*

For patients with *normal* and *good* muscle strength, testing is conducted with the patient lying prone on the plinth. The posterior hip and gluteal area are stabilized by the therapist. The patient flexes his knee while the therapist applies resistance in an opposing direction at the posterior ankle, rotating the leg outwardly. In this manner the biceps femoris is tested. To test the gracilis, semitendinosis and simimembranosis, the therapist rotates the patient's leg inwardly as he flexes his knee.

Patients with muscle grades below *normal* and *good* lie in pronation while the therapist stabilizes the thigh. The patient flexes his knee through its range of motion. If the gastrocnemius is weak, the knee may be flexed to ten degrees as a starting position for the motion. If the biceps femoris is stronger, the lower leg will rotate outwardly, while if the semitendinosis and semimembranosis muscles are stronger, the lower leg will rotate inwardly during flexion.

Patients who have less than *fair* muscle strength are tested in a side-lying position, with the therapist supporting the upper leg and stabilizing the thigh of the extremity being examined. The patient is instructed to flex his knee through its range of motion. Uneven muscular pull will result in a rotation of the lower leg.

When a patient has *trace* or *zero* muscle strength he lies face downward with the knee partially flexed and the lower leg supported by the therapist. He attempts to flex his knee. Palpation can be performed on the tendons of the knee flexor muscles at the back of the thigh near the knee joint.

In attempts to determine whether or not the popliteus muscle is active, the patient is seated on the edge of the plinth with his knees flexed over the sides. He is asked to maximally rotate his leg, first outwardly and then inwardly.

The length of the hamstrings may be determined as the therapist raises the patient's leg straight up while he is lying in supination. The opposite leg is held stabile on the plinth.

Defects of Structure and Function Resulting from Abnormality of Major Knee Flexor Muscles

Weakness of the popliteus muscle can result in hyperextension of the knee and external rotation of the lower leg on the femur. Such weakness is usually found when the outer hamstring muscles are strong but the inner hamstrings are weak.

Shortness of the popliteus results in a slight knee flexion and internal rotation of the lower leg on the femur.

Weakness of the inner hamstrings and gracilis produces a loss in internal-lateral stability of the knee. It permits a knock-knee position with a tendency toward external rotation of the lower leg on the femur.

Weakness of the outer hamstrings results in a tendency toward loss of lateral stability of the knee, permitting a thrust in the direction of a bow-legged position during weight-bearing. When both inner and outer hamstrings are weak, hyperextension of the knee results. If this weakness is bilateral, there is a forward pelvic tilt into a position of lordosis of the lumbar spine. The consequence of unilateral weakness is a pelvic rotation.

Contracture of both inner and outer hamstrings results in a position of knee flexion, and extreme contracture adds to this a posterior pelvic tilt and flattening of the lumbar spine. A patient with this type of contracture is unable to assume a standing position.

Shortness results in restriction of knee extension when the hip is flexed, or restriction of hip flexion when the knee is extended. Hamstring shortness permits standing, but the patient's posture will be characterized by a posterior tilting of the pelvis and a flattening of the lumbar spine.

EXTENSION OF THE KNEE. The muscle involved in knee extension is the *quadriceps* muscle (m. quadriceps femoris), which is composed of four muscle segments. These are: the *rectus femoris,* which extends the leg and flexes the thigh; the *vastus medialis,* the *vastus lateralis* and the *vastus intermedius,* all of which extend the leg.

There are two test positions which can be employed in evaluating the quadriceps muscle. The patient may either sit with his knees flexed over the edge of the plinth, or he may lie in a supine position with his knees flexed over the edge of the examination table. (Note: Strength of contraction of the rectus femoris can be estimated by comparing the strength of the extensor group in both test positions.) The therapist stabilizes the involved extremity by fixing the thigh above the knee joint as the patient extends his knee through the range of motion. Resistance is applied over the lower tibia.

Patients with below functional muscle grades have their knees initially flexed to about 120 degrees prior to attempting knee extension. For grades of *poor,* the position may be one of side-lying with support being given to the upper leg. The patient extends his knee through its range. In patients with *trace* or less muscle strength, the position is one of supination with the knee flexed and supported by the therapist. The patient is asked to try and extend his knee. Grading below functional strength is based upon the active range of motion. In the lowest grades, palpation of the tendon between the patella, or knee cap, and the tuberosity of the tibia and fibers of the muscles is used to determine contraction of the quadriceps. Testing of the quadriceps in knee extension is performed with a pad placed under the patient's knee so that the therapist can palpate various areas of muscle.

Defects of Structure and Function Resulting from Abnormality of the Quadriceps Muscle

Weakness of the quadriceps interferes with stair climbing, ambulating up an incline and rising from and lowering down to a sitting position. The weakness requires that the patient lock the knee joint in slight hyperextension for function. Continuous thrust, however, in the direction of hyperextension, may result in a marked deformity in growing children.

Contracture of the muscle results in knee extension.

Shortness restricts knee flexion. (A shortness of the rectus femoris results in a knee flexion restriction when the hip is extended, or in a restriction of hip extension when the knee is flexed.)

Muscles of Ankle Motion

DORSIFLEXION OF THE ANKLE. The muscles of ankle dorsiflexion, or backward flexion, include the following: the *tibialis anterior,* which provides dorsiflexion of the foot with inversion of the forefoot; the *extensor hallucis longus,* a toe muscle whose continued action also assists in foot dorsiflexion; the *extensor digitorum longus,* a muscle of the toes which acts, when the toes are stabilized, to dorsiflex the foot and draw it into partial forefoot eversion; and the *peroneus tertius,* which acts for dorsiflexion of the foot and eversion of the forefoot.

In patients with functional muscle grades the test for ankle dorsiflexion is conducted with the subject either sitting with his knees flexed over the edge of the plinth, or in pronation with his heel over the end of the table. He is directed to dorsiflex his foot completely, without eversion or inversion. The therapist provides resistance in a downward direction at the medial dorsum, or top of the foot. Palpation is employed to the tendons across the anterior ankle joint while the patient strongly activates it into dorsiflexion. Next, the foot is dorsiflexed and the forefoot is brought into partial inversion with the toes flexed and relaxed. Resistance is applied over the first metatarsal bone.

The *extensor digitorum longus* is tested by having the patient dorsiflex his foot and evert the forefoot slightly. Resistance is given over the dorsum of the four lateral metatarsals toward plantar flexion and slight inversion.

Below functional muscle grades require that the patient lie on his side for testing, with the involved extremity resting on its lateral surface. The heel is lifted and the tibia is externally rotated by the therapist. The patient slides his forefoot along the table through the range of motion of inversion and dorsiflexion. Grading depends upon the amount of active motion present. For the lowest grades of muscle strength, evaluation is made by tendon palpation.

Defects of Structure Resulting from Abnormality of Major Ankle Dorsiflexor Muscles

Weakness of the tibialis anterior results in a drop-foot condition in which the foot hangs in a plantar-flexed position with eversion and a tendency toward collapse of the longitudinal arch.

Contracture of this muscle causes as calcaneo-varus position of the foot, a form of bent foot.

Weakness of the peroneus tertius contributes to a drop-foot in the direction of plantar flexion and inversion.

PLANTAR FLEXION OF THE ANKLE. The primary muscles involved in ankle plantar (forward, downward) flexion are these: the *gastrocnemius,* which plantar flexes the ankle and provides weak knee flexion; and the *soleus,* which plantar flexes the ankle.

The accessory muscles include the following: the *tibialis posterior,* which inverts the foot with ankle plantar flexion; the *peroneus longus* and *peroneus brevis,* which can weakly assist in plantar flexion; the *flexor hallucis longus,* which assists in plantar flexion of the ankle; the *flexor digitorum longus,* also assisting in ankle plantar flexion; and the *plantaris,* which is an external rotator of the femur and an internal leg rotator.

The test for the primary ankle plantar flexors is conducted with the patient who has muscle grades of *fair* or better in a standing position whenever possible. The patient keeps his knee straight and balances by grasping the therapist's hand. He is required to raise his heel from the floor—i.e. stand on tiptoe. A single such elevation receives a grade of *fair.* A grade of *good* is assigned when this act can be performed five to ten times in succession. A *normal* rating means that the patient is able to raise his heel from twenty to forty times.

When the patient cannot be tested in a standing position, non-weight-bearing tests are conducted. The subject lies prone on the plinth with his knee extended and his ankle at the edge of the table, foot extended over the edge and pointing downward. The therapist stabilizes the lower leg as the patient plantar flexes his foot. Resistance is given on the posterior surface of the calcaneus, or heel bone, or against the metatarsal heads towards dorsiflexion.

Patients who have *poor* or less muscle strength are examined in a side-lying position with the leg being tested resting on its lateral surface. The knee is extended and the foot is in mid-position. The leg and ankle may or may not be supported by the therapist. The patient plantar flexes his ankle through its range of motion. Grading depends upon the amount of active motion. With the very lowest grades of muscle strength palpation is employed.

In evaluating the soleus muscle alone, the above tests are given with the patient keeping the knee of the involved extremity in flexion as he plantar flexes his ankle.

Defects of Structure and Function Resulting from Abnormality of Major Ankle Plantar Flexor Muscles

Weakness of the gastrocnemius muscle allows for a calcaneous position of the foot if there is also soleus weakness, and a hyperextended knee during non-weight-bearing. In standing, it produces hyperextension of the knee and an inability to rise up on the toes. There is also an inability to transfer weight normally, which in ambulation produces what is called a "gastrocnemius limp."

Contracture of the gastrocnemius results in an equinus position of the foot, in which the foot is plantar flexed, causing the patient to walk on his toes, and also knee flexion.

Gastrocnemius shortness restricts ankle dorsiflexion when the knee is extended and knee extension when the ankle is dorsiflexed. Muscular tightness limits the normal flexion of the lower leg in relation to the dorsum of the foot as in weight-transfer while taking a step, and it results in a tendency toward toeing out during ambulation.

Soleus weakness permits a calcaneous foot position and a predisposition toward a cavus, in which the longitudinal arch of the foot is abnormally high. It makes the patient unable to rise on his toes and permits a forward displacement of body weight during standing. The deviation resulting from soleus weakness results in an anterior displacement of body weight from the normal plumb-line distribution, as is observed when a plumb line is hung slightly anterior to the outer malleolus, the rounded protuberance on the lateral surface of the ankle joint.

Contracture of the soleus produces an equinus of the foot during both weight-bearing and non-weight-bearing.

Shortness of this muscle results in a tendency toward hyperextension of the knee in the standing position.

INVERSION OF THE FOOT. The prime mover of foot inversion is the *tibialis posterior muscle,* which inverts the foot with plantar flexion of the ankle. Accessory muscles are the *flexor digitorum longus,* the *flexor hallucis longus* and the *gastrocnemius,* which have been previously described.

The tibialis posterior is tested with the patient either sitting with his knees flexed over the edge of the examining table or lying on the table in supination. The latter is the more frequently employed position and is the one discussed herein.

The patient with *normal* or *good* muscle strength is tested lying on his back with his foot in plantar flexion. He moves his foot through the range of motion for inversion, maintaining plantar flexion, while the therapist stabilizes his lower leg. She adds resistance on the medial border of the forefoot in the direction of ankle dorsiflexion and foot eversion.

A patient with *fair* muscle strength lies on his side with his foot plantar flexed and resting on its lateral border. The lower leg is stabilized by the therapist while the patient raises his foot through the range of motion for inversion while maintaining plantar flexion.

If muscle strength is *poor,* the task is performed by the patient in supination with his foot over the edge of the plinth.

The lowest grades of strength are arrived at by palpation of the tibialis posterior between the medial malleolus, the rounded protuberance on the medial surface of the ankle and the navicular bone, or above the malleolus.

Defects of Structure and Function Resulting from Abnormality of Major Foot Inversion Muscles

Weakness of the tibialis posterior produces pronation of the foot, collapse of the longitudinal arch and forefoot valgus, a deformity in which the heel is turned outward from the midline of the leg. It tends to result in a gastrocnemius limp and it interferes with the ability to rise up on the toes.

Contracture causes an equinovarus position during non-weight-bearing, where the heel is turned inward from the midline of the leg and the foot is plantar flexed. During weight-bearing, contracture results in a supination of the heel with anterior foot varus.

EVERSION OF THE FOOT. Foot eversion muscles are primarily the *peroneus longus* and *peroneus brevis,* which act to evert the foot.

Other involved muscles are the *extensor digitorum longus* and the *peroneus tertius,* which have already been discussed.

As with foot inversion procedures, testing for foot eversion may be performed with the patient either sitting on the plinth, knees flexed over the edge, or lying on the plinth. The latter is the position more often used and is the one discussed at present.

The patient with muscle strength better than a grade of *fair* lies in supination with his foot in plantar flexion. The therapist stabilizes the lower leg while the patient everts his foot from plantar flexion and depresses the head of the first metatarsal.

In order to test the peroneus brevis, the therapist gives resistance on the lateral border of the foot, while to test the peroneus longus, resistance is applied against the plantar surface of the first metatarsal head. The extensor digitorum longus should remain relaxed during testing.

Patients with *fair* muscle strength lie on their side with their foot in plantar flexion and resting on the medial border. The therapist fixes the lower leg and the patients evert their foot while depressing the first metatarsal.

A patient with *poor* muscle strength performs the task in supination with his foot extended over the end of the plinth. Muscle grading depends upon the amount of active motion.

The lowest muscle grades are evaluated by means of palpation. The tendons of the peroneus brevis are found proximal to the base of the fifth metatarsal on the lateral border of the foot. Contraction of the peroneus longus may be determined by light upward pressure under the head of the first metatarsal.

Defects of Structure and Function Resulting from Abnormality of Major Eversion Muscles

Weakness of these muscles permits a varus position of the foot, inflare of the forefoot and an inability to rise up on the toes. In addition, it results in a decrease in the lateral stability of the ankle.

Contracture of the peroneus longus produces a valgus, or pronated position of the foot with the head of the first metatarsal pulled downward during non-weight-bearing. In weight-bearing the forefoot is drawn into outflare.

Muscles of Toe Motion

FLEXION OF METATARSOPHALANGEAL JOINTS. The most important muscles for this action include the following: the four *lumbricales,* which flex the metatarsophalangeal joints of the toes and extend the distal phalanges; the *flexor hallucis brevis,* which flexes the metatarsophalangeal joint of the big toe; and the *flexor digiti minimi brevis,* which flexes the metatarsophalangeal joint of the small toe. (Note: The metatarsus is the anterior portion of the foot between the instep and the toes. The phalanges are the long toe bones.)

Other muscles which are involved are as follows: the *dorsal interossei,* which abduct and flex the toes; the *plantar interossei,* responsible for toe adduction and flexion; the *flexor digiti quinti brevis,* which flexes the small toe; and the *flexor digitorum longis* and *flexor digitorum brevis,* both of which provide toe flexion.

Testing is carried out with the patient lying on his back. In testing the lumbricales, the therapist stabilizes the metatarsals while the patient flexes the four lateral toes. Resistance is provided beneath the first phalangeal heads toward toe extension. To test the flexor hallucis brevis, stabilization is provided by the therapist at the first metatarsal and the patient is directed to flex his hallux, or big toe. Resistance is given beneath the proximal phalanx. Below functional muscle grades are evaluated by observation of motion.

Defects of Structure and Function Resulting from Abnormality of Major Metatarsophalangeal Joint Flexor Muscles

Weakness of the lumbricales with an active flexor digitorum longus results in hyperextension at the metatarsophalangeal joints. The distal joints flex, causing a hammer-toe position of the four lateral toes. There is also a diminution of the support of the anterior arch.

Weakness of the flexor hallucis brevis muscle permits a hammer-toe position of the big toe and lessens the stability of the longitudinal arch. Contracture of this muscle causes a restriction of dorsiflexion and a flexion of the proximal phalanx of the big toe.

EXTENSION OF METATARSOPHALANGEAL JOINTS. The muscles of metatarsophalangeal joint extension are: the *extensor digitorum longus,* which extends all joints of the four lateral toes, but particularly the metatarsophalangeal joints, and also strongly dorsiflexes the foot and partly everts the forefoot with continued action; and the *extensor digitorum brevis,* which extends the metatarsophalangeal joints of all but the small toe.

The patient may be tested in either a prone or a sitting position with his knee bent over the end of the examining table. The therapist stabilizes the metatarsal area of the foot. The patient extends all toes while resistance is applied at the dorsum of the proximal phalanges of the toes toward metatarsophalangeal flexion.

Defects of Structure Resulting from Abnormality of Major Metatarsophalangeal Joint Extensor Muscles

Weakness of these muscles results in a tendency toward drop-foot and anterior foot varus. Furthermore, the strength of foot eversion and dorsiflexion is diminished.

Contracture results in a position of eversion and dorsiflexion of the foot.

FLEXION OF INTERPHALANGEAL JOINTS. Interphalangeal joint flexion requires strength in the following muscles: the *flexor hallucis longus,* which flexes the big toe and assists in ankle plantar flexion; the *flexor digitorum longus,* which flexes the toes and assists in ankle plantar flexion; the *flexor digitorum brevis,* additionally responsible for toe flexion; and the *quadratus plantae* (m. flexor accessorius), which assists in toe flexion and stabilizes the tendon of the flexor digitorum longus.

The patient being tested lies supinely on the plinth. In testing the flexor hallucis longus muscle, the proximal phalanx of the big toe is held stabile while the distal phalanx is flexed by the patient. Resistance is given toward extension.

The flexor digitorum longus is tested with the therapist stabilizing the middle phalanges. The patient's foot is maintained in a neutral position while he flexes the distal phalanges of the lateral digits.

To examine the flexor digitorum brevis, the therapist stabilizes the proximal phalanges and maintains the patient's foot and ankle in neutrality. The patient must flex the middle phalanx of the four lateral toes. Below functional grades are assessed by observing active motion in the involved muscles.

Defects of Structure and Function Resulting from Abnormality of the Interphalangeal Joint Flexor Muscles

Weakness of the flexor hallucis longus muscle permits, during weight-bearing, a tendency toward pronation of the foot as a result of loss of medial stability which this muscle normally provides. Weakness also produces a gastrocnemius limp and interferes with the patient's ability to rise up on his toes.

Contracture of this muscle results in a hammer-toe position of the big toe.

Weakness of the flexor digitorum longus during weight-bearing permits a tendency toward pronation of the foot because of loss of medial stability of the ankle. It also tends the patient toward a gastrocnemius limp and inhibits rising on the toes.

Contracture of this muscle produces a flexion deformity of the distal phalanges of the four lateral toes with restriction of dorsiflexion and foot eversion.

Weakness of the flexor digitorum brevis reduces the muscular support of the longitudinal arch and the transverse, or metatarsal arch of the foot.

Contracture restricts toe dorsiflexion.

ABDUCTION OF THE TOES. There are four *interossei dorsalis pedis* muscles which abduct (and flex) the second, third and fourth toes. In addition, toe abduction is a function of the *abductor hallucis muscle,* which abducts the big toe, and the *abductor digiti minimi,* which abducts the small toe.

The patient being tested lies on the plinth in a supine position and abducts his toes. Resistance is given on the lateral side of the third, fourth and fifth toes, on the medial side of the hallux, and on both sides of the second toe. The fibers of the abductor hallucis and the abductor digiti minimi can easily be palpated on the medial and lateral borders of the forefoot.

Weakness of the abductor hallucis allows anterior foot valgus, hallus valgus and medial displacement of the scaphoid, the most lateral bone in the proximal row of tarsal bones. Contracture pulls the foot into anterior foot varus with abduction of the big toe.

ADDUCTION OF THE TOES. Toe adduction is accomplished by the *adductor hallucis,* which adducts the big toe, and the three muscles of the *interossei plantares,* which adduct the third, fourth and fifth toes.

With the patient in supination or in a sitting position, he adducts his toes. The therapist provides resistance medially to the big toe and laterally to the third, fourth and fifth toes.

The Evaluation of Range of Motion

The term "range of motion" refers to the range within which a joint can move. Limitation of range limits a patient's functioning. Range of motion is measured in degrees, usually with a instrument known as a goniometer which is described in the section on occupational therapy.

There are primarily two types of range of motion. *Active range of motion* is the range through which the patient is able to move the joint without assistance. *Passive range of motion* refers to joint movement performed by the therapist on the patient without active participation by the patient.

The physical therapist is primarily interested in range of motion in the lower extremities, although many of the tasks of physical therapy require good range in the upper extremities as well. In such cases, the functions of the physical therapist overlap with those of the occupational therapist. This is also true for those tasks of occupational therapy which require good range in the lower extremities.

Hence, the distinction presented herein is more academic than practical.

This chapter has been concerned mainly with but one phase of the physical therapy evaluation, manual muscle testing. There are other procedures for assessing muscle strength and several other phases tothe general evaluation of a patient. These are described in the following chapter.

———————

Chapter 5

EVALUATION PROCEDURES—PART 2

A COMPLETE EVALUATION of a patient's muscle strength will often require the use of electrodiagnostic methods. The necessity for these techniques may be noted during the initial evaluation and in such cases electrodiagnosis will be included as a routine part of the physical therapy screening. In other cases, electrodiagnostic testing will be conducted, after the patient has been admitted to an active rehabilitation program, because of the need to investigate the integrity of some portion of the neuromuscular system as a result of changes observed in the patient's condition or lack of expected change following therapy.

ELECTRODIAGNOSIS

Electrodiagnosis is usually employed to objectively determine whether a neuromuscular lesion exists, the extent of the lesion, the nature of the defect and the prognosis for spontaneous recovery or the need for surgery.

Current electrical tests are most useful in the diagnosis and prognosis of peripheral nerve lesions, but are also of much value in the study of other neurogenic diseases as well as in some myopathic disorders and a variety of central nervous system diseases with motor dysfunction.

The physical therapist generally does not conduct the electrodiagnostic testing herself, but assists the physician in this work.

Basic Concepts of Electrodiagnosis

The techniques of electrodiagnosis depend upon the activation and display of the electrical activity of the motor unit. This is the physiologic unit of the nervous system. It is comprised of the anterior horn cell, the motor cell of the spinal cord, its axon and terminal branchings, and all of the muscle fibers which it innervates.

The motor unit is activated in an all-or-none fashion. That is, it responds to stimulation with all of its potential or it does not respond at all. The activation, or response, consists of an electrical disturbance passing from the anterior horn cell down the axon and its branches to the myoneural junction where a chemical mediator is released initiating a wave of excitation along each muscle fiber. The contraction of the muscle fiber occurs approximately one millisecond following the action potential. The summated muscle fiber action potentials represent the motor unit potential, and thus, the electrical activity displayed by the electromyograph.

Each motor neuron has a threshold of stimulation. The reciprocal of this threshold is its excitability. The speed with which the wave of excitation passses along the axon is its conduction velocity. This velocity varies almost directly with the diameter of the axon and is favorably influenced by a myelin sheath. This is a sheath which surrounds the axon of the nerve fiber, consisting of myelin, a fatlike substance, alternating with a spirally wrapped neurolemma, a thin membrane. In humans, the nerve fibers which conduct the fastest are termed the "A" fibers. These are the large myelinated fibers which go to the skeletal muscles. Their conduction velocity varies between forty-five and seventy meters per second in the normal adult.

A muscle fiber's action potential represents a change from a potential of one hundred millivolts positive to fifteen millivolts negative external to the cell membrane. Immediately following the wave of excitation the fiber proceeds to recover to the resting state. The brief delay immediately prior to recovery is called the refractory period. The initial two-tenths milliseconds of this delay time is termed the absolute refractory period, so called because no stimulus, regardless of its intensity, can excite the cell. Following this there is a longer period known as the relative refractory period, during which a stimulus which is stronger than normal is required to produce excitation. If an exploratory electrode is placed near a cell membrane which is undergoing a change in polarization, the resultant electrical disturbance can be detected, amplified and displayed by the electromyograph.

Properties of irritability and conductivity are possessed by both nerve and muscle fibers, but are far more highly developed in nerve fibers.

Living tissue is a volume conductor, and thus, the resultant wave form depends upon the location of the electrode tip with relation to the wave of excitation. Action potentials can be monophasic, biphasic or triphasic depending upon this relationship. Usually, the motor unit action potentials are biphasic (or diphasic) or triphasic.

In normal individuals, less than ten per cent are polyphasic. The excitation disturbance sweeps along the cell membrane of the muscle at a rate of from four to five meters per second. The rate, amplitude, duration and shape of the displayed action potentials are influenced by the electrical characteristics of the tissue as well as those of the electromyograph.

Instrumentation

The basic components for electromyography and nerve stimulation are a set of electrodes, a pre-amplifier, an audio-amplifier and loudspeaker, an oscilloscope and a physiologic stimulator. If the displayed electrical activity is to be stored, a magnetic tape recorder and a camera are also included.

There are four types of electrodes. *Surface electrodes* vary from one-half centimeter to several centimeters in diameter. These are very useful for kinesiologic electromyographic studies and also for recording muscle action potential during nerve stimulation procedures. The active electrode is placed over the middle of the muscle and the reference electrode is placed over the tendon.

A *coaxial electrode* is a hollow needle with a wire, which is insulated except for the tip, placed in the barrel to act as the active, or exploring electrode. It has a sharp, bevelled tip and it responds to a small sphere of influence, which is directional as related to the bevel. It requires a ground electrode placed centrally to the muscle under study.

Monopolar electrodes are sharp pieces of stainless steel wire which are coated with an insulating material, such as Teflon®, except for a fraction of a millimeter at the tip. A surface electrode is placed on the skin over the muscle as a reference electrode.

A *bipolar electrode* has two insulated wires inserted in a hypodermic needle acting as active and reference electrodes. The barrel serves as a ground. Bipolar electrodes are employed in the investigation of very restricted areas.

The pre-amplifier should have a uniform response for frequencies ranging from sixteen to sixteen thousand cycles per second with an input impedance of several megohms. It should be a differential amplifier so that the common mode signal will be rejected at a rejection ratio of at least 100,000 : 1 for hospital use. A convenient gain adjustment and provisions for the insertion of high and low frequency filters are also necessary.

The oscilloscope provides a visual display of the electrical signal so that observation is made possible of the amplitude, duration and shape of the potentials. Sweep speeds for motor nerve conduction velocity should include two to one hundred milliseconds per inch.

The physiologic stimulator should have sufficient output to insure a supramaximal stimulus under all clinical conditions. It is necessary to have step adjustments and vernier adjustments for the intensity and the duration of stimulating voltage and step adjustments for the frequency and delay of the stimulus. An isolation transformer is used to isolate the stimulator from the ground. The stimulator triggers the sweep for nerve conduction velocity measurements, and it can be coupled to a one kilocycle oscillator so that the time base is locked to the start of the sweep. A satisfactory time base for nerve conduction studies is usually provided by the crosshatching on the face of the oscilloscope which corresponds to the known sweep speed.

An intramuscular needle thermometer is useful to indicate tissue temperature since changes in temperature can alter the conduction velocity. The thermometer is inserted in the muscle near the middle third of the peripheral nerve being studied.

Electrodiagnosis requires that the subject have a clean skin. The electrodes must be placed securely and electrode jelly used sparingly. Firm pressure is used with stimulating electrodes.

Procedures

Percutaneous Stimulation of Peripheral Nerves

At certain points in the body peripheral nerves are quite accessible to electrical stimulation. Since nerves typically have a low excitation threshold, a stimulus of short duration can be used to elicit a response. Stimulation of this type is not painful and is well tolerated by the patient even at relatively high voltages. Percutaneous nerve stimulation produces a visible contraction in each muscle which is so innervated. It is valuable in determining partial denervation, sensory loss, tendinous disruption, and the functional integrity of surgical repair of a severed tendon.

Muscle Stimulation

The response of skeletal muscles to electrical stimulation may be studied by applying a current to the skin area which overlies the point of entry of the nerve into the muscle belly, the motor point of the muscle.

FARADIC CURRENT STIMULATION. This form of testing uses the electrical outflow from the secondary of an inductance coil. It has a sharp spike of one millisecond duration on break of current. It is this duration which provides the value of faradic current in electrodiagnosis.

Normal muscle has an average maximal time requirement for stimulation of one millisecond and will contract if faradic current of adequate intensity is applied. If, however, there is denervation present, the chronaxie is increased and the faradic current's effective duration will then be too short to elicit a tactile response. Faradic current, then, is useful for the gross detection of denervation. (Note: Chronaxie is the minimal length of time for which a stimulus must be applied in order to elicit a muscle contraction when the stimulus is twice the threshold value. In denervated states the chronaxie is higher than for normal muscle and can rise to fifty milliseconds or more. With regeneration it progressively decreases, reaching a normal value after clinical recovery. It is believed that the progressive fall in chronaxie values during regeneration provides an index of the increasing maturity of the newly regenerating nerve fibers.)

GALVANIC CURRENT STIMULATION. When an electrical stimulus is applied to a muscle which has an intact nerve supply, the muscle is activated by impulses arriving from the motor nerve. Conversely, if a muscle has lost its nerve supply the muscle fibers must be stimulated directly, and since they have a higher threshold of stimulation than nerve tissue, the flow of current must be longer at similar intensities to produce a muscle contraction. Galvanic current permits current flow of prolonged duration. (Note: Reaction of degeneration [RD] is a reaction of muscle responding to galvanic stimulation.)

Galvanic current stimulation uses direct current of known polarity with which stimulation can be obtained through the negative elec-

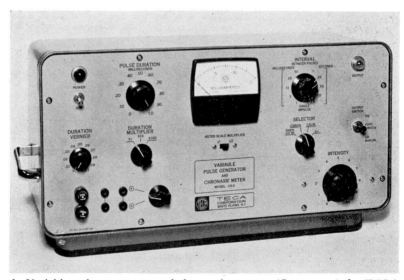

FIGURE 1. Variable pulse generator and chronaxie meter. (*Courtesy of the TECA Corp.*)

trode. Most types of apparatus in use today permit accurate control of the stimulus duration and intervals between stimuli, allow for rapid changes in polarity, and deliver a square-shaped wave with a rapidly attained maximum and minimum intensity. The current can be employed to determine muscle rheobase and chronaxie, the quality of electrical response, and the effect of polar reversal.

In galvanic testing, the quality of the muscle contraction provides the most informative observation from direct muscle stimulation. Normal muscle contracts rapidly and sharply, while denervated muscle responds with a relatively slow contraction, a slower relaxation, and a tendency for the contractions to spread to contiguous fibers.

The cathode closing current (CCC) is the most effective for exciting nerve tissue, but is has no such property for denervated muscles. In the classic Erb's test, the RD consists of absence of response to faradic stimulation, increased intensity requirements for or lack of response to galvanic current, a sluggish, wormlike contraction, and reversal of the polar formula so that anode closing current (ACC) at least equals or is greater than CCC.

Erb's test, however, is generally considered to be outdated and somewhat obsolete, and the term RD is felt to be a poor one since concern is not with degeneration, but rather with denervation. Furthermore, Erb's test does not take into consideration the fluctuation in rheobase which occurs with reinnervation following nerve injury. In addition, the concept of reversal of polar formula is no longer considered valid. Despite these limitations RD is still widely used in testing. (Note: Rheobase is the minimal amount or intensity required to stimulate or produce a contraction of a muscle when a current is permitted to flow for a prolonged or indefinite period of time.)

While a characteristic finding in denervated states is a slow contraction of muscle fibers, this is most easily observed in complete lesions. Partial lesions pose greater diagnostic problems and often require special tests to indicate the presence of denervation. Most applicable to such cases are stimulation away from the motor point and the use of a progressive current to demonstrate the lack of ability of the denervated fibers to accommodate.

To determine chronaxie the rheobase is obtained, then doubled, and the duration of its flow required to produce the same minimal visible contraction is the chronaxie. The determination of the rheobase is subject to procedural errors and to variables such as temperature of the extremity, presence of adipose tissue, presence of scars and unusually high skin resistance. Some of these factors may be obviated by using chronaxie determinations. These are accurate, reproducible studies which are highly significant in the detection and prognostication of the course of denervated states.

Normal chronaxie values vary from 0.04 to 0.8 sigma, with a rough normal value of less than one millisecond for any skeletal muscle. The variation in normal value is dependent upon whether the muscle is proximal or distal and whether it is a flexor or an extensor muscle. In denervation there is, characteristically, an elevation of chronaxie while reinnervation produces a progressive fall in chronaxie to normal. Frequently there is a terminal lag with a somewhat elevated chronaxie persisting for a short time following re-establishment of valuntary motor function.

Special Tests

The Strength-Duration Curve

When stimuli of progressively shorter durations are employed, increasingly greater intensities of current are required to elicit the standard motor contraction. Eventually, a stimulus may be so brief that it will not effectively result in muscle contraction unless intolerable current intensities are employed. There is, then, a minimal time factor which must be exceeded in the same sense as the minimal current threshold if the standard muscle contraction is to be produced. This minimal time factor may be viewed as an indirect relationship between the muscle and its nerve supply, in that when the nerve fibers are functionally intact the time factor is short, while when the nerves are degenerated the time factor is long. When the nerve fibers are regenerating the time factor lies somewhere between the two. Plotting the duration of current flow against the intensity of the applied current results in the strength-duration curve.

Chronaxie determinations depend upon a formula which relates muscle response, stimulus duration and stimulus intensity. The formula is: $K = k$ (intensity x duration), where k is the local excitatory state. The stimulus duration must fall within the utilization time limits for the inverse relationship to intensity to be valid.

Strength-duration curves are actually determined by the same formula, but instead of a single chronaxie reading, multiple intensity and duration values in relation to K are established and plotted. This provides a statistical advantage over unitary determinations and the shape of the curve may yield prognostic data. Adequate results can be obtained by utilizing between eight and sixteen determinations of K.

The normal strength-duration curve is relatively flat with a rise only at the zero end of the time abscissa. Denervation is characterized by a sharply progressing shift of the curve to the right, a decrease in the rheobase and an increase in the chronaxie. Reinnervation is typified by a shift of the curve to the left with a fall in chronaxie and an increase in rheobase with the appearance of plateaus. These plateaus represent regions where the serial determinations remain steady.

The Galvanic Tetanus Ratio (G.T.R.)

When denervated muscle is stimulated, exciting it requires a high intensity of current. A very slight further increase in intensity will tetanize the muscle, or throw it into a condition of continuous spasm. Very little current is required to excite a normal muscle, but much more is needed to tetanize it. The G.T.R., then, relates the intensity of the current necessary to elicit a simple muscle twitch (the rheobase) to the intensity required to bring this same muscle into a sustained, or tetanic, contraction. In a normal individual this ratio is approximately from 3.5:1 to 6:1. During regeneration the ratio increases from the value near unity to several times normal before dropping back to the normal level, as functional recovery takes place or as regenerating fibers mature. The G.T.R is thus a valuable test as an index of nerve regrowth. Changes in the G.T.R. are probably the earliest signs of changes in the nerve.

Neurotization Time (N.T.)

A peripheral nerve which has been severed or otherwise injured distal to its cell body has the innate ability to regenerate. After a time period following the injury the reparative ability of the nerve begins to operate and, if circumstances allow, growth of the nerve fiber down its old pathway tends to take place. The rate of regrowth varies with the size of the fiber and its cell body, with the distance over which growth must occur, and with the severity of damage to the peripheral or distal segment of the nerve. Even under ideal conditions the rate of regrowth of the fibers probably does not exceed approximately five millimeters per day, and the usually accepted rate of regeneration is about one millimeter per day. With these time limitations known, if the site of the nerve injury is also definitely known, it is possible to arrive at a rough estimate of how long it will take for regrowth to occur, and to estimate whether or not a nerve has had time to reconnect with the muscle tissue fibers which it normally innervates.

Neurotization time is an index which represents a ratio of the duration of the neuropathy to the theoretical time necessary for rein-nervation to occur. It is arrived at through computation of the fol-lowing formula:

$$\% \ N.T. = \dfrac{\dfrac{\text{Days since injury} - 10}{\text{Distance in mm from site of injury to motor point}}}{\text{Rate of regeneration in mm/day}}$$

Ten days are subtracted from the numerator as an arbitrary repre-sentation of the time for reparative forces to begin actual regrowth.

The formula can actually be stated more simply as:

$$\% \ N.T. = \dfrac{\text{Elapsed time since denervation} \times 100}{\text{Theoretical time for reinnervation}}$$

When the neurotization time exceeds 250 per cent with no electro-diagnostic evidence of regrowth, prognosis is poor and surgical inter-vention is considered.

Response to Repetitive Stimuli of Varying Frequency

If a muscle is normal the application of rapidly repeated stimuli produces a tetanic contraction. The required intensity for this is relatively stable regardless of the frequency of the applied current. Denervated muscle, however, shows an inverse relationship of inten-sity to frequency. Early in the reinnervation process this relationship reverses and returns to normal.

Progressive Current Ratio

The basis for this test is the loss of accommodation of denervated muscle. It relates the threshold of contractile response to stimulation with progressive current to the rheobase. The test is valuable for detecting partial denervation.

Electromyography

Electromyography deals with the detection, recording and inter-pretation of the electric voltages generated by skeletal muscle. Since measurement is made in milliseconds and microvolts the apparatus must be able to record these minute quantities. The electrical output of a muscle is detected with either surface or needle electrodes and is fed into an amplifier system. From the amplifier the electro-motive force is directed to a cathode ray oscilloscope and also to a loudspeaker where the electrical energy is converted into audible sound. Thus, both visual and auditory observation of muscle po-tentials is possible. Usually, the apparatus also contains some perma-nent recording device. The recording of electromyograms is typically carried out in a well shielded room so that extraneous noise is not picked up as interference.

Normal Electromyographic Patterns

A normal muscle is electrically silent when at rest. Upon contraction, either voluntary or reflex, an electrical potential is generated. When the needle electrode is moved the result is a burst of electrical activity, the duration of which is at least partially dependent upon the characteristics of needle insertion, which usually lasts from ten to thirty milliseconds. This is a consequence of the acitivation of muscle fibers with the mechanical stimulus of electrode movement. If this insertional activity is absent, it is an indication that either there are no functioning muscle fibers or that the electrode is not correctly placed in muscle tissue. If the tip of the electrode is stimulating an intramuscular nerve, the result is a sputtering burst of electrical activity against a background of high frequency, low amplitude electrical disturbance.

If the patient being tested is asked to think of contracting a designated muscle and the electrode is carefully moved as close to the firing unit as possible, a single motor unit action potential will result. As the tip of the needle approaches the activated motor unit, the sound grows louder and the amplitude increases.

Maximal muscle contraction is demonstrated when the patient contracts the muscle against maximal resistance. When the face of the oscilloscope is obscured by motor unit action potentials the interference pattern is normal. Normal motor units begin activating at five per second and, as the force of the contraction effort increases, they increase their rate of firing. Additional motor units are simultaneously recruited. Maximal firing rates range from thirty to fifty per second and the patient's contraction effort is estimated from the rate of firing. The amplitude ranges from about two hundred to two thousand microvolts. Sound is highly important in determining the duration. The number of action potentials is compared with the strength of contraction.

Pathological Electromyographic Patterns

Examples of electromyographic patterns for a number of specific disorders are presented below.

Peripheral Nerve Injuries. When the nerve supply to a muscle has been disrupted the denervated muscle will exhibit fibrillation, or small, local contractions, after a period of approximately eighteen to twenty-one days following injury. In the denervated muscle,

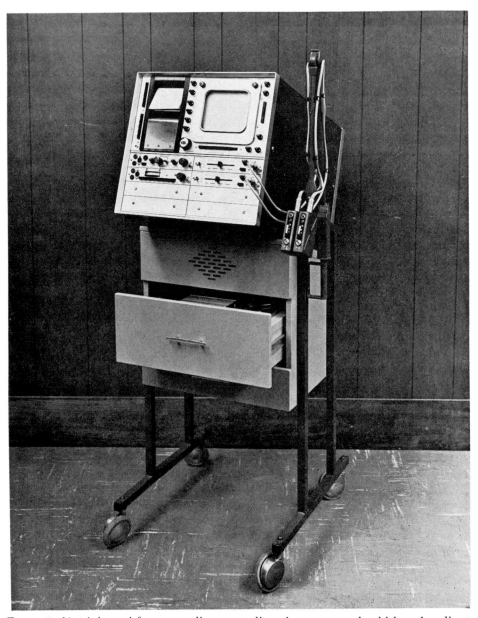

FIGURE 2. Multi-channel four trace direct recording electromyograph which makes direct graphic records for immediate evaluation of all displayed information. The model shown contains facilities for nerve conduction and reflex studies, muscle stimulation, direct latency time indication and a two channel magnetic tape recorder. (*Courtesy of the TECA Corp.*)

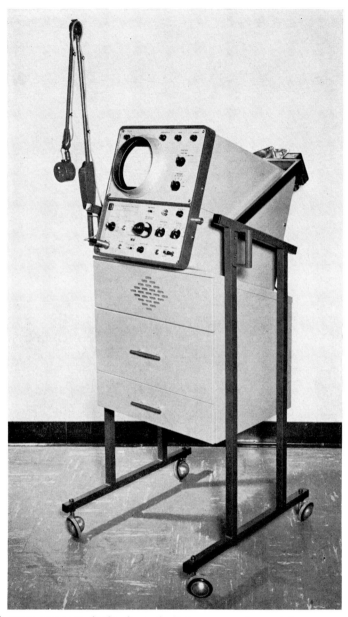

FIGURE 3. A more compact single channel electromyograph, used for sensory and motor nerve conduction studies. (*Courtesy of the TECA Corp.*)

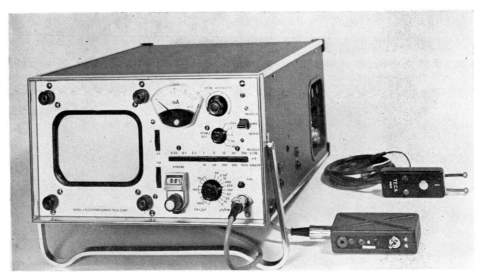

FIGURE 4. A portable electromyograph, useful in examination of bedridden patients. (*Courtesy of the TECA Corp.*)

needle insertion results in prolonged runs of electric potentials. Furthermore, fibrillation will also be present at rest. The magnitude of these waves varies up to several hundred microvolts. Their duration is from one to two seconds and the repetitive frequency varies from five to thirty per second. The form of these waves is typically diphasic with an initial positive deflection followed by a negative, equally high deflection.

These fibrillary potentials exist until reinnervation occurs or until the muscle undergoes complete loss of contractility and fibrosis, the formation of fibrous tissue. Reinnervation is electromyographically displayed by progressively decreasing fibrillation, by polyphasic potentials and, finally, by the appearance of normal motor unit discharge.

PERIPHERAL NEUROPATHY. The electromyographic records of the peripheral neuropathies differ from those of peripheral nerve injuries. Frequently there is complete electrical silence during both voluntary attempted contraction and in resting states. Fibrillation is observed less often. In the recovery period some motor units may discharge at very low frequency rates without regard to the intensity of effort. Reduplication of action potentials may also occur. There have been, in addition, descriptions of large, rhythmic action potentials with voltages which are six to eight times those of normal, as well as decrementing types of fasciculations, which are small, local muscle contractions, visible through the skin, representing a spontaneous discharge of a number of fibers innervated by a single motor nerve filament.

DIABETIC NEUROPATHY. The typical case is one of reduction of motor nerve conduction velocity, seen first in the peroneal nerve, then in the facial nerve and, finally, in the ulnar and median nerves. When the onset of the disorder is insidious, abnormal electromyographic patterns are minimal, if present, while there is a reduction in velocity of twenty to thirty per cent. Conduction velocity may be assumed to be reduced earlier in sensory fibers than in motor fibers.

ACUTE IDIOPATHIC POLYNEURITIS. This disorder exhibits reduced motor nerve conduction velocity and a neuropathic electromyelogram. Motor unit action potentials are usually of normal amplitude. There are fasciculation potentials, fibrillation potentials, and reduction in the number of voluntary potentials of which the proportion of polyphasic potentials is increased. A rise in conduction velocity follows, but lags behind clinical recovery.

POLIOMYELITIS. Fibrillation potentials appear from eighteen to twenty-one days following the death of the anterior horn cell. There is a decrease in the amplitude of motor unit potentials and in the number of impulses fired per second. Polyphasic potentials are observed early in the course of acute poliomyelitis. Fasciculation potentials are frequently seen in anterior horn cell disease. It has been found that muscles which show one hundred per cent fibrillation between the twenty-first and the sixtieth day after onset of the disease will recover motor power at the end of one year.

Synchronous discharge of motor units in different locations in the partly functioning muscles and their antagonists has been reported.

The rate of nerve conduction in patients with poliomyelitis is normal.

ROOT COMPRESSION SYNDROME. Irritative lesions of spinal nerve roots may result in a spontaneous discharge of simple or complex voltages and produce and involuntary contraction of either a single muscle fiber or of the complete motor unit. Involved muscles characteristically demonstrate sustained spasm, even during rest. Simple fasciculation voltages are of normal motor unit size and configuration. They may be continuously present during both activity and rest. Complex fasciculation potentials resemble polyphasic potentials.

While fasciculations are significant for diagnostic purposes it is also important to note fibrillation potentials. These appear, often about eighteen days following onset, in the para-spinal muscles.

CARPAL TUNNEL SYNDROME. Noted here is a delay in conduction from the proximal wrist crease to the thenar eminence of greater than five milliseconds (the normal conduction rate) with an average delay of eight and one-half milliseconds. If the compromise is severe the electromyogram will be neuropathic. Fibrillations are rare but have been known to occur.

AMYOTROPHIC LATERAL SCLEROSIS. The electromyogram of a patient with this disease is neuropathic despite normal conduction velocity. There are numerous fasciculation potentials which may be polyphasic or simple, short-duration potentials. Voluntary motor unit action potentials are increased in amplitude to ten millivolts and in duration to nine to eighteen milliseconds. Fibrillation potentials, while often difficult to demonstrate, are present. There are always positive waves and prolonged insertional activity. Electromyographic abnormalities are generalized despite the fact that the clinical findings of weakness may be localized.

PROGRESSIVE MUSCULAR DYSTROPHY. The electromyogram is myopathic, or indicative of muscle disease, showing fibrillation potentials due to disintegrating muscle fibers and positive waves. There is an increased proportion of low amplitude, short duration polyphasic potentials. Some of these are disintegrated potentials. Insertional activity is reduced, and late in the disease there is an increased resistance to needle advancement as a result of fibrosis and fat infiltration.

In cases of restrictive muscular dystrophy the electromyogram is myopathic but fewer fibrillation potentials are found because of the slower course of these forms of the disease. Insertional activity is reduced as muscles fibrose.

MYOTONIA. Electromyographic tracings show that the electric phenomena associated with the characteristic tonic muscle spasms of the disease is an output of high frequency potential with a rate varying between twenty-five and one hundred spikes per second. Individual spikes may resemble fibrillation potentials and may persist for one minute following cessation of voluntary effort.

MYASTHENIA GRAVIS. The electromyographic record of a patient with this disease characteristically reveals large spikes followed by a progressive diminution of motor unit output. The decline from large to small spikes is very rapid and beyond this point the fall is slower. In the latter period of discharge motor units drop out singly but before they do so there is a fluctuation in the amplitude of the spike. In a region where unit failure has occurred there is no recovery while effort is being maintained but even momentary relaxation will produce new firing followed by failure.

THE EVALUATION OF POSTURE

Good posture is important not only for disabled persons but for the non-disabled as well. Whatever postural position we assume, we are constantly subjected to the force of gravity. This force is utilized in equilibrium and movement while at the same time it places much stress on the bodily structures which are responsible for maintaining the upright position. Thus, postural defects are common and a large number of persons suffer acute distress and disability as a consequence of strain and injury to anti-gravity structures.

For persons who are disabled to the extent that intensive rehabilitation is required, appropriate posture is important for performing the necessary therapeutic exercises and for ambulation. In order to plan for effective treatment it is necessary to assess the patient's status regarding posture and, in general, body alignment.

The basic criterion employed in the evaluation of body alignment is the standing posture. While this has its limitations in that standing is a static position and is only one of many postures which an individual assumes during a day, it is nonetheless a useful method of judging several points quickly and accurately.

There are some fundamental concepts of which the physical therapist must be aware while conducting her examination. A body's center of gravity is a point located at the exact center of the mass of the body. Its location varies according to physique, and in a given individual it moves upward, downward or sideways according to changes in the position of body segments during movement. A body behaves as though its entire mass were centered about this point. Although the human body is comprised of several movable segments, each with its own center of gravity, when standing posture is considered the entire body may be viewed as a whole, with a single center of gravity located in the region of the second sacral vertebra.

Most daily postures involve the maintenance of the body in an upright position which is continually being opposed by the downward pull of gravity. If extensive muscular effort is employed to maintain these positions the result will be extreme fatigue. This is avoided by supplementary supporting structures such as ligaments and fasciae which assist in this work and conserve energy. When an individual is standing, the suprafemoral mass is supported on the segmented lower extremities so that gravity itself is utilized to promote stability.

The line of gravity is a vertical projection of the center of gravity with the individual upright. It is viewed as if an imaginary plumbline were passing through the center of gravity of the body. In order for the standing position to be stable the line of gravity must fall well within the base of support. The placement of the feet will influence the stability of the standing position by providing a base of variable size.

Another factor in standing posture is the constant, slight swaying of the body over the feet. The magnitude of these oscillations varies from 0.9 to 2.7 centimeters, and is largely anteroposterior in direction. The sway is characteristic for each individual.

A weight-bearing joint will be mechanically balanced and in equilibrium only if the line of gravity of the mass it supports falls exactly through the axis of rotation. If the line falls anterior to the axis the upper segment tends to rotate forward. If the line falls posterior to the axis the upper segment tends to rotate backward. In either case, there is a tendency towards rotation of the upper segment about the axis of the supporting joints.

There is a tendency at the ankle joint for the tibia to rotate forward about the ankle. Prevention of this is accomplished by the action of the plantar flexors which pull the tibia in the opposite direction. When the knee is flexed the ankle may be dorsiflexed through about thirty degrees of additional range of motion. Standing balance, therefore, needs to be maintained by muscle activity. Considerable support is provided by the gastrocnemius muscle.

In considering general stability various joints must be taken into account.

The stability of the ankle joint lies at a slight angle to the frontal plane, passing backward from the medial to the lateral sides of the joint. Some measure of standing ability is provided by the obliquity of this axis, especially if the feet are pointed outward. An individual with weak plantar flexor muscles can maintain equilibrium by keeping his weight farther back than normal and balanced directly over the ankle joints.

At the knee the weight line in standing is anterior to the axis. Forward rotation of the femur on the tibia is prevented by strong posterior collateral and cruciate ligaments and by muscles which pass over the posterior aspect of the joint. Knee extensor muscle activity is not a requisite for standing. An individual with weak quadriceps muscles has no difficulty if he keeps his knees fully extended and his center of gravity well forward.

At the hip the weight line usually passes posterior to the joint axis. Thus, the trunk tends to fall backward. Posterior trunk rotation is prevented by the structures which cross the anterior aspect of the hip joint, namely the iliofemoral ligament, a very strong, triangular-shaped band which covers the anterior and superior portions of the hip joint, and the hip flexor muscles.

In prolonged standing, the average person shifts position frequently, assuming asymmetrical and symmetrical attitudes, although the former predominate.

The Evaluation of Body Alignment

An analysis of body alignment serves several purposes. It acquaints the therapist with postural deviations of the individual patient, it serves as a guide in planning a treatment program, and it provides a record for future reference from which progress can be measured.

Posture is usually the first variable which is evaluated. Postural malalignment is based on the concept of a "normal" standard. The overall balance of the body is observed. The body should be evenly supported in an anteroposterior direction. The patient's weight should be carried evenly on both feet. Deviations from the sagittal plane, or in an anteroposterior direction from the vertical gravity line, or observed from the side. They are judged from external bony landmarks. The therapist visualizes a hypothetical vertical gravity line starting at the floor and passing upward anterior to the outer malleolus, just posterior to the patella, through the greater trochanter of the femur, the middle tip of the shoulder and the lobe of the ear.

Deviations in the frontal plane, or laterally from the midline, are assessed from an anterior or posterior view. The gravity line ideally bisects the body into two symmetrical halves. Since certain lateral displacements are best seen from certain views the observations are usually made from both aspects.

Observations and measurements of body and body part alignments are made of the following:

Body type	Lithe, Medium or Stout.
Anteroposterior balance	Consistent presence of forward or backward shifting of body weight.
Lateral balance	Forward, left or right tilt, or rotation.
Chest	*Hollow,* or concave appearance of anterior thoracic wall; *Funnel,* or pectus excavatum, a marked depression of the anterior thorax; *Barrel,* or rounded thorax; *Pigeon,* or pectus carinatum, a thoracical misalignment in which the anteroposterior diameter is increased and the sternum is displaced forward; and *Harrison's*

	groove, a transverse depression across the lower thorax.
Shoulders	High left or right if there is a scapular height difference.
Scapulae	*Abduction*, an abnormal degree of separation from the midline; and *Projection*, which is prominence of the inferior angle of the scapulae or of the entire vertebral border.
Hip level	High left or right as judged from the relative heights of the anterior superior iliac spines.
Abdomen	Habitual relaxation or weakness as seen in protrusion of the abdominal wall; segmental deviations as noted in flaring of the lower ribs; anterior pelvic tilt and lordosis; and grooving of the upper abdominal wall to an extreme degree.
Spine	Kyphosis, Lordosis, Scoliosis, rounded back or flat back (decrease in, or absence of normal anteroposterior spinal curves).
Legs	Knock knees (*genu valgum*), bow legs (*genu varum*), back knees, hyperextended knees (*genu recurvatum*) and tibial torsion.
Feet and toes	Pronation; depression, or flattening of the long arch; calluses; papillomas, which are benign tumors arising from the epithelium; and other skin conditions of the metatarsal area; presence and degree of toe deviations, such as overlapping toes, hammer toes, corns and *hallux valgus*.

GAIT

Any physical examination of disorders which involve the locomotor system must include an analysis of the patient's gait pattern. Despite the fact that most individuals ambulate without awareness of the skeletomuscular actions involved in such activity, human locomotion is a complicated process. It involves transforming a series of controlled, coordinated angular movements occurring simultaneously at various joints in the lower extremities, into a smooth path for the center of gravity of the body.

It should be kept in mind that there are six basic determinants of locomotion. They are knee-ankle interaction, knee flexion, hip flexion, pelvic rotation about a vertical axis, lateral tilting of the pelvis, and lateral displacement of the pelvis.

Normal Gait

If the therapist is to recognize pathological gait patterns she must be familiar with the mechanisms of normal gait.

Locomotion is a cyclic activity. The gait cycle consists of two main parts, a stance phase and a swing phase. The stance phase begins with the foot in the forward position, heel on the ground, and the leg partially or fully weight-bearing. It ends when the toe pushes off and the foot leaves the ground. The swing phase begins at this point. The foot is not touching the ground and the body weight is borne by the contralateral leg. It lasts until the heel touches the ground again. One foot and leg bear the weight, while the opposite foot and leg swing forward and in their turn take over the body weight. The stance phase is longer than the swing phase.

There is also a period when both feet are simultaneously on the ground. This is known as the period of double support, or the double support phase.

A more detailed analysis of the gait cycle shows that the stance phase begins when the heel strikes the ground and terminates when the toe rises at the end of the stride. The stance phase has three parts—heel strike, midstance and push-off. The swing phase begins when the toe leaves the floor and ends when the forward swing of the leg has stopped. It too has three parts—acceleration, swing-through and deceleration.

While the leg plays the most obvious role in locomotion, other body elements—such as the trunk, pelvis, and even the upper extremities—have their functions. All must be carefully observed in an extensive gait evaluation.

Pathological Gait

Pathological gait patterns are typified by excessive or asymmetric movements of body parts or of the body's center of gravity.

Paralysis, or marked paresis of the pre-tibial group of muscles, results in slapping of the forefoot immediately after the heel strike

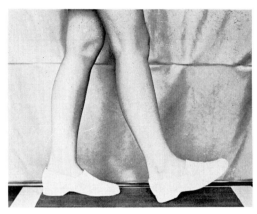

FIGURE 5. Normal gait pattern, stance phase: The heel strike part.

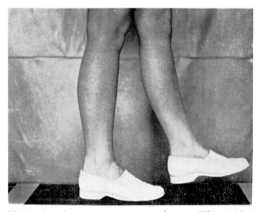

FIGURE 6. Normal gait pattern, stance phase: The mid-stance part.

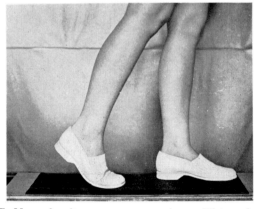

FIGURE 7. Normal gait pattern, stance phase: The push off part.

and in a foot-drop during the swing phase of ambulation. The foot-drop is compensated for by excessive knee and hip flexion producing what is known as steppage gait.

In the more extensive lower motor neuron forms of lower extremity paralysis, the foot may be dropped with rotation of the entire leg. This gait form is typical of patients with plantar flexion spasticity for whom a steppage gait is unfeasible because of extensor spasticity involving the entire lower extremity.

Moderate weakness of the dorsiflexors of the foot may not result in foot-drop during the swing phase, but there will still be a definite foot slap. If the dorsiflexors exhibit only a mild weakness, foot slapping will be observed only when the patient is ambulating rapidly or is fatigued.

Paralysis or paresis of the muscles of the calf may be characterized by both dropping of the pelvis on the affected side and by slowing of its forward movement at the last instant of the stance phase. At moderate speeds a patient can compensate for both characteristics by contracting the abductors and rotators of the contralateral hip at the period of double support. In the calf muscle limp the drop and lag of the hip occur on the same side as the defect. With rapid ambulation the limp is accentuated.

In the case of quadriceps paralysis, knee extension during weight-bearing is produced by hip extensor muscle contraction which drives the distal femur and, hence, the knee, backward. The quadriceps limp is typified by forcible knee extension at heel strike concomitant with the forward drive of the involved hip. If there is a constant hyperextension of the knee as a mechanism of stability and compensation in the early stance phase, the usual result is a *genu recurvatum*.

Isolated weakness of the gluteus maximus muscle is rare. The term "maximus gait" refers to weakness or paralysis of hip extensors as a muscle group. This type of gait is characterized by an anterior protrusion of the involved hip immediately after the heel of the affected extremity strikes the ground. A tightly extended knee in midstance is also typical of a maximus gait.

Weakness of the hip flexors is characterized by a sudden backward thrust of the trunk and pelvis just prior to and during the swing phase of the involved extremity. If the patient cannot shorten the affected leg during the swing phase, the backward thrust of the trunk is preceded and reinforced by a lateral trunk movement toward the unaffected side, which permits the patient to clear the ground with the involved leg during the swing phase.

Weakness of the hip abductor muscles results in the gluteus medius gait. This gait, when not compensated for, is seen as a greater than normal dropping of the pelvis on the unaffected side during the swing phase, a lateral protrusion of the involved hip during weight-bearing and a distinct lateral sliding of the upper two-thirds of the trunk and head toward the affected side produced by movement of the lumbar spine. There may also be a slight steppage gait and a forward swinging of the shoulder on the uninvolved side accompanying the stance phase of the involved extremity. The shoulders' swing substitutes for the absent, or reinforces the weak, rotary functions of the medius by carrying the unaffected hip forward at the end of the arc of stance of the involved lower limb.

A compensated gluteus medius gait is observed in patients with a severely weakened gluteus medius muscle. It is marked by a medial deviation of the hip on the affected side in weight-bearing to bring the axis of rotation of the supporting hip beneath the main mass of the body. This medial deviation simultaneously occurs with a marked bending of the entire trunk downward and sideways over the affected hip during weight-bearing, and a consequent lowering of the shoulder on the involved side.

The Gait Evaluation

In examining a patient's gait the therapist requests the patient to demonstrate his ambulation several times so that she may determine the main abnormal features. It is essential for the patient to change his pace of ambulation several times since some disorders may be detected only during rapid walking while others can be pronounced only at very slow speeds. In like fashion, standing up, sitting down, walking up and down inclines, or climbing stairs may bring out gait abnormalities. As the patient ambulates, each joint is carefully observed and comparisons are made between the gait of the individual patient in question and known normal gait patterns. Attention is also directed to the swing of the upper extremities. The patient is asked, in addition, to stop suddenly, make turns, pass objects and other persons, and to pass through a doorway.

It is possible for a patient to have an accumulation of imbalance during consecutive steps, and the therapist must determine whether or not a patient who requires only slight assistance during ambulation will be able to walk without such help if he stops after every other step.

A patient may be directed to hop on one leg, since this is a rather sensitive test of ability to recover balance.

During the evaluation the patient will be instructed to ambulate with his eyes closed or covered. Such a task provides information about the patient's orientation in space and enables differentiation between various ataxias.

Having a patient walk on his toes or heels is a useful screening technique for muscle strength evaluation. The therapist also checks the soles and heels of the patient's feet for areas of marked wear as the patient ambulates barefooted.

A patient's gait is analyzed under two conditions—ambulation while being relaxed as possible and ambulation when concentration is given to the best performance possible. Patients having certain disorders may, when asked to concentrate, be able to eliminate some gait abnormalities, such as shuffling, be able to shorten the swinging leg properly, or be able to dorsiflex a foot in which a tendon transplant has recently been performed.

In patients with central nervous system dysfunction it is necessary to determine whether differences exist between their performance of particular motor functions while they are lying down and while they are ambulating, and if any differences are present, what these are. It is important to know the degree to which postural reflexes and patterns aid and reinforce the patient's ability to ambulate and to what extent they may possibly actually hinder ambulation. A hemiplegic patient, for example, may show no voluntary active hip flexion while reclining, but during walking he may be able to initiate the swing of his leg with his hip flexor muscles. Another patient may, while reclining or sitting, be able to dorsiflex his involved foot, but during the swing phase of ambulation he may drag this same foot in a plantar-flexed position.

Patients who cannot ambulate either unassisted or with assistance from the therapist, will be required to walk between horizontal parallel bars. This also helps the therapist ascertain the degree of the patient's awareness that he is not maintaining the upright position during ambulation.

If a patient routinely uses assistive devices such as canes or crutches, or orthotic devices such as braces, or wears a prosthesis, he is requested to walk with and, within reason, without these aids.

The therapist records the type, extent and severity of deviations from normal gait patterns, strength of certain muscles and muscle groups, limitations in range of joint motion, length of lower extremities, fatigability, and localization and severity of pain or discomfort. These data are all essential in planning a program of ambulation training and for referral of the patient to the physician for neurological or other examination if such appear to be warranted.

THE PHYSICAL THERAPY RE-EVALUATION

Approximately every four to eight weeks, each patient on an active rehabilitation program is re-evaluated as to his progress. Each therapy service re-assesses the patient's status and compares it with his condition at the time of admission and/or with his status at the previous re-evaluation. A re-evaluation conference is held at which the various staff members of the rehabilitation team report on the patient's activities and improvement or lack of improvement observed in the areas of treatment. Based upon their findings, the physician who heads the team will modify a patient's therapy program, increasing or decreasing it, prescribe new activities, eliminate active rehabilitation, or plan for discharge from the hospital.

Following a medical summary report of the patient's current health the first discipline to state its findings is usually physical therapy. In preparation for this report the therapist has retested the patient in some, many, or all of the areas of function in which he was initially evaluated. The extent of this re-evaluation procedure depends upon the disabilities of the patient. Patients with arthritis, multiple sclerosis and muscular dystrophy, for example, may be given the entire series of tests for muscle strength, range of motion, balance and gait. The patient's scores on each test are recorded and compared with his previous scores, and thus, the therapist is able to state whether or not improvement has occurred, where it has occurred and where more intensive therapy is needed. Other patients, such as those with unilateral hip fractures or amputations, or senile gait patterns, may be evaluated only in regard to specific problems which pertain to their particular disorder. Most physical therapy re-evaluations will include at least a general screening of all functions, with emphasis on particular problems.

It must be recognized that the physical therapist who performs the re-evaluation has been working with the patient on a daily basis for a long period of time, and thus, is familiar with his condition and the changes which have occurred in it through therapy. Her re-evaluation is a formal procedure in which scores are obtained in each area of function, so that an objective record is maintained and so that the patient's current status can be compared to his previous condition.

Depending upon her knowledge of the patient and his progress and upon her findings during the re-evaluation testing, the physical therapist will, after reporting to the rehabilitation team, make certain suggestions concerning the patient's future program. She may feel that the current program is too strenuous and wish to reduce it, or she may feel that the patient can tolerate an increased exercise program. She may suggest that a patient is ready for ambulation training, or for a prosthesis, or for ambulation without assistance, or for a particular form of exercise. A patient's report of pain or discomfort may lead her to request the application of therapeutic heat. A therapy modality such as radiation, ultrasound, or hydrotherapy may be suggested as applicable for a patient. The therapist might recommend that a patient be taken off a physical therapy program, either because he is not yet ready, for one or more reasons, or because his progress has been at a plateau for a long time and no further gains are expected, or because he has completed his program and, from her point of view, is now ready for discharge.

The physician will listen to the therapist's report and suggestions and then will prescribe for the patient's future therapy program. It has been this author's experience that when recommendations for program changes are made by a therapist who has been working regularly with a patient, they are usually accepted by the physician. At times, he may wish to examine or observe the patient himself before prescribing future treatment and, rarely, he may decide not to follow the therapist's suggestions, but the general procedure is for the physician to act in accord with the report presented by the physical therapist.

Chapter 6

THE EXERCISE PROGRAM

THERE ARE SEVERAL DEFINITIONS of the term "therapeutic exercise," but they all have the same basic elements in common. The one offered here has been compounded from those in general use in the rehabilitation field.

THERAPEUTIC EXERCISE AND MUSCLE RE-EDUCATION

Therapeutic exercise may be defined as the scientific application of bodily movement for the purpose of treatment of disease or disorder. Its aim is the correction of dysfunction or impairment, improvement of musculoskeletal function, and the improvement of balance, body stability and coordination of body movements, or the maintenance of a physical state of well being.

Muscle re-education is the term used to designate the phase of therapeutic exercise which is devoted to the development or recovery of voluntary control of skeletal musculature. Its objectives are the development of motor awareness and voluntary responding, and strength and endurance in patterns of movement which are necessary, effective, acceptable and safe.

Types of Therapeutic Exercise

Therapeutic exercises are designed to utilize the natural basic motions of the body. These motions are passive, active and forced.

Passive Exercises

Passive exercises are those which are performed by the therapist, or by some kind of apparatus, on the patient without any active contraction of the involved body part by the patient.

The primary purpose of passive exercise is to prevent contractures by maintaining the normal range of motion in the joints. It is most frequently used with patients who have either paralyzed or severely paretic muscles. The therapist must stabilize the proximal joint and support all distal segments. Movement is kept within the pain-free range and the therapist moves the patient's affected part slowly and smoothly through its entire range.

Passive exercise prevents contractures and the formation of adhesions, increases proprioceptive sensation, maintains the resting length of the muscle, stimulates reflexes of flexion and extension, and prepares the patient for active exercise.

Active-Assistive Exercises

Active-assistive exercises are accomplished by active contraction of the part by the patient with the assistance of the therapist or some mechanical agent.

This form of exercise is the initial step in a program of muscle re-education. Only active contraction of muscles by the patient can result in muscle strengthening. The therapist must support the weight of the distal segment to eliminate the resistance of its weight or the pull of gravity. In this way the patient is able to maintain an active contraction through the greatest possible range of motion. Mechanical or hydrotherapeutic modalities are often prescribed during this phase of treatment.

The therapist explains the task to the patient and indicates the point of insertion and the line of pull of the involved muscle. She provides only enough assistance to insure a smooth movement. She also prevents the patient from substituting other muscles for the affected one during the exercise. When a program of active exercises is initiated, proper guidance and assistance strengthen muscles and establish the correct patterns for coordinated movement.

Active Exercises

Active exercises are performed solely by the patient without any external assistance or resistance. They represent a progressive increase of active-assistive exercises, and their prescription is a positive sign that the patient no longer requires assistance.

Exercises are presented to the patient movement by movement in proper sequence—i.e. starting position, movement to the farthest point, return to the starting position and rest. Exercises are scheduled so that they present the patient with the correct grade of difficulty for his level of ability. The patient is supervised by the therapist to insure that he is performing the motions smoothly and correctly, and is not using substitute movements.

A program of active exercises improves function and increases strength. It also tends to improve bodily function in general through assisting in increasing cardiac reserve, respiratory reserve and body conditioning.

Resistive Exercises

Exercises which are performed by the patient against resistance supplied by either the therapist or apparatus are termed resistive exercises.

In doing resistive exercises the patient moves the body part through its arc of motion and external resistance is applied against his movement. This resistance may be only that provided by gravitational force or it may be given by the therapist or by some type of equipment. Manual resistance, as applied by the therapist, varies from slight to marked, depending upon the patient's muscle strength and the position in which the part is placed for exercise. While resistive exercises are ordinarily instituted when a muscle has *good* to *normal* strength, they may be used with *fair* muscles if the part is placed in a way that gravity is either eliminated or assists in the movement.

The least amount of resistance is usually given at the beginning and at the end of the range of motion, while the greatest resistance is applied during the middle one-third of the range. Resistance is applied at a point distal to the joint which is involved in the motion.

The major outcome of a program of resistive exercise is the development of strength.

Progressive resistive exercises are used primarily to strengthen a muscle group by means of applying progressively increased mechanical resistance. The strength and endurance of the exercised muscle are increased by resistive exercises employing weights. A system of pulleys is devised so that there will be a sufficient counterbalancing load to offset the weight of the body part until the weakened muscle can complete the arc of motion.

Stretching Exercises

Stretching exercises are accomplished by either active or passive forced motion. The force may be supplied by the therapist or by a device or by the patient himself using the contraction of antagonistic muscle groups.

Motion is never forced if there is acute pain. If pain persists or the range decreases, the amount of force employed or the duration of treatment is reduced.

Stretching is done gently and gradually over a long period of time. The distal segment is supported so that force is applied in the desired place. Stretching should not become an active-resistive type

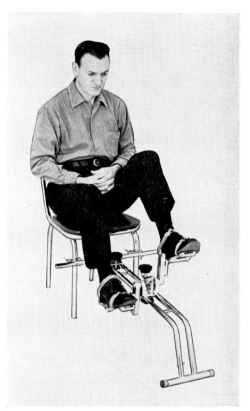

FIGURE 8. Patient using a Restorator® in exercising his lower extremities. The Restorator® can be attached to a chair, tubular bed or wheelchair and provides active or resistive exercises in a controlled manner for re-establishing muscle power, range of motion and coordination. (*Reprinted by permission of J. A. Preston Corp., 1971*)

of exercise and thus, the involved muscle should be as relaxed as possible during the work. If a part is weak or paralyzed, active motion or supporting devices must be used to maintain increases obtained through stretching or the gains will be temporary.

Stretching is aimed at restoring the normal range of motion where limitation in range is due to loss of elasticity of soft tissue and not to bone malalignment.

Functional Exercise

As stated earlier in this text, the goal of any rehabilitation program is to enable the patient to function as fully as possible within the limits imposed by a physical disability. Unfortunately, sometimes the patient is taught functional skills before a foundation of exercise is laid. This may be analogous to teaching a physician surgery prior

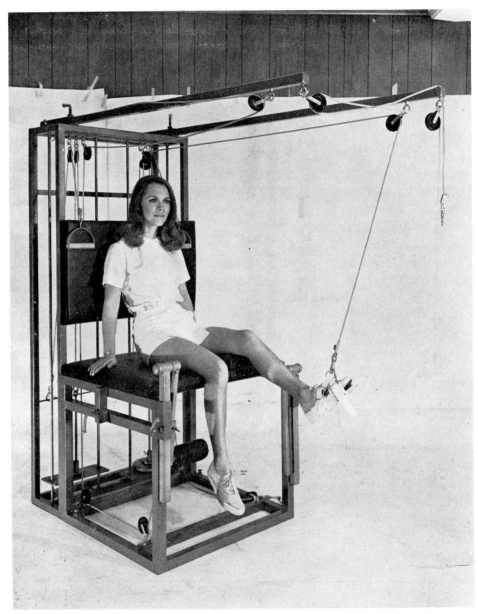

FIGURE 9. Multiplex Exerciser®. This unit provides quadriceps exercises, hamstring stretching, shoulder and elbow exercises, shoulder adduction and abduction, shoulder depression, reciprocal arm and shoulder motion and hip exercises. (*Courtesy of La Berne Manufacturing Co., Inc.*)

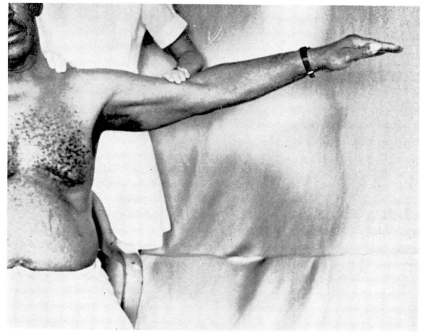

FIGURE 10. A resistance exercise. The therapist is resisting the middle deltoid muscle to stabilize the patient's shoulder.

to his learning anatomy and physiology, and thus, the probability of success is small. In physical therapy, exercise must precede function.

Exercises may be carried out by the patient in his bed, on special exercise mats, within upright parallel bars, or on crutches. They may be conducted on an individual basis or with groups of two or more patients. All exercises prepare the patient for future training in functional activities.

Mat Exercises

Mat exercises are performed on large padded mats in the physical therapy gymnasium or other specially designated area. They have many purposes which can be listed as follows: to teach changing of body position from pronation to supination to sitting; to teach sitting balance while moving body parts such as the trunk and upper extremities; to teach movement in all directions while sitting on a level surface; to teach handling of the affected extremities; to strengthen muscles; to teach active or passive stretching; and to teach coordination and skill in preparation for standing, ambulation and activities of daily living.

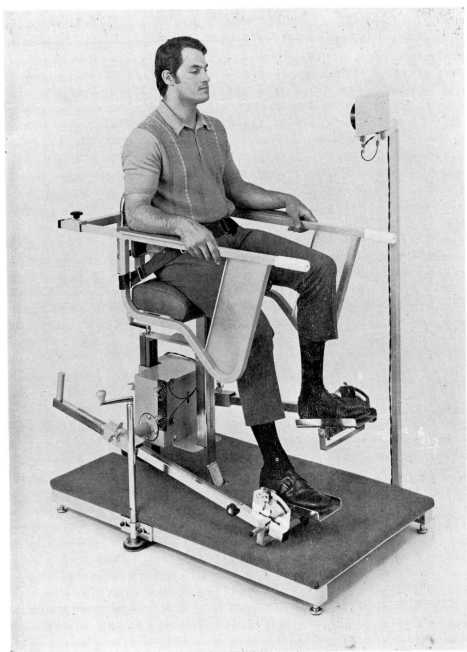

FIGURE 11. An exercise and training system unit designed to provide automatic accommodating resistance to active extension and flexion movements performed by the patient. It is employed to develop the fundamental dynamic weight-bearing requirements of ambulation-weight-bearing strength, speed, endurance and weight transfer skills. (*Courtesy of Lumex, Inc.*)

Parallel Bar Exercises

These exercises are designed for patients with or without braces. They are preliminary to independent ambulation and are aimed at the following: developing tolerance for the standing position and for weight-bearing on affected lower extremities; teaching standing balance while moving the trunk and upper extremities; strengthening the upper extremities through push-ups so that they will be able to carry the weight of the body; teaching pelvic control; teaching locking and unlocking of braces while in sitting and standing positions; teaching rising to a standing position and sitting down while holding onto the bars; and teaching basic ambulation patterns and rhythm preparatory to crutch walking, climbing and activities of daily living.

Crutch Balancing

Crutch balancing is also feasible for patients who function either with or without braces. The objectives of crutch balancing exercises include the following: to teach standing balance while on crutches; to teach pelvic control; to teach the placement of crutches in different directions and positions; to teach locking and unlocking of braces while standing on crutches; to teach pre-climbing exercises; and to teach pre-falling exercises preparatory to crutch walking, climbing and activities of daily living.

Ambulation

Basic gait techniques are taught to patients who do or do not wear braces or use crutches. They are designed to provide the patient with good, safe gait patterns in preparation for independent walking.

Independent practice in ambulation techniques is for patients with or without orthotic devices or prostheses. They are designed to teach independent ambulation, one rapid and one slow gait, individually prescribed, in all directions and on different indoor floor coverings, to develop endurance and speed, and to train the patient in outdoor ambulation on a variety of ground surfaces.

Climbing techniques are also prescribed for patients who do or do not require orthotic and/or prosthetic aids. They are taught in order that the patient learn independent navigation of ramps, curbs and stairs with or without railings.

There are also special exercises and exercise programs for patients with respiratory problems resulting from diseases such as empyema, emphysema, asthma and tuberculosis, or which are a result of postural deformities, weak or paralyzed diaphragm and/or abdominal muscles, athetoid cerebral palsy, post-surgical difficulties, scoliosis or posture or trunk stability problems. A detailed description of these special programs is beyond the scope of this book.

Prescribing Therapeutic Exercise

Following the medical examination by the physician, and after completion of the physical therapist's evaluation, the prescription is written for a rehabilitation program.

The word "prescription" is usually interpreted as pertaining to medication and in rehabilitation pharmaco-therapy is often an important part of a patient's total therapeutic regimen. However, the use of the word is not restricted to drugs and can refer to any written order for treatment by a physician. In physical rehabilitation prescriptions are written for all of the therapy services, for foot care, dental care, orthotics, prosthetics, wheelchairs and, in fact, for any aspect of the total range of possible patient care.

During the medical examination the physician will note certain points in particular for patients who are to be given therapeutic exercises. He pays special attention to cardiac status and blood pressure, to defects of the thoracic and abdominal walls, to hernias, to joint status, to sensation, to areas of pain, to respiration, and to specific problems of the skeletomuscular, genito-urinary and nervous systems.

The physician's prescription, based upon his findings and on the physical therapist's report, includes the following: precautions; weekly and daily frequency of exercise; number of sets of exercises; frequency of medical examinations and progress re-evaluations; purposes of the exercises; a list of exercises; a statement as to whether exercises should be unilateral or bilateral, and if bilateral, whether they should be performed on both sides simultaneously or alternately; method of administration; and whether exercises should be performed in bed, on a stretcher, in a wheelchair, sitting or standing.

The therapist carries out the prescription and reports to the physician as changes in the patient's status occur which might warrant modifications in the original orders.

Fundamentals of Therapeutic Exercise

Strength is usually defined as the maximal tension able to be exerted by a muscle during a contraction.

Endurance is the term used to describe the ability of the muscle to contract and exert tension for a prolonged period of time.

Power may be defined as distinct from strength. It is the rate of doing work or the amount of work done per unit of time. Repetitive muscular contractions, even at far less than maximal tensile strength, will produce fatigue when continued for a few minutes. Since activities are normally repetitive, an assessment of muscle power may be the most useful predictor of performance.

The tension which is generated during contraction of a muscle fiber is considered to be the stimulus which produces hypertrophy and an increase in the strength of the fiber. Maximal or near maximal tension has been found to be most effective for increasing strength. Studies have reported that the most rapid increase in strength occurs when an exercise exceeds two-thirds of the maximal strength of the muscle. One maximal contraction of each muscle fiber is the adequate stimulus to cause the alteration of metabolism which leads to an increase in tensile strength of the fiber. It is easier to attain maximal tension during an isometric contraction than during a concentric contraction.

With respect to power, work per unit time which exceeds metabolic capacity is felt to be the stimulus resulting in muscular hypertrophy, increased strength, increased ability to recruit motor units, and increased ability to withstand discomfort associated with heavy exercise.

Muscular endurance is related to factors of muscle strength circulation, muscular metabolism, central nervous system fatigue, and to the patient's motivation to continue an activity.

A direct relationship exists between the maximal tension that a muscle is able to exert and its ability to contract repeatedly against a constant load. As the muscle increases in strength, working against a constant load requires proportionately less of the muscle to be contracting at any moment and leaves a greater recovery time for muscle fibers following contraction. Tension during muscular activity is sustained because of the irregular contractions and relaxations of many motor units which fuse into a smoothly sustained contraction of the entire muscle. During great effort or fatigue the precision of muscular contraction is reduced because larger motor units are activated and these provide less precise responses than do the smaller units which have a lower excitation threshold. After each contraction voluntary motor fibers undergo relaxation and metabolic recovery. If the rest period between successive muscle contractions is not of sufficient duration to allow for full metabolic recovery, the muscle fiber fatigues.

The cardiovascular capacity to sustain work increases as a consequence of repeated, prolonged effort. Metabolites produced in the muscle during work are effective in increasing local circulation, car-

diac work and respiration. As circulatory capacity improves in response to exercise, the duration of the activity can be increased.

Alternating isotonic contractions of antagonistic muscle groups
aid venous and lymphatic flow. Compression of the vessels by the
contracting muscles produces centripetal flow and the valves in the
vessels prevent retrograde flow. Muscles are ischemic, or have a
diminished blood supply, during strong isometric contractions, and
metabolites which are accumulated during ischemic contraction act
reflexly to directly increase circulation to the active muscle.

The metabolic changes which are associated with prolonged muscular activity result in an increase in the cellular stores and in the
cellular metabolic capacity. Exposure of muscle fibers to moderately
fatiguing activity for progressively longer time periods with appropriate rest intervals, permits these changes to occur without exposing
the cell to the detrimental effects of exhaustion. The development of
tolerance for discomfort, of motivation to continue the activity for a
prolonged period, and of readjustments in neuronal metabolism are
also built up by periods of tiring activity for increasingly long periods of time.

There are two general classes of active exercise which are of
clinical value. In *monometric exercise* there is no shortening of the
muscle upon contraction, while in *polymetric exercise* there is both
shortening and lengthening of the muscle during exercise. Both
monometric and polymetric exercises are given either with or without resistance. If resistance is employed the amount depends upon
the therapeutic objective for the muscle. If the objective is increased strength, then heavy resistance is applied for a few repetitions. This is the phase of resistive exercises described earlier in this
chapter.

Monometric exercises are utilized clinically in cases of joint immobilization or where joint motion is contraindicated. Resistance
may or may not be used against the contractions. Monometric exercise produces little fatigue and, hence, can be performed several
times daily with good results. A daily program of monometric exercises may consist of ten to fifteen isometric contractions performed
two or three times per day or even hourly.

Polymetric exercises are administered through manual, mechanical
or automatic counterbalancing procedures. These also accomplish
little work when not resisted and can be prescribed for frequent daily
performance.

In active resisted exercises, resistance can be provided by the
weight of the extremity alone against gravity, by only a part of the

extremity's weight through counterbalancing, or by the weight of the extremity plus additional weight. When a resistance exercise program is planned, the resistance-repetition combination is determined which will produce the desired quality in the muscle. A purely repetitive exercise will increase endurance, while a purely resistive exercise will improve strength. The typical procedure in rehabilitation is to use strength-building exercises until maximum functional strength is developed and then initiate a program of endurance exercises.

Exercise Techniques

Increasing Strength

There are several techniques which the physical therapist can employ to increase muscle strength, and within the main methodologies there are a number of modifications.

PROGRESSSIVE RESISTIVE EXERCISE. The first step in a program of this type is the determination of the *10 R.M.*, or *10 repetition maximum*. This is the maximal resistance which the muscle can lift ten times through the range of motion. The 10 R.M. is determined by contracting the muscle to the shortened position against a light load for ten contractions and progressively increasing the weight of the load for bouts of ten contractions each, until the maximum load which can be lifted ten times is reached.

For each exercise, five days per week, the patient performs bouts of ten contractions. These begin at ten per cent of the 10 R.M. and increase by deciles to the final ten repetition maximum. A brief rest period of about two to four minutes is permitted between bouts. The ability to exceed 10 R.M. is tested each week to assess gains made in muscle strength and to establish a new 10 R.M. for the following week.

One modification of these exercises involves beginning with the ten-repetition bout at fifty per cent of the 10 R.M. and progressively increasing this by quartiles until the 10 R.M. is reached. A second modification of the basic procedure has the patient begin with a ten-repetition bout at twenty-five per cent of the 10 R.M. and progress by quartiles until the 10 R.M. is achieved. A third modification begins the patient at a five-repetition bout at fifty per cent of the 10 R.M. and then proceeds to a ten-repetition bout at one hundred per cent of the 10 R.M.

PROGRESSIVE ASSISTIVE EXERCISE. In cases where the affected muscles cannot raise the body part against the force of gravity, progressive loading is used, with gravity either eliminated entirely or counterbalanced.

Exercises performed horizontally can be carried out against progressive resistance if the extremity is suspended or supported on a skate board or powder board, a small, wooden board covered with powder so as to make movement on it less difficult and less abrasive.

Exercises can be performed in the vertical position by counterbalancing the weight of the body part with a pulley system and gradually increasing the resistance to the muscular contractions by decreasing the counter-balancing weight. The general principle of increasing the resistance against which the muscle must contract in successive bouts of exercising is the same as for progressive resistive exercises.

REGRESSIVE RESISTIVE EXERCISE. The initial step is the determination of the 10 R.M. Then, for each exercise, five days per week, the patient performs bouts of ten contractions each, beginning at one hundred per cent of the 10 R.M. and decreasing the number by deciles to a final bout of ten per cent of the 10 R.M. Strength is tested weekly, beyond the 10 R.M., so as to determine the maximal load for the next week. In this procedure resistance is decreased as the patient fatigues. Thus, muscles perform maximal work for the entire exercise session.

A modification of the above procedure involves having the patient begin with a ten-repetition bout at one hundred per cent of the 10 R.M. and then decrease the percentage of R.M. by quartiles.

BRIEF MAXIMAL EXERCISE. The first step consists of establishing the maximal load that can be raised from the dependent position to the anti-gravity position and held for five seconds. This is done progressively and on each succeeding day a standard increment is added to the weight of the previous day. One successful lift constitutes the exercise for the involved muscle group for that day.

Should the patient be unable to lift the scheduled weight for five seconds, he is retested again after a four-minute rest period with the weight minus one increment. If he is still not able to raise the weight this is repeated, but even if he fails at minus two increments, that weight is maintained as the exercise load for the day. On the following day the patient is exercised with either one increment added or one increment subtracted, depending upon whether or not he was successful on the previous day. The standard weight increment varies for particular muscle groups from 0.625 pounds for the shoulder abductors to 2.5 pounds for the ankle plantar flexors.

BRIEF MAXIMAL ISOMETRIC EXERCISE. In this form of muscle exer-

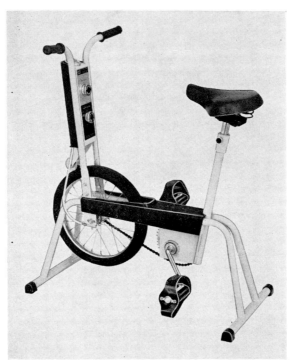

FIGURE 12. A bicycle exerciser. *(Reprinted by permission of J. A. Preston Corp., 1971)*

cise the patient contracts a given muscle against a fixed resistance and maintains the contraction for five seconds. The force he exerts is monitored by some type of isometric tension gauge, such as a cable tensiometer, which measures the amount of tension in the effort, or a strain gauge, which measures the force by means of changes in the electrical resistance of a wire loop as it is bent.

Increasing Endurance

Endurance exercises are of the low resistance-high repetition type. A muscle performs them many, even hundreds of times per day, which results in fatigue of the muscle at the end of the exercise period. The load on the muscle is set between fifteen and forty per cent of maximal strength so that the patient can perform many repetitions of the exercise, and the cardiovascular system can be stimulated to respond before the activity is terminated by fatigue. Endurance will not develop unless some fatigue is produced by the exercises. Great endurance is the consequence of marked fatigue.

Weight lifting or pulley exercises can be used as endurance tasks. The muscles are loaded so that fatigue begins to set in after about twenty or thirty repetitions or contractions. Whenever it is possible, multiple muscles are exercised in the same endurance activity. Thus, rowing or bicycling is ideal. Stair climbing is useful for increasing the endurance of the lower extremities as well as of the cardiovascular system, barring medical contraindications.

To avoid boredom and loss of motivation for the activity the exercises are made as interesting as possible. Thus, some craft work or competitive group activities are often integrated into the program.

Developing Coordination

Coordination is developed through constant repetition of a precisely performed pattern of activity, producing an integration of sensory stimuli with the motor behavior. Training in coordination is conducted at a rate which is slow enough for the patient to become aware of the sensations which are related to the various components of the acts. As the therapeutic activity is repeated exactly many times, a habit pattern is formed which then enables the activity to be performed with less effort. Less attention to the act is required, and the spread of excitation to neurons external to the activity pattern becomes decreased. Eventually, the activity is performed with little cerebral perception of its individual components. It is then termed *automatic.*

Coordination training is begun by using simple patterns and then proceeds to those of greater complexity. Resisance given against an involved muscle is slight in relation to the strength of the muscle. Increasing muscle strength and endurance can contribute to improved coordination.

Frenkel's exercises are a series of exercises of progressive difficulty which are designed to improve proprioceptive control in the lower extremities. They begin with simple motions with gravity eliminated, and gradually progress to complex movements utilizing simultaneous hip and knee motions against the pull of gravity. Initially, the emphasis is placed on slow, precise movement and positioning. Each exercise is performed only about four times per therapy session to avoid fatigue. As the patient gains the ability to do each exercise he is instructed to practice it every three or four hours.

Frenkel's series of exercises are conducted while the patient is lying supinely on a plinth, while he is sitting and while he is standing.

In the supine position they consist of the patient flexing his hip and knee and abducting and adducting his leg to various degrees. They are carried out first unilaterally and then bilaterally and reciprocally. Some examples are as follows: the patient flexes the hip and knee of one extremity, sliding the heel along in contact with the plinth, returns to the original position and then repeats the task with the contralateral extremity; the patient flexes the hip and knee only halfway, returns to the original position and adds abduction and adduction; the patient flexes both lower extremities simultaneously and equally, and adds abduction, adduction and extension; the patient flexes one extremity at the hip and knee with the heel held two inches above the table, and returns to the original position; the patient flexes the hip and knee with the heel held two inches off the plinth, places the heel on the opposite patella, and slides it down the crest of the tibia to the ankle and down the crest of the opposite tibia, over the ankle to the foot and toes; the patient reciprocally flexes and extends the lower extremities, both with the heels touching the plinth and with the heels held two inches above the plinth, and follows the movements of the therapist's fingers with his toes.

Exercises performed while the patient is seated can include the following: practice maintaining correct sitting posture for two minutes in a chair that has arms and back support and in a chair which lacks these supports; marking time to the therapist's count by raising only the heel of the foot off the floor; alternately gliding the feet over a chalk cross-mark on the floor in all planes of the cross; practice rising from and sitting down on a chair in time with the therapist's cadence count.

Some examples of standing exercises are as follows: walking sideways to a counted cadence; walking forward between parallel lines on the floor with emphasis on correct foot placement; walking on footprints traced on the floor, practiced in quarter-steps, half-steps, three-quarter-steps and full steps; turning exercises.

Maintaining and Increasing Range of Motion

MAINTENANCE. Twice daily all joints are carried through their entire range of motion three times. If the patient is very weak or experiences much pain, assistance is given. Joints are moved gently and slowly, and as the patient improves the range is gradually increased, leading to active-assistive and then active exercises.

IMPROVEMENT. The main technique for increasing range of motion is stretching. A tight muscle can be vigorously stretched unless there is inflammation present. With patients who have poliomyelitis or Guillain-Barré syndrome, stretching is carried out past the point of pain, but there should be no residual pain after completion of the exercise.

When joints are tight, stretching is done less vigorously. The motion employed is slow and gentle with the patient relaxed, and

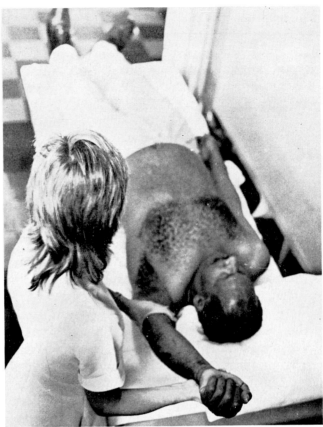

FIGURE 13. A range of motion exercise. The therapist is performing passive shoulder flexion on the patient.

it stops short of the point which causes joint pain. Prolonged, moderate stretching is more effective than brief, vigorous stretching.

Some examples follow of exercises for increasing the range of motion in certain joints.

To increase range of motion in the hip flexors, the patient lies in pronation and is strapped to a board the width of the pelvis by a strap at the level of the ischial tuberosities. A sling under the distal end of the thigh is attached by a rope through overhead pulleys to a weight which provides a constant tension. A stretching weight of from twenty to forty pounds is added to the weight to counterbalance the lower extremity. One hip is stretched at a time because it is impossible to immobilize the pelvis adequately enough to stretch both hip flexors simultaneously. The contralateral knee and hip are flexed and the leg is supported on a chair or cushion of appropriate height. This stretch is maintained for twenty minutes each day.

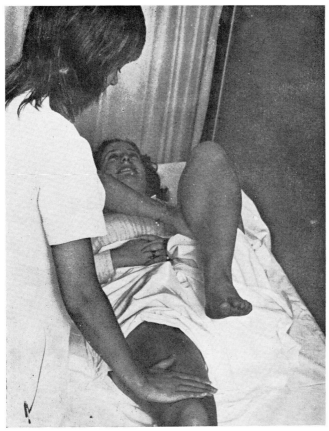

FIGURE 14. Stretching of the hip flexor muscles.

Knee flexion contractures are stretched with the patient lying in a prone position on a firm surface with a pad of some type placed under the knee and the leg extending without support. A sandbag, or a weight of from five to fifteen pounds, is placed across the heel for approximately twenty minutes. Alternatively, the patient sits with the knee extended, the heel supported at seat level, and the thigh and leg unsupported while a sandbag of from fifteen to twenty pounds is placed across the knee for twenty minutes.

To stretch the triceps surae muscle, the patient sits on an Elgin exercise table, or DeLorme table, to which an exercise boot with a toe extension can be attached. (Note: This is a padded, adjustable, center-break table with a pulley housing at one end through which several cables are threaded. Weights of gradual increments are placed on a pan attached to the cable which passes over a pulley.) The foot is strapped to the exercise boot, and ten to thirty pounds of tension is exerted at the end of the toe extension bar for twenty minutes.

Alternatively, to dorsiflex the ankle, the patient stands at arm's length from a wall with his feet on a wedge-shaped board which elevates the front of the foot twenty degrees. He leans forward against the wall for a period of from one to five minutes, three to five times per day. The same stretch can be accomplished by placing the patient on a tilt table, or standing table. (Note: The tilt table is a treatment table having either manually operated or motor-driven mechanisms which permit changing the pitch of the surface. A footboard at one end allows the patient to bear weight as the table is brought head-upward toward a right angle with the floor. Wide belts or straps secure the patient firmly to the table.)

Neuromuscular Re-Education

Neuromuscular re-education is aimed at developing or recovering voluntary control of skeletal musculature. It consists of training or retraining the patient to use muscles, first in executing simple, and later, complex motor acts. Through proper exercise, abilities which have been lost through disease or injury may be regained. Re-education is begun as soon as the clinical course of the pathologic condition permits.

Two principles which are adhered to in muscle re-education are these: (1) the more difficult the exercise is to perform, the more the patient must concentrate on the act; and (2) the harder a muscle contracts, the greater is the proprioceptive response.

If a patient is unable to voluntarily contract a portion of a muscle, a single muscle or a group of muscles, the re-education program must begin by applying certain techniques which will activate these lower motor units. Such stimulation may be arbitrarily and roughly divided into two groups, focusing procedures and proprioceptive stimulation.

Focusing Procedures

At first, the patient is informed regarding the location of the muscle to be controlled and the results of contraction. Demonstrations are given as the patient must be clear as to what is being done and what is expected of him during these procedures.

Passive motion attempts to activate the lower motor unit. The patient is instructed not to assist or resist the movements carried out by the therapist. These movements may be simple one-joint, one-plane excursions, or multiple joint movements in single or multiple planes.

Passive motion is designed to make the patient aware of desired movements by feeling and seeing them as they are carried out. These

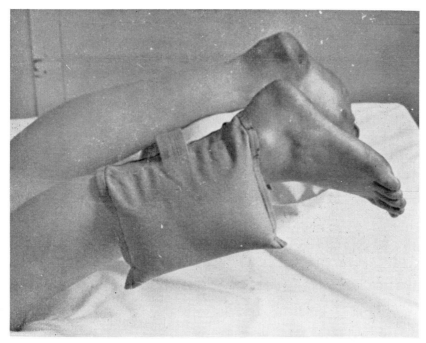

FIGURE 15. Using sandbags to stretch a knee flexion contracture.

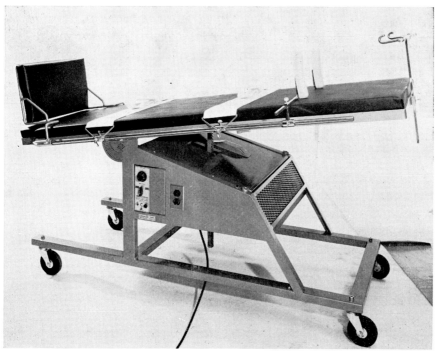

FIGURE 16. Variable speed electric tilt table. (*Courtesy of La Berne Manufacturing Co., Inc.*)

movements also stimulate proprioceptive reflexes of flexion, extension and stabilization.

The arc and the speed of movement must continually be altered by the therapist until the desired results are either achieved or proven to be impossible to attain.

Passive motion usually begins with movement of a single joint through an accustomed range, within limits set by pain and contractures, and proceeds to multiple joints and multiple planes.

Cutaneous stimulation is designed to assist the patient in concentrating upon the areas of treatment so that he can better see and feel contractions in specific muscles. The therapist can use her fingers to stroke or tap the muscle or tendon, or she may use a brush, ice, or a rubber hammer. Basic massage methods are also useful in producing adequate stimulation.

Electrical stimulation may aid the patient in seeing and feeling muscular contractions by causing contractions in muscles. The unpleasant sensations resulting from electricity may be of some value in sensory reflex stimulation. Proprioceptive stimulation is provided by the tension produced by proper muscular contraction with electricity.

Electromyographic apparatus which has both visual and auditory output can be employed to assist the patient in gaining awareness of contractions of skeletal muscles. Since contractions can often be too slight to be detected by the therapist's palpations and observations, the electromyograph will be useful for such cases. Attempts by the patient to increase the sound or the heights of the changes in electrical potential can aid him in focusing on the desired muscles.

Proprioceptive Stimulation

This activation methodology is designed to stimulate skeletal muscles to contract through excitation of proprioceptive receptors in the musculoskeletal system. These receptors can be stimulated by passive motion and by positioning body segments in a variety of postural positions. Any position in which a body segment attempts to support itself by the stabilizing tension of muscle—e.g., balancing in sitting, crawling, kneeling and standing position—will induce proprioceptive stimulation.

Stretching-and-resistance is useful since muscle tissue responds best when it is extended or put under some tension. Muscles must be made to contract against resistance when partially elongated. Active responding is also facilitated by sudden stretching of muscles or sudden release of tension.

Reflex stimulation can be used to initiate muscle contraction if the reflexes can be consistently elicited. If the muscle responds to reflex action, this response may be useful as a focusing and facilitating mechanism to assist the patient's own voluntary efforts.

Once the patient has become aware, through a program of activation exercises, of the muscles of his body and their functions, and has learned to voluntarily control them, the re-education program shifts in its emphasis to tasks which develop strength, endurance and coordination. The former two have previously been discussed.

Coordination is the ability to employ the appropriate muscles at the correct time and with the correct intensity to best achieve desired movement. Coordinate patterns of movement are those with which the normal musculoskeletal and neuromuscular system can function most efficiently and with the greatest safety. Coordination is achieved through reflex training. Most of the components of coordinated movement take place without the awareness of the individual and without voluntary control. The therapist sets up patterns of movement which are normal and which will lead to successful accomplishment of the desired act. The patient performs these patterns while the therapist attempts to analyze movements and change patterns as faults are observed.

It is to be remembered that all muscle re-education programs are based upon the premise that the balance and strength sufficient for functioning will eventually be regained. Thus, the therapist must be alert to any substitution patterns since these can become permanently ingrained habits unless corrected, and can limit the best utilization of muscles which may later regain strength.

In summary, proprioceptive neuromuscular facilitation means promoting or hastening the responses of the neuromuscular mechanism by means of methods which stimulate the proprioceptors. (Note: *Facilitation* specifically means the effect produced in nerve tissue by the passage of an impulse. The term *proprioceptive* refers to stimulation received within body tissue.) The techniques are related to the normal responses of the neuromuscular system. The physical therapist places certain demands on the system which have a facilitating or therapeutic effect, thereby reversing the patient's limitations.

AMBULATION TRAINING

Walking must be preceded by training in proper standing and balance. Early ambulation training is usually begun by having the patient walk between upright parallel bars while holding onto the railings. This develops security in stance, shifting of weight, and perception of balance. If a patient is severely disabled, a tilt table can be employed to attain the upright position initially, and provide

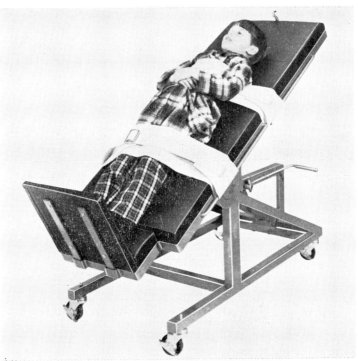

FIGURE 17. Patient on a child size tilt table. (*Reprinted by permission of J. A. Preston Corp., 1971*)

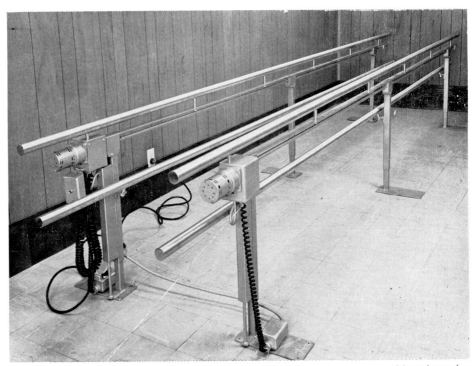

FIGURE 18. Electrically operated parallel bars. (*Courtesy of La Berne Manufacturing Co., Inc.*)

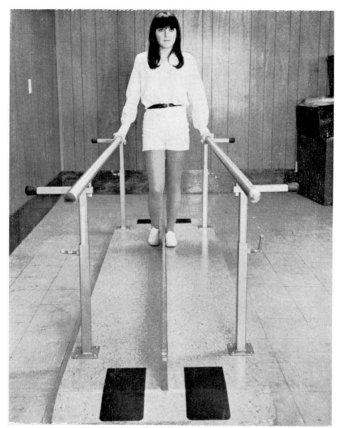

FIGURE 19. Platform mounted parallel bars. (*Courtesy of La Berne Manufacturing Co., Inc.*) The bars are adjustable in height.

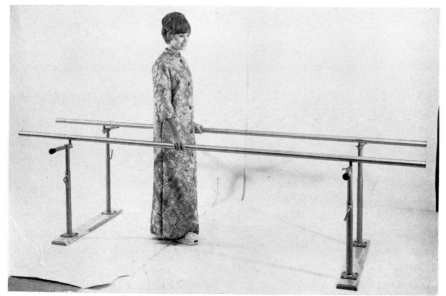

FIGURE 20. Folding parallel bars. (*Courtesy of La Berne Manufacturing Co., Inc.*)

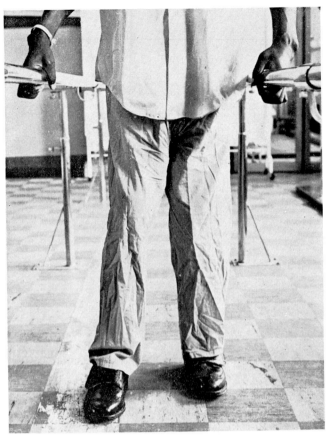

FIGURE 21. A patient demonstrating the four point position while ambulating in the parallel bars.

security while he is strapped in this posture. Then, as stability of the trunk develops, transfer can be made to the parallel bars.

Prior to actual ambulation, drills are given which develop good balance. These include removing one hand at a time from the railing, balancing with one hand, shifting weight from one leg to the other, shifting backward and forward, unlocking and locking the knees, raising one foot and replacing it, and forward and backward placement of the feet.

Should the use of crutches be anticipated for a patient, crutches may be substituted for the parallel bars once balancing techniques are mastered. Patients who use prostheses, braces, walkers, walkerettes or canes are taught the proper management of these devices and are taught to ambulate with them if their use is anticipated in the future. The final chapter of this section deals with this aspect of ambulation in detail.

Chapter 7

TREATMENT MODALITIES

IN ADDITION TO THERAPEUTIC EXERCISE, the physical therapist possesses a large and varied armamentarium of techniques which are employed to bring about improvement of a patient's function.

THERAPEUTIC HEAT AND COLD

The skin is possessed of great adaptability in order to furnish protection for the body against the external environment. This adaptability is a result of the skin's physical and chemical composition and its physiologic activities. These variables can be altered by regulatory mechanisms within the skin and within the interior of the body. The blood vessels of the skin are a reservoir which is capable of holding one quarter of the total blood volume which markedly increases or decreases in accord with local and general needs. The automatic nervous system transmits the impulses which regulate changes in blood volume. Changes are also produced by the action of nerves and nerve endings, lymph channels, sebaceous and sweat glands, and metabolic responses such as pigment formation and Vitamin D production. The skin also possesses a far greater specific reacting capacity for antigen than does muscle, plasma or the brain. These and other changes which occur in the skin are important for an understanding of the therapeutic value of physical methods whose influence is totally or primarily limited to the integument, or skin.

There is a great deal of variation in the temperature of different areas of the body. Therapeutic effectiveness of conductive heating may be a consequence of protective physiological responses of the body, either as a mechanism for avoiding thermal damage at the surface, or as reflexive adjustments required for the maintenance of thermal homeostasis. In a cold environment the temperature of an extremity decreases. The direct local action of cold upon the blood vessels produces immediate vasoconstriction of the minute vessels of the skin which then may be followed, after a brief period, by vasodilation. This cyclic phenomenon is most marked in the digits. In a warm environment the temperature level of the skin rises to that of the skin surface of the torso, and the entire skin surface temperature may continue to increase. When the surrounding temperature is higher than that of the body heat loss by conduction ceases and further heat loss occurs through perspiring and consequent evaporation of perspiration from the surface of the body.

Wider variations in temperature can be tolerated by localized portions of the body than by the body as a whole. The limits for several hours appear to be 110 degrees F. (Fahrenheit) and 40 degrees F., with considerably higher temperatures tolerated for shorter periods. Therapeutic applications of hot packs or melted paraffin can be applied at temperatures far higher than other modalities, such as water baths or electric pads, which are maintained at constant temperatures. Thus, repeated applications of hot packs of high temperatures may induce reflex responses more effectively than prolonged, continuous heating at a lower temperature.

Through conductive transfer of heat, changes in body surface temperature produce changes in the thermal gradient extending from the skin to deeper structures within the body. These changes are modified by vascular reflexes which increase or decrease arterial blood flow to the surface and subcutaneous tissue. As external conditions approach the extremes of hot and cold, the difference between skin and external temperatures becomes greater. Although the skin can be cooled or heated externally, it is simultaneously being cooled or heated by the blood circulating within the body. Local application of cold results in an intense initial vasoconstriction of the small vessels of the skin and subpapillary vessels. The application of heat, on the other hand, produces an active hyperemia, or increased amount of blood in the part as a result of increased afflux of arterial blood in the dilated capillaries at the skin surface, and this serves as a cooling mechanism by means of which the venous blood returning from the surface is warmed and transfers heat to other areas.

Reflex actions occur within the structures beneath the surface when heat or cold is applied at the surface. The benefits of localized thermal stimulation of an inflamed joint or of a local cutaneous area of irritation depend upon the reflexive vasodilation which is produced. Temperature changes also affect vasomotor tone. The cyclic variations which occur in normal individuals at normal environmental temperatures are abolished by extremes of temperature which produce vasodilation or vasoconstriction. There is, furthermore, marked increase in blood flow with temperature elevation for a period of approximately sixty minutes, after which there is a decrease in blood flow. Capillary pressure also rises with an increase in heat at the skin, and local application of cold acts as a pressor stimulus resulting in increase of both systolic and diastolic blood pressure.

A fall in environmental temperature will result in a fall in metabolism. The metabolism of tissue is increased by heat. In addition, the effect of direct heat is an increase in the tone of the endothelial vessels which line serous cavities, blood vessels and lymphatics, while direct cold will decrease the tone of these minute vessels.

In summary, applications of cold and heat produce a wide variety of physiological effects on the body. Of the two, heat is most frequently employed in physical therapy. When heat is externally applied it produces an increase in tissue temperature, vasodilation, and an increase in circulation. The rise in the temperature of the tissue increases metabolic activity, adding to increased temperature and further vasodilation. Some heat is conducted to underlying tissues. Excessive local heat is controlled by blood flow to other areas of the body. As sweat glands are stimulated moisture appears on the skin, the evaporation of which produces cooling. Local heating of an area of inflammation results in an increase in phagocytosis, or cellular ingestion and digestion. If the general temperature of the body is significantly elevated for some hours there is a marked rise in the leukocyte, or white blood cell count.

Techniques of Application in Thermal Therapy

There are three classes of therapeutic application of heat. *Conductive heating* is achieved by direct application of heat in the form of heated or moist air, heated water, heated paraffin, or electrically heated pads. *Radiant heating* involves the use of the infrared and ultraviolet portions of the electromagnetic spectrum. Short wavelengths range from 7,700 Angstroms to 14,000 Angstroms (one millimicron to ten millimicrons), and long wavelengths vary between 14,000 Angstroms and 120,000 Angstroms (ten millimicrons to one millimeter). *Conversive heating* is an indirect type of heating which results from the conversion of various forms of primary energy into heat in the body tissues. This is medical diathermy.

The present section will be concerned with conductive heating while the other forms of therapeutic heat will be discussed in subsequent sections.

Conductive Heating

THE ELECTRIC HEATING PAD. This device maintains a constant temperature during usage. Most electric heating pads have three grades of heat—low, medium and high. Caution must be taken to guard against burns, particularly if the patient lies on the pad rather than under it.

THE HOT-WATER BOTTLE. The hot-water bottle can deliver about thirty thousand gm-cal. to its environment by the time heat transfer to the patient ceases. Much caution is required because water which is too hot can cause serious skin damage. A hot-water bottle of 118 degrees F. can be tolerated next to the skin for several minutes, but at this temperature only about one-half of a thirteen thousand gm-cal. heat delivery will go to the patient.

There is a special type of hot-water bag known as the "Elliot" which is designed for use in body cavities. A heater and thermostat maintain the water at a constant temperature while a pump circulates it through the apparatus maintaining a pressure of two pounds per square inch. The pressure distends the bag which acts as the applicator, permitting good contact with the heated surface.

Chemically heated bags are also available in special forms, depending upon the body area to which they are applied.

Therapeutic heating bags can also be filled with hot salt or hot sand.

HOT PACKS. There are two main types of hot packs which are widely utilized today. The *moist hot pack* provides little heat because, as the water which gives heat evaporates, less and less heat is delivered and for an increasingly shorter time. A wet towel is most frequently employed. The *Kenny wool pack* is usually steam heated and then spun dry. It typically has an inner hot pack covered by a layer of waterproof plastic and an outer layer of insulating wool. There is little danger from burns. A hot wool pack can have a temperature as high as 140° F. at application but this falls rapidly to about 40 degrees F. within a few minutes. It is most effective in the relief of tenderness and muscle spasm. Usually, a series of three or four packs of this intense heat is left on the part for five or ten minutes each.

A third form of hot pack is the *hydrocollator pack,* which retains heat for a longer time. Hydrocollator packs are canvas-enclosed packs of silica gel which come in several sizes. They are heated in water to approximately 140° F. to 160° F. and are applied to the skin with several layers of toweling as insulation. They are valuable for the relief of muscle spasm and pain, and also aid in the absorption of inflammatory products, produce sedation and relaxation, and increase perspiration. Because of their weight, extreme tenderness and the possibility of ischemia often preclude their use.

PARAFFIN. The typical paraffin mixture used for therapy consists of about one part mineral oil to seven parts paraffin. The melting point of the wax is then approximately 126° F.

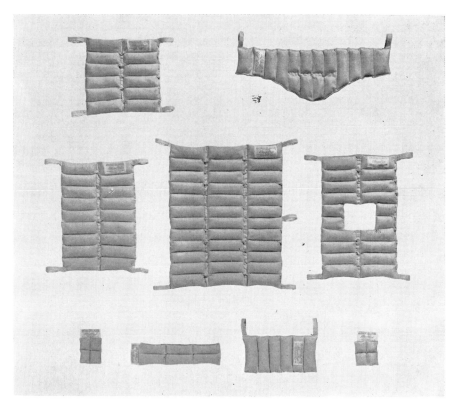

FIGURE 22. Hydrocollator® steam packs. Pictured above, from left to right, are: Top-Standard size steam pack, neck contour steam pack; Center-spinal size steam pack, over-size steam pack, knee-shoulder steam pack; Bottom-eye size steam pack, OB size steam pack, half size steam pack, eye pack. (*Courtesy of Chattanooga Pharmacal Co.*)

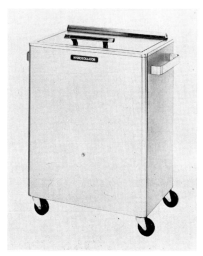

FIGURE 23. Hydrocollator® master heating unit. (*Courtesy of Chattanooga Pharmacal Co.*)

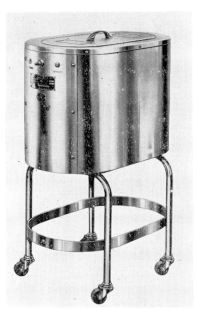

FIGURE 24. Mobile hand, wrist, elbow, foot and ankle paraffin bath. (*Courtesy of Ille Electric Corp.*)

The part to which the melted paraffin is to be applied is washed and dried. The paraffin can then be applied either by brush or by dipping the body part into the wax. The initial sensation may be hot but as an insulating layer of wax is formed the sensation of heat is greatly diminished. After several applications a thick coating forms on the part and the part can then be left in the paraffin bath or removed, with the coating remaining on for about fifteen to thirty minutes. Paraffin baths are most often used for the hands and feet while paraffin packs, which are brushed on, have a wider application.

Heat is transferred from the paraffin to the skin mainly by conduction. Following removal of the paraffin the body part will be red, soft and moist, and easily manipulable and well suited for massage.

Paraffin is an excellent method for providing heat in cases of arthritis, bursitis, fibrositis, tenosynovitis, stiff joints following fractures, weakness or stiffness following nerve injury, and scar tissue which limits range of motion. It should not be placed on open surfaces nor used with aged and debilitated patients, nor where a patient has little ability to tolerate heat.

The term *hydrotherapy* refers to the external application of water in the treatment of disorder. Water is an excellent medium for conductive heating and cooling in that it readily absorbs and gives off heat. In addition, the buoyancy of the water provides gentle support without hindering movement to an appreciable extent. Thus, movement can be performed more effortlessly in water than in air. Water is also versatile, as it can be applied to specific areas of the body or can be used to heat or cool the entire body.

Partial Immersion Baths

THE WHIRLPOOL BATH. This bath is given in a metal tub filled with water which is kept in constant agitation. It thus provides both water temperature control plus the mechanical effects of water in motion.

The water is kept in agitation by an ejector, a turbine or compressed air. The bath provides heat, gentle massage, debridement (the excision of contused and devitalized tissue from the surface of the wound), relief from pain and muscle relaxation. It also permits active or assistive exercise of the part which is immersed in the tub.

The tub's temperature is maintained constant by a thermostat. Typical temperature settings are 90 to 100° F. for the entire body, 100 to 102° F. for the legs, and 105° F. for the upper extremities. Often, 110° F. to 115° F. are used for therapeutic effects. When the patient has impaired circulation, temperature should not exceed 105° F. Treatment usually is of twenty minutes' duration.

Whirlpool baths are employed in the treatment of chronic traumatic disorders, inflammatory conditions, joint stiffness, pain, adhesions, neuritis, tenosynovitis, sprains, strains and painful stumps following amputations. Adding a small amount of sodium sulfathiazole to the water hastens the healing of infections. The bath may be used preceding, or instead of massage or other mechanical applications to injured extremities.

THE CONTRAST BATH. Contrast baths involve sudden, alternate immersions of upper or lower extremities in hot and then cold water. They increase circulation because of the contraction and relaxation of the blood vessels as a result of the alternating temperature extremes. One bath container is filled with water at a temperature of 100 to 110 degrees F., and the other holds water of 50 to 65 degrees F.

The body part being treated is immersed in the baths in a definite, systematic manner. While authorities differ slightly on the actual length of time a limb should be immersed in each tub, there is still fair general agreement. A typical contact sequence might be as follows:

> hot for four to ten minutes, cold for one to two minutes;
> hot for four minutes, cold for one minute;
> hot for four minutes, cold for one minute;

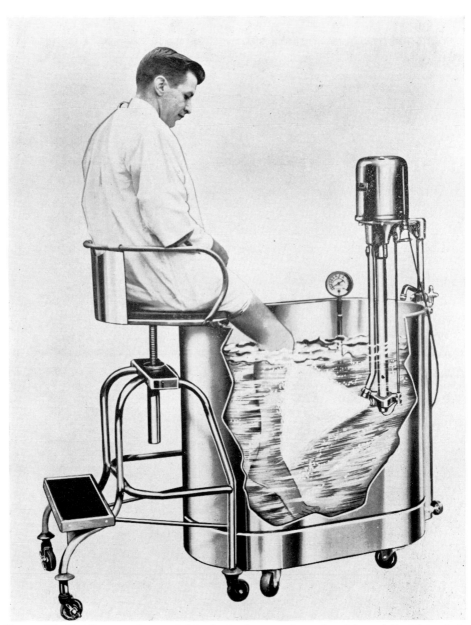

FIGURE 25. Mobile arm, leg and hip hydrotherapeutic tank with mobile high chair. (*Courtesy of Ille Electric Corp.*)

hot for four minutes, cold for one minute;
hot for five minutes.
Treatment always begins and ends with immersion in hot water.

Contrast baths are therapeutically effective for headaches, arthritis, fractures, peripheral vascular disease, and as a precedent to massage and exercise in cases of sprains and contusions. When treating patients with peripheral vascular disease, care must be taken to avoid great extremes of temperature.

In addition to the above there are a variety of other partial immersion or localized baths. These are as follows: the *hot full wet pack,* in which the patient is wrapped from neck to feet in a sheet which has been immersed in water of about 80 to 90° F. and wrung out; *cold, hot or neutral baths for the extremities,* which vary by temperature; *douches and showers,* in which streams of water at controlled pressure and temperature are directed at the surface of the body; *ablutions,* or sponge baths; *leg, foot, arm* and *hand baths,* which require immersion of the involved body part in small baths of controlled temperature; *half-baths,* in which the patient sits, the water level being at about the level of the navel: *affusions,* where the water is poured on the patient from a basin or a pitcher at approximately 60 to 80 degrees F. of temperature; *sitz baths,* in which the torso but not the extremities is immersed in water; *Hauffe baths,* which provide a constantly increasing water temperature; and a number of other kinds. The particular form of bath employed depends upon the disorder being treated, the body part or parts involved, the patient's physical condition, and the purposes of the hydrotherapy.

Full Immersion Baths

THE HUBBARD TANK. The Hubbard tank is a full-body therapeutic pool with a water temperature of 98 to 104 degrees F. The water is usually agitated and aerated, providing both heat and gentle massage. The patient lies on a canvas plinth and is lifted to and from the pool by means of electrically-driven overhead cranes. Some tanks have a grating on the floor which permits the able patient to stand. Partial weight-bearing and ambulation can be initiated in the pool which may be prescribed when gait exercises are indicated, but the stress of weight is contraindicated.

The Hubbard tank is useful where the patient's disease or disability is manifest in many joints, such as in chronic arthritis or in burn cases when débridement and active exercise are desirable.

EXERCISE IN WATER. Water exercises are performed in a pool large

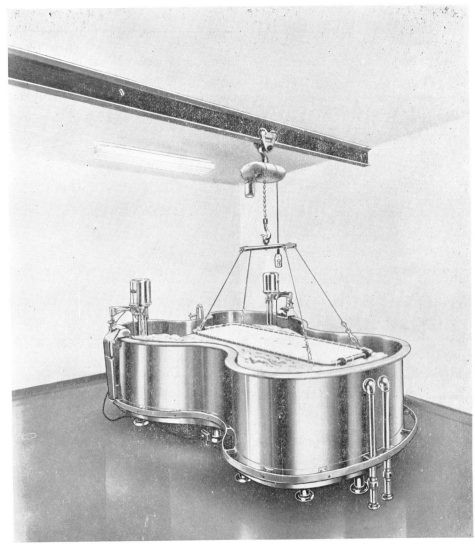

FIGURE 26. Full body immersion hydrotherapy tank unit, commonly referred to as the Hubbard tank. (*Courtesy of Ille Electric Corp.*)

enough to permit abduction of the extremities. Temperature is thermostatically maintained at a neutral level. The pool often has an indented center portion so that the therapists can easily approach the patient. Patients are transferred in and out of the pool as they are with the Hubbard tank. The advantage of the pool is that it permits freer motion of the extremities due to the buoyancy of the fluid medium.

Exercise in water is indicated for the following conditions: spastic paralysis, as in paraplegia; marked muscle weakness with the possibility

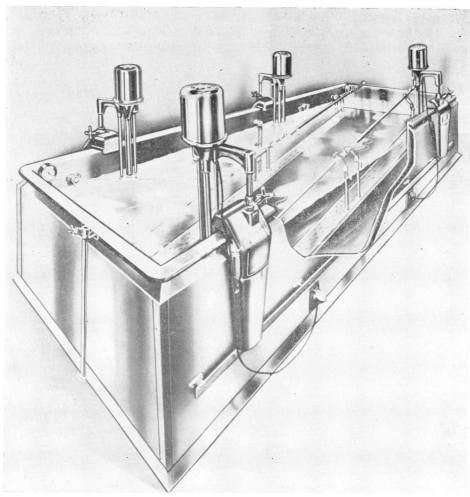

FIGURE 27. Therapeutic tank and pool. (*Courtesy of Ile Electric Corp.*)

of increasing strength through voluntary motion, such as in partial
peripheral nerve lesions, e.g. polyneuritis; poliomyelitis; following amputation when muscle strengthening and stretching of contractures in
the involved extremity are indicated; chronic arthritis; following joint
injuries; for mobilization in the aftercare of plastic and joint operations
and tendon transplants; after abdominal fascial transplants; in certain
cases of cerebral palsy; extensive skin burns; muscular incoordination;
some neurologic disorders; and disorders requiring metabolic stimulation.

Water activities are contraindicated for cases of acute joint inflammation or other acute infections, febrile disease, acute neuritis, active
pulmonary tuberculosis, and acute stages of poliomyelitis.

Other types of full immersion hot baths include: *full-body hot baths,* with water temperature at 96 to 105 degrees F., used for brief periods of time in treating chronic, rheumatic joint manifestations, and for the relief of muscle spasm and colic; *chemical baths,* usually involving the introduction of carbon dioxide gas into the water for therapy with patients suffering from chronic heart disease; *oxygen baths,* which pump oxygen into water of about 90 to 95 degrees F. used for hypertensive and advanced cardiac disease cases; *brine* or *salt baths,* using sodium chloride, primarily for treatment in cases of osteomyelitis, fractures, dislocations, arthritis, myositis, fibrositosis, gout and chronic sciatica; *foam baths;* and *sponge baths.*

The Therapeutic Use of Cold

COLD BATHS. Cold baths are used following acute injury as a means of reducing pain and swelling through the vascular constriction and analgesic effects of cold. Local cold applications are effective in reducing spasticity in multiple sclerosis, reducing the knee-jerk reflex in hemiplegia (although effects do not last beyond the treatment period), as a metabolic stimulant and for atonic states. The temperature varies from 50 to 70 degrees F. and the bath is used for short periods of time, accompanied by vigorous rubbing of the patient's body by the therapist.

COOL BATHS. The cool bath may be used for longer periods of time at a water temperature of about 70 to 90 degrees F. A *cool ablution* of 70 to 85 degrees F. is useful for reducing temperature in acute febrile disease, for neuritis, arthritis and functional nerve disorders.

COLD COMPRESSES. Compresses are usually made of several thicknesses of linen, gauze or towels. They are immersed in water of from 60 to 65 degrees F., wrung out and applied locally.

Cold applied to the region of the precordium, or in front of the heart, is valuable in the treatment of functional arrhythmias, tachycardia and cardiac decompensation.

DOUCHES. A douche can be cold as well as hot or warm. The cold douche varies from 50 to 80 degrees F. It is applied briefly, for from five to thirty seconds, with a pressure of from five to thirty pounds.

The *Scotch* douche alternates cold water with hot water.

Radiant Heating

One of the oldest and most frequently employed uses of heat is that derived from radiation. Man has utilized the effects of solar radiation for centuries, deriving benefit from its ultraviolet, visible and infrared energies.

When an object such as a piece of metal is heated to beyond 5400

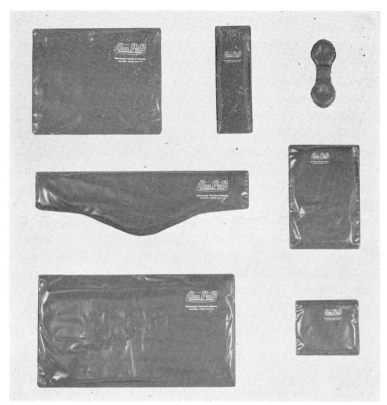

FIGURE 28. Cold packs. Shown above, from left to right, are: Top-standard cold pack, throat pack, eye size cold pack; Center-neck contour cold pack, half size cold pack; Bottom-oversize cold pack, quarter size cold pack. (*Courtesy of Chattanooga Pharmacal Co.*)

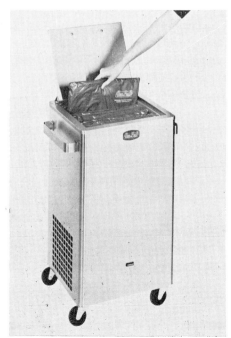

FIGURE 29. Hydrocollator® master chilling unit. (*Courtesy of Chattanooga Pharmacal Co.*)

degrees F., wavelengths are produced of from .39 to .18 microns which are too short to be perceived by the naked human eye. These are termed "ultraviolet" because they lie beyond the violet end of the electromagnetic spectrum. They were first discovered by Ritter in 1801 when he noted the changes which they produced on silver chloride.

In 1800 Herschel discovered that radiations whose wavelengths were longer than those which could be seen by the human eye, caused an elevation of temperature which could be registered on a thermometer. As these rays lie beyond the red end of the spectrum, they are called "infrared."

Today, we are aware of the therapeutic properties of both ultraviolet and infrared radiation and they are in wide use for the treatment of a variety of medical and physical conditions.

Infrared Radiation Therapy

PENETRATION AND PHYSIOLOGIC EFFECTS. There is some disagreement as to the penetration depth of infrared energy. Until recently it was believed that near infrared energy penetrated tissues to a greater depth than did far infrared energy. Recent studies have demonstrated that both near and far infrared rays penetrate tissue to the same extent. Many authorities, however, still maintain that near infrared energy penetrates to a depth of about three millimeters and far infrared rays penetrate to a depth of about one millimeter. Definite conclusions have not been reached.

Infrared energy seems to produce some photochemical reactions, as the skin pigment will become mottled after prolonged exposure, but the mechanisms of these changes are unclear.

Vasodilation of the vessels of the skin and subcutaneous tissues also occurs, but the cause of this is not fully understood. Heating of localized body areas does not produce a change in pulse rate, nor in arterial blood pressure, although some elevation of venous pressure has been found by investigators. Local heating does not affect rate or depth of respiration, renal plasma flow, or glomerular filtration. Sweating is increased, and tissues become receptive to massage and to active or passive motion.

In small doses, infrared rays cause an analgesia of the skin while greater intensities produce marked counterirritation.

APPARATUS. There are two types of infrared units which are ordinarily used for therapy—luminous and nonluminous.

LUMINOUS RADIATION is emitted from lamps which are heated to incandescence or to a lesser degree by means of electric current. The bulbs may vary from a few to 150 watts input, and are made of glass,

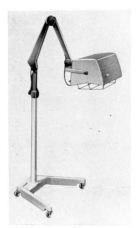

FIGURE 30. An infrared lamp. *(Courtesy of Burdick Corp.)*

either completely evacuated or filled with an inert gas, such as argon or nitrogen. Their filaments are made of either carbon or tungsten. Carbon filament lamps burn at a lower temperature and are yellow because they emit rays which are mostly from the red end of the spectrum. Tungsten filament lamps emit a white light and burn at a temperature of 4350 degrees F. Both types of bulbs are placed in a proper reflector to concentrate the heat in the desired area. The lamp and its reflector can be housed in stands of various sizes and shapes so that they can be placed on the floor, clamped to a chair, set on a table, etc.

Nonluminous radiation is emitted from heating elements of resistant materials placed in a suitable reflector. The heating unit can be made of coils of resistant wire wrapped around a cylindrical or cone-shaped piece of porcelain or steatite. Some units are made of circular discs of resistant metal or of Carborundum® rods.

One commonly employed type of generator is made of one bar, covered with silicon and carbon compound, permitting a large radiating surface, with maximum output in proportion to the current input.

Lamps come in sizes ranging from 75 to 1500 watts input and are placed in reflectors which can be moved about easily on stands.

Carbon arc lamps which are primarily sources of ultraviolet radiation also emit infrared rays. When they are heated to a temperature of over 6300 degrees F., the spectral energy distribution is mainly in the near infrared region. Carbon arc lamps, because of a variety of disadvantages, are not used often for infrared radiation.

For infrared heating of fairly large areas of the body, such as the back, or both thighs, the *heat cradle* or "baker" is employed. It con-

sists of several sixty-watt tungsten or carbon filament bulbs backed
by a semicircular metal reflector. It is supported on adjustable legs and
is usually covered with a sheet to reduce the loss of heat due to air
currents. A variable number of bulbs may simultaneously be lighted.

Thermostatically-controlled heat lamps can be used to treat peripheral vascular disease. Two carbon filament tubes are connected
to a thermostat and fastened onto a frame, or cradle. The frame is
placed over the lower extremities and covered with a blanket. One
disadvantage to this is the difficulty in controlling the heat under the
hood.

Electric light cabinets are also employed as a means of infrared
radiation. In one type of cabinet the patient is seated, and in the other
type he reclines. The cabinet contains several sixty-watt tungsten
filament bulbs and it is lined with mirrors or polished chromium. Such
a facility is large, and thus is seldom seen in a general hospital setting.

Technique and Dosage. The size of the lamp used depends upon
the size of the area to be treated. The dosage is dependent upon the
tolerance of the patient.

The patient is placed comfortably on a plinth. The skin area to
be treated is cleansed. A time clock is used to measure accurately the
duration of treatment. The lamp is placed over the part to be treated
and is turned on. Some burners do not reach maximum heat for ten
minutes and therefore, after this period has elapsed, the therapist tests
the amount of heat reaching the surface. This testing is usually done
on the flexor surface of the forearm since it is sensitive to heat, and
the therapist must always be on guard against the danger of skin burns.

The distance of the patient to the lamp varies depending upon
the apparatus being used. Smaller non-luminous lamps of 250-watt
input can be placed from twelve to sixteen inches from the surface.
Tungsten filament lamps of 250-watt input may have to be placed from
sixteen to twenty-four inches from the skin. The type of filament and
reflector are the major considerations in determining distance. Larger
lamps should be at a distance of from twenty-four to thirty inches from
the body. It is to be remembered that the quantity of radiation varies
inversely with the square of the distance from its source. Thus, if
the lamp distance is doubled, the radiation reaching the body is one
quarter of its previous intensity, and if the distance is halved, the
energy at the skin is quadrupled. In addition, radiation is more intense if the rays are at a right angle to the treated surface than if they
are at an acute or obtuse angle.

Infrared radiation can generally be applied for from twenty to
thirty minutes. With large areas of the body the therapist may start

with a five to ten minute period of treatment and gradually increase the exposure time. Radiation is most effective if carried out daily for approximately twenty minutes per session.

INDICATIONS AND CONTRAINDICATIONS. Infrared radiation is useful for cases of sprains, strains, fibrositis, bursitis, tenosynovitis, arthritis, arthralgia, some neuralgia, some upper respiratory infections, relief of pain, relaxation of skin and muscles prior to massage, passive or active motion, relief of spasm, increasing circulation, and peripheral vascular disease.

Care must be taken to avoid burns in patients with a lack of normal thermal sensation, such as those with syringomyelia, peripheral vascular disease, scars and certain peripheral nerve lesions.

Goggles or moist cotton over the eyes are usually prescribed for patients receiving infrared treatments, particularly of the luminous type.

Ultraviolet Radiation Therapy

PHYSIOLOGIC EFFECTS. The systemic effects of ultraviolet radiation vary as a function of extent, intensity and duration of exposure. In general, ultraviolet radiation can cause blood changes, metabolic changes, erythema, or skin inflammation, pigment formation, photosensitivity of various types, and germicidal effects.

Blood changes which are a result of ultraviolet radiation include increased red cell, white cell and platelet count, lowered blood sugar, increased sugar tolerance, increased blood calcium, relative lymphocytosis, in which there is an increased number of leukocytes, and eosinophilia, a form of relative leukocytosis in which the greatest proportionate increase is in the eosinophils.

Metabolic changes which result from irradiation by ultraviolet light are seen in the formation of Vitamin D from the activated provitamins in the skin, in an increase in endogenous nitrogen metabolism and in cholesterol, the fat content of the blood, and in increased uric acid excretion.

After about four hours following exposure of the Caucasian skin to ultraviolet radiation, a skin erythema will appear which gradually increases for approximately twenty-four to forty-eight hours and then recedes for the next forty-eight to sixty hours. If the radiation intensity is weak no reddening of the skin results. This dosage is termed suberythemal. If radiation is intense, edema and vesiculation, or blistering, may follow the erythema. Pigmentation changes in the form of tanning are produced by repeated exposure to ultraviolet light, due primarily to the deposit of melanin in the basal layer of the skin.

Among certain light-skinned persons, slight and brief intensities of ultraviolet radiation produce a reaction known as photo-allergy, characterized by urticaria (hives), itching and systemic signs. These usually subside with the removal of the radiation. Cases of hay fever, asthma, angioneuro-edema, which is edema due to vasomotor disorder, and eczema have been linked to photo-allergy, and many skin diseases show increased sensitivity to ultraviolet energy.

Many substances, including certain foods of animals, such as buckwheat, clover and maize, and human pharmaceuticals, such as barbituates and sulfanilamide, become sensitizers. Some substances, such as Vaseline® and eau de cologne, when rubbed into the skin, will sensitize it to ultraviolet radiation. Removal of the individual from the source of the rays results in rapid cessation of these effects.

Ultraviolet radiation has the ability to kill or attenuate a large number of bacteria, including B. diphtheria, B. coli, Staphylococcus and Vibrio cholerae.

APPARATUS. There are several types of ultraviolet energy generators in use today.

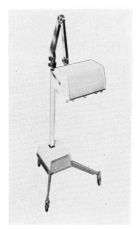

FIGURE 31. An ultraviolet lamp. (*Courtesy of Burdick Corp.*)

Carbon arc lamps produce a continuous spectrum ranging from the far ultraviolet to the infrared and thus, of all artificial sources of ultraviolet light, most closely resemble the spectrum of the sun.

The relative intensity of the ultraviolet radiation can be altered by using carbon rod electrodes with different metallic salt cores. The electric current passing across the arc creates intense heat which volatilizes the carbon and the mixture in the core. The positive electrode of the carbon arc has a temperature of approximately 6,000 degrees F.

Radiation comes mainly from the luminous vapor produced by volatilization and the crater of the positive electrode.

It is important for the lamp to have an automatically adjusting feed mechanism so that the size of the gap is kept fairly constant as the carbons are burned away.

The carbon arc lamp is of clinical value for treating wounds, tuberculosis and high blood pressure. Its main disadvantages lie in the continual need for changing the carbons as they are consumed and in the production of ozone and ashes during operation of the lamp.

Mercury-vapor arcs include four types of lamps—the hot quartz lamp, the cold quartz lamp, the sun lamp and the high pressure, or activated, electrode. The general principle underlying their operation involves activation of mercury vapor within a quartz envelope by electricity. While the arc emits a continuous spectrum of energy, more intense emanations occur at various points in the ultraviolet and blue end of the spectrum.

In the *hot quartz lamp* tilting of the burner breaks away the layer of mercury between the electrodes. The heat developed by the current as it extends across the gap which is thus produced, vaporizes the mercury, permitting the current to flow across the tube. After about ten minutes the flow of current becomes stable and the lamp is ready for use. The radiation is produced by the incandescence of the mercury vapor.

The lamps may be cooled by air or circulating water so that they can be used close to body surfaces. Quartz rods attached to the lamps permit direct transmission of the radiation to wounds and sinuses. Air-cooled burners are housed in reflectors which increase the radiation.

The *cold quartz mercury vapor lamp* has a relatively low mercury pressure and also contains a gas, such as argon or neon, to activate the arc. Sufficient heat is developed by electricity to vaporize the mercury in the tubes. The lamp itself remains relatively cool, the envelope being warmed only to about 60 degrees C. (Centigrade). Radiation reaches its maximum within approximately one minute.

The tube can be shaped to irradiate wound interiors or body orifices. When it is coiled into a spiral and backed by a reflector it is used on large body areas.

A *sun lamp* (mercury vapor tungsten filament) essentially consists of a glass envelope with a tungsten filament. The glass permits rays with wavelengths not shorter than 2800 Angstroms. A small amount of mercury is contained in a vacuum. The filament's heat vaporizes the mercury which becomes incandescent and thus produces ultraviolet radiation.

When the internal pressure of the mercury vapor arc is raised to about one atmosphere or more above that of the cold quartz lamp, the spectrum develops the characteristics of the hot quartz lamp but operates at a temperature of 1800 degrees F. instead of at 500 degrees F. The *high pressure tube* is a quartz envelope in which a few drops of mercury and argon at a few millimeters of pressure are introduced after degassing. When the current is activated, electrodes which are covered with barium oxide become incandescent under ionic bombardment. As the temperature of the argon gradually increases, greater amounts of mercury become vaporized resulting in a high mercury pressure which carries most of the current and shows the spectrum of the high pressure arc.

TECHNIQUE AND DOSAGE. Both patient and therapist must be shielded from the ultraviolet source except during the actual therapeutic exposure time. The therapist typically wears glass goggles during application and the patient may wear goggles or have pieces of wet gauze or cotton placed over his eyes.

The therapist must know the minimal erythema dose (M.E.D.). (Note: The *M.E.D.* is defined as the dose of ultraviolet radiation which will produce, in a few hours, a minimal erythema in the average Caucasian skin.)

The timing device which is employed must be capable of precise measurements of the time units being used for treatment.

The distance of the source from the patient must be accurately measured, and the angle of incidence has to be considered, since the intensity of the radiation is greatest when the rays are perpendicular to the surface they strike.

Portions of the patient's body not designated for treatment must be covered, and the treatment room itself should be well ventilated and maintained at a temperature of approximately 70 degrees F.

The single most important criterion for establishing dosage is the reaction of the patient's skin to the radiation. This reaction varies in different individuals. Furthermore, different areas of the body react differently to the radiation. It is believed that the best method of determining dosage is by observation of the reactions of the patient to the radiations from a particular apparatus. Small areas of the skin, the inner forearm, the groin, or the back are covered with a piece of paper in which ten small holes have been cut. The lamp is placed at a distance of about thirty inches from the surface and is allowed to shine through these openings for varying periods of time. After a period of from four to twenty-four hours following this procedure the radiated portions of the skin are examined to determine the effects of the radiation and the treatment dosage is set accordingly.

INDICATIONS AND CONTRAINDICATIONS. Ultraviolet radiation has therapeutic application for the following: skin disorders, such as acne vulgaris, psoriasis, erysipelas and adenoma sebaceum; decubiti and indolent ulcers; wounds; the arthritides; forms of tuberculosis and empyema; disturbances of calcium and phosphorous metabolisms, such as rickets, osteomalacia, infantile tetany and spasmophilia; bone diseases—e.g., osteomyelitis; painful conditions, such as sciatica, fibrositis and lumbago; cardiac dyspnea; colitis, pylorospasm and pyloric stenosis; treatment of tissues of the eye in a variety of conditions; and several other disorders.

Ultraviolet therapy is contraindicated or used with great caution with individuals who are markedly sensitive and develop reactions in the form of headaches, elevation of systemic temperature, vesicular skin eruptions, etc., in cases of diseases such as hyperthyroidism, diabetes, decompensated heart disease, nephritis, pulmonary tuberculosis, advanced bilateral tuberculosis, and with certain skin diseases, e.g. acute aczema, lupus erythmatosis and herpes simplex.

Conversive Heating

Diathermy methods involve techniques which employ electric currents of high frequency for heating the deep tissues of the body.

There are three forms of diathermy treatment. *Long wave diathermy* consists of the use of currents at frequencies of one megacycle. *Short wave diathermy* employs a frequency of from ten to one hundred megacycles. *Microwave diathermy* uses a frequency of 2,450 megacycles.

Since July 1, 1952 the Federal Communications Commission has forbidden the use of long wave diathermy unless treatment is given in a thoroughly screened room because of the interference it causes in radio and television communication. As a result of this ruling long wave diathermy is no longer used as frequently as it once was, and clinical usage of these deep-heating procedures has been fairly well restricted to short wave and microwave techniques.

Short Wave Diathermy

Despite the claims made by some physicians for therapeutic benefits of short wave diathermy other than those from purely thermal reasons, it is generally concluded that a special nonthermal effect is not exerted by the short wave current.

As the high frequency current enters the body it spreads, enabling a fairly large area to be heated. Fatty tissue reaches a greater temperature than muscle. The maximal depth of temperature increase is about from two to three centimeters over a period of thirty minutes.

APPARATUS. Basically, a short wave diathermy machine operates in the following manner: A filament is heated to incandescence by an auxiliary circuit. An oscillatory circuit, or tank circuit, consisting of an inductance and a condenser is magnetically coupled to the filament through an inductance and the filament is connected to the grid of the tube. When the generator is connected and the filament is lighted, current flows to charge the condenser and produce a magnetic field around the tank inductance. This causes the grid coil to become momentarily negative. The flow of current from the generator is interrupted by this negative grid and the condenser discharges into the inductance, resulting in an undamped oscillation. Due to the grid-excitation voltage the grid becomes positive during the next oscillation, permitting current to flow from the generator through the tube. The oscillations are maintained by means of a boost, once each cycle, by the generator through the tube. The loss of energy in the tube is converted into heat.

The patient's circuit can be inductively coupled into the tank circuit with no direct connection between the patient's circuit and the current source.

The part to be treated is placed in the field between two condenser plates, which are metal plates covered by a non-conducting substance such as glass or rubber. In another arrangement, an induction cable is wound around the part of the body under treatment. This is considered the most satisfactory technique for administering short wave diathermy.

TECHNIQUE AND DOSAGE. There are a variety of devices which can be used to administer short wave therapy.

In the *condenser field method* the electrodes are generally placed on either side of the body part being treated, parallel to each other. If rigid electrodes are used, they are covered with a material such as hard rubber. Rigid electrodes are held in place by supports and are separated from the skin by an air space which permits surface temperature to remain low relative to the deep tissues. Electrodes may also be placed at right angles to each other, as against the back of the calf or on the plantar surface of the foot, or they can be aligned in the same plane on one surface of the treated area.

When using rigid electrodes the patient can be seated on a wooden chair or placed on a wooden table so that electrodes may be applied in an anteroposterior position. If the patient is lying supinely, one elec-

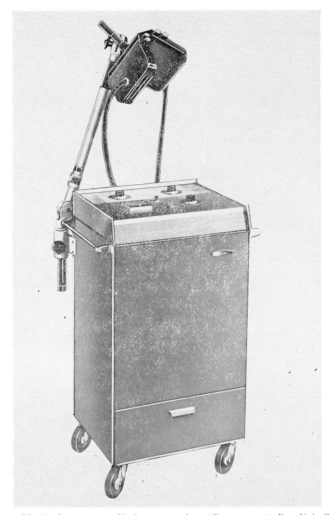

FIGURE 32. A short wave diathermy unit. *(Courtesy of Burdick Corp.)*

trode may be placed under the table. The surfaces of flexible electrodes can be manipulated to conform to the body contours of the patient. The electrodes need not be of equal size. A smaller electrode placed on the body part being treated is termed the active electrode, and the larger electrode placed on another part of the body is called the inactive electrode.

The *coplanar technique*, which has been found to be successful, involves placement of both electrodes on the same surface with the nearest edge of the plates in parallel position to each other. They can be arranged so that the current flows either longitudinally or transversely.

Cuff electrodes vary in size from a width of from one to two inches and a length of from fifteen to twenty inches. The length is determined by the size of the area being heated. Cuff electrodes are covered with insulation and are employed primarily in the treatment of the extremities.

Coil electrodes make possible very effective heating of the tissues. The coil is wrapped around the extremity being treated, with the windings as equidistant as possible from each other and from the surface of the skin. Toweling or other material is used between the induction cable and the skin. If a large body area is to be heated, the coil can be shaped into the form of a long U. The cable can also be coiled to make a flat applicator surface.

With a proper circuit, metal electrodes can be placed directly into contact with the skin. These are called *direct contact electrodes*.

Orificial electrodes are used for the heating of body cavities.

Dosage is dependent upon the comfort of the patient. The therapist must be certain that the patient possesses a thermal sense, especially important to be aware of in disabilities such as hemiplegia, nerve injuries, syringomyelia, etc., where sensory disturbances often exist. If sensation is impaired or lost caution must be taken during application of the heat. The therapist generally has to rely on the patient's report of his sensation, and he is instructed to inform her of discomfort.

In acute conditions or in the early phase of treatment, when a patient's reaction is not yet known, duration of heat application should be about ten minutes. The average treatment period ranges from twenty to thirty minutes, and may often be extended to forty minutes. Initially, applications are made daily or every other day and the intervals are later increased.

INDICATIONS AND CONTRAINDICATIONS. Short wave diathermy has been found valuable in the treatment of the following: inflammations; subacute and chronic arthritis; soft tissue injuries; sprains; bursitis; inflammation of fibrous and muscular tissues, as in fibrositis and myositis; bronchitis; bronchial asthma and pleurisy; arteriosclerosis; some cases of thromboangitis obliterans; diseases of the gastrointestinal tract—e.g. cardiospasm and pylorospasm; spastic conditions of the gallbladder and bile ducts; pain, as in sciatica, intercostal neuritis and trigeminal neuritis; local infections; and osteomyelitis.

Diathermy is inadvisable in cases of acute bursitis, acute arthritis, recent cerebral hemorrhage, during menstruation or pregnancy in females, or when the patient reacts adversely.

Microwave Diathermy

The energy for microwave diathermy is composed of radiated electromagnetic waves. Current microwave machines radiate wavelengths of twelve and two-tenths centimeters at a frequency of 2,450 megacycles per second.

Physiologic Effects. Upon exposure to microwaves there is a marked elevation of temperature in the muscular, cutaneous and subcutaneous structures of the body. There also seems to be an increase in blood flow. Bone growth appears to be unaffected. Testicular damage may be produced.

Apparatus and Dosage. The high frequency currents are produced by vacuum tube triodes placed in oscillating circuits. The frequency is increased by reducing the length of the coils and the size of the condensers. To produce wavelengths shorter than one meter with enough energy to be therapeutically valuable, a magnetron, which is a self-contained oscillator, must be employed. The only circuit is that which carries the generated microwaves to the patient. The energy is led to the patient by means of a coaxial cable which ends in an electrode called a director. Directors come in the form of four- to six-inch hollowed hemispheres. There is also an angulated electrode known as a corner director.

Spherical directors are used on irregular surfaces and angular directors are employed for the heating of smooth and concave body contours.

Dosage is determined by the patient's comfort and the experienced judgment of the therapist. Treatment duration is usually fifteen minutes.

Indications and Contraindications. In general, the patients who benefit from short wave diathermy will also benefit from microwave therapy and the contraindications are similar.

Its use should particularly be avoided with non-draining infections, active or potential hemorrhage, tuberculosis, cancer, pregnancy, areas of anaesthesis, areas of organically blocked circulation, areas of effusions, edema, and areas covered by plaster casts, adhesives or moist dressings.

ULTRASOUND

The term *ultrasound* is used to describe sound waves which are of a higher frequency than those heard by the human ear, namely, twenty thousand cycles per second in the young adult.

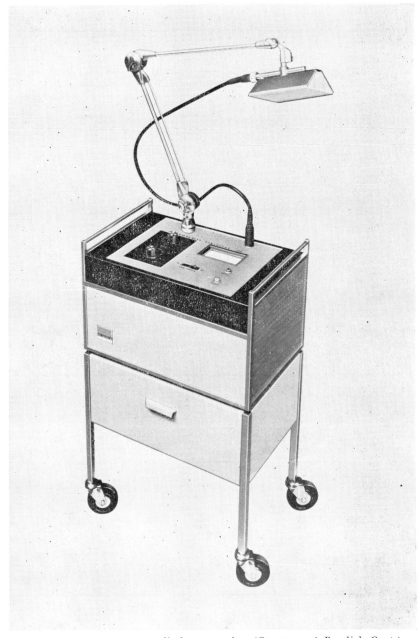

FIGURE 33. A microwave diathermy unit. (*Courtesy of Burdick Corp.*)

Basic Principles

The energy for therapy using ultrasound comes from mechanical vibrations with a frequency range of from seven-tenths to one megacycle. When a properly cut quartz crystal is placed in an attenuating electrical circuit, mechanical vibrations are produced at the frequency of the alternating current in the circuit. Since these ultrasound waves do not travel through air, a conductive medium such as heavy mineral oil or water is used between the head of the applicator and the surface of the skin.

Physiologic Effects

Ultrasound application produces a rapid rise in tissue temperature.

It also rapidly changes the state of colloids from a gel to a sol, and inactivates or destroys enzymes (such as pepsin), hormones (such as adrenalin, pituitrin and insulin), and vitamins (such as ascorbic acid).

Studies on the effects of ultrasound in a variety of different organisms have found that it can damage the spinal cord, damage or destroy bone, destroy living cells in the spleen, halt urine production, produce albumin, red cells and granular casts in urine, and slow kidney circulation. It has been experimentally demonstrated to damage testicular cells and it is known to destroy bacteria of many types and the smallpox virus.

Technique and Dosage

The ultrasound generator appears to resemble a short wave diathermy generator. The high frequency oscillating circuit activates a quartz crystal, however, and the energy is not transmitted directly to the patient.

The crystal is mounted in a water-cooled applicator head and is protected by a thin layer of aluminum. Treatment is given either by slightly moving the sound head back and forth over the body area, or by stroking massage, or by immersion of both the sound head and the body part in water. The last is used primarily for treatment of the extremities, and when used underwater the sound head is kept at a distance of from one-half inch to two inches from the skin.

Energy is usually applied at one megacycle (one thousand kilocycles) per second. The sound intensity is measured in watts per square centimeter. The dosage is a function of the intensity and the duration of the application. Depth of penetration relates to the frequency. At a frequency of one megacycle, fifty per cent of the energy reaches a depth of two inches, and twenty-five per cent reaches a depth of four inches.

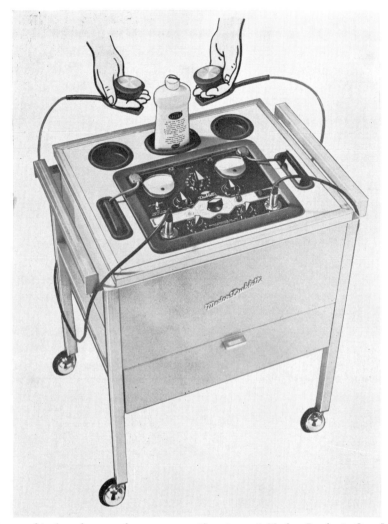

FIGURE 34. An ultrasound generator. (*Courtesy of Medco Products Co., Inc.*)

Indications and Contraindications

Ultrasound therapy has been found to be effective in the following: rheumatic conditions, such as Marie-Strümpell disease, arthritis, idiopathic sciatica, myalgias and osteochondriasis; in skin conditions—e.g., varicose ulcers, scleroderma and neurodermatitis; peptic ulcer; vascular diseases; chronic prostatitis; and in respiratory diseases, such as asthma.

Contraindicating conditions include malignancies and acutely inflamed joints. In addition, ultrasound is not applied to the head, eyes, cervical ganglia, heart, pregnant uterus, gonads, anaesthetic skin or juvenile bone.

ELECTROTHERAPY

Because electric currents are highly effective in stimulating nerve and muscle, and can be accurately measured and finely gradated, they are well suited for producing muscular contraction, either directly or by way of nerves for therapeutic purposes.

Basic Principles

The effectiveness of a stimulus is influenced by several variables, including the magnitude, rate and duration of the change it produces. The minimal effective stimulus for muscle is far longer than that for nerves.

There are two types of electric currents which can be employed for therapy. High frequency-high voltage currents are used in diathermy, and low voltage currents are utilized for stimulation of nerves and muscles. This latter type, which is discussed herein, includes direct, or galvanic, current and a variety of low frequency alternating currents.

Direct Current

Direct, or galvanic, current is a unidirectional current with distinct polarity, low amperage and low voltage. Amperage is below fifty milliamperes and voltage is less than one hundred volts. The current flows while the circuit remains closed. When direct current passes through an electrolyte, there is a movement of ions toward the two poles of the circuit.

Iontophoresis, or *ion transfer,* refers to a procedure which utilizes the polarity effects of direct current to introduce certain ions into the body through the skin by an electromotive force. Positive ions are driven through the skin at the anode, or positive pole, and negative ions are introduced at the cathode, or negative pole. The greatest concentration enters the skin along sweat glands, pores and hair follicles.

The ions lose their electrical charge rapidly and remain in the superficial tissues as soluble or insoluble compounds. The velocity of movement of the transferred ions is directly related to the voltage applied. The amount which is transferred depends upon the current flow and its duration. Current usually flows at the rate of from one to three milliamperes per square inch of the electrode surface. Treatment duration is typically fifteen minutes. The current is slowly turned up to the desired level, maintained there for the length of treatment, and slowly turned off.

Ion transfer concentrates a relatively large amount of a drug in a local area. The drug is not delivered to structures deeper than the skin, but may be taken up by the circulation. The two most frequently employed drugs are histamine and Mecholyl®, both of which produce prolonged vasodilation thought to be beneficial in the treatment of arthritis, chronic ulcer and certain vasospastic conditions of the limbs.

Low Frequency Alternating Currents

This group of currents has a frequency below ten thousand per second, a voltage which is low and constantly changing, and the ability to stimulate sensory and motor nerves.

There are five currents which have the ability to stimulate nerves. Two of them, the *interrupted direct current* and the *faradic current* are used mainly in diagnosis. The remaining three currents produce stimuli which will cause a contraction in both innervated and denervated muscle which closely resembles the normal.

The *surging faradic current* has a smoothly increasing and decreasing rise and fall in intensity and will stimulate muscles having an intact nerve supply. The *modulated alternating*, or *rapid sinusoidal*, *current* has a frequency of sixty cycles per second and may range up to three times that amount. This form of current can either be surged or modulated and will only stimulate muscles which have their nerve supply intact. The *surging uninterrupted direct current with alter-*

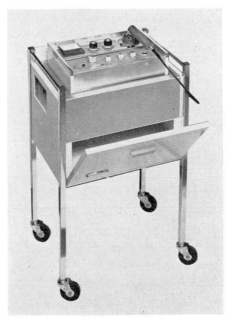

FIGURE 35. Combination electrical stimulator and ultrasound unit. (*Courtesy of Burdick Corp.*)

nating polarity, or *slow sinusoidal current,* has the form of a gradual rise and fall of direct current with a reversal of flow at a rate of from two to ninety cycles per second. It is the current which is best suited for stimulating denervated muscles.

Technique

While devices may differ from each other in certain respects, there are several general steps which the therapist follows in the techniques of electrical stimulation.

She insures good contact between the electrodes and the skin. A conductive solution, or jelly, or sodium chloride solution, or electrode jelly, or other conducting substance, is often used to decrease resistance at the point of contact.

Usually, "active" and "indifferent" electrodes are used in a mono-polar technique. The density of current flow at the larger indifferent electrode is less than at the smaller active electrode, and stimulation can be selectively produced at the latter. When stimulating innervated muscle, the therapist places the active electrode over the motor point of the muscle. In the stimulation of denervated muscle which has no motor point, the electrode may be placed at the point giving the best response, or two equally-sized electrodes may be placed with one at each end of the muscle. In this way the current will pass through the muscle and stimulate it in its entirety. Both electrodes are usually placed on the same side of the body.

Clinical Applications

Electrotherapy has its clinical use in the stimulation of muscle. The object of stimulation of denervated muscles is the maintenance of the muscles in as normal a condition as possible. This means retarding the progress of atrophy, decreasing intrafascicular and interfascicular agglutination and sclerosis of areolar tissue, and improving the circulation and the nutrition of the muscles. Electrical stimulation is helpful, but it will not completely prevent the effects of denervation on muscles.

Stimulation is done with either a direct current or a slow sinusoidal alternating current at a frequency of from two to thirty-two cycles per second. Three or four brief treatment sessions per day comprises a typical schedule. Heat, applied prior to stimulation, is useful.

Contractions produced by stimulation should be strong. Usually, only about twenty-five to thirty strong contractions can be achieved per session because of the rapid fatigability of denervated muscle. If resistance is applied against the contraction even greater benefits may be obtained. Once the patient is able to produce good, active muscle contractions, electrical stimulation is discontinued.

Innervated muscle is stimulated through its nerve supply. Electrical stimulation is useful when anatomic reinnervation has occurred, but maximal contraction of the muscle in a coordinated manner is not possible. Such would be the case where the patient has not yet learned to use the reinnervated muscle properly. It results from weakness and past use of other muscles as substitutes for the denervated ones.

The minimal effective stimulus duration is approximately three one-hundredths of a millisecond, and innervated muscle can be stimulated by impulses of one millisecond in duration.

Indications

Stimulation of innervated muscle is of value for the following: conduction deficit without denervation; relaxation of muscle spasm following trauma; prevention of atrophy due to disuse in muscle which the patient cannot voluntarily contract well; muscle re-education; reducing spasticity in spastic paralysis secondary to spinal cord injury; stimulation of the abdominal wall and diaphragm as an aid to respiration; and others.

MASSAGE

Massage is perhaps the oldest known form of physical therapy. It is generally defined as systematic and scientific manipulation of body tissues for therapeutic purposes. While there are a number of machines on the commercial market which provide massage, they are of limited value. Manual techniques, performed by a trained and skilled professional, are by far the most satisfactory.

The General Effects of Massage

There are two main classes effects of massage—mechanical and reflex.

Mechanical Effects

The mechanical effects of massage include an increased venous and lymphatic flow, increased interchange of substances between the bloodstream and tissue cells, increased peripheral blood flow, increased level of red blood cells, and an increment in the renal output of water. In addition, massage removes excess lymph from tissue spaces, thus decreasing the possibility of fibrosis. Massage also decreases excess fluid in the tissues by forcing it into venous and lymphatic channels and by moving the fluid along these vessels, lowering their pressure so that they can receive the excess fluid.

Mechanical stretching and disruption of fibers in connective tissue can be accomplished through forms of massage. Massage also improves the nutrition of muscle fibers and removes extravascular fluid.

Reflex Effects

Reflex effects of massage are produced in the skin by stimulation of the peripheral receptors which transmit impulses to the brain via the spinal cord.

The effects include dilation or constriction of arterioles, relaxation of involuntary muscle contraction, raising of the threshold for pain, sedation, and accommodation of tissue to pressure.

Massage cannot prevent atrophy or loss of muscle strength due to disuse or denervation, nor can it increase muscle strength. Furthermore, contrary to much popular belief, massage will not reduce local deposits of fat regardless of the vigorousness of the application.

Techniques and Clinical Application

Stroking
(*Effleurage*)

Superficial stroking massage consists of light, slow and gentle passage of the hand over the surface of the skin. The direction of the stroke is not important since only reflex effects are obtained by this type of massage, and the only pressure required is that for good contact.

In *deep stroking massage* the direction of force is important because the aim of this form of massage is improved blood and lymph flow. Thus, the force of the stroke is centripetal. Excessive pressure or rapid movement is not necessary. Proximal body segments are massaged in advance of distal segments.

Compression
(*Pétrissage*)

There are three compression techniques—kneading, friction and vibration.

Kneading refers to the method in which a portion of soft tissue, or of a muscle or group of muscles, is lifted up between the thumb and fingers and is manipulated, or compressed, from side to side in an alternating manner. One or both hands may give this massage.

Kneading is used for its circulatory benefits, for stretching retracted muscles and tendons, and for stretching adhesions. The patient is relaxed and the movements are performed slowly and rhythmically by the therapist. Sometimes the word "squeezing" is employed to designate muscle manipulation and kneading is reserved for soft tissue massage, but this is an unnecessary distinction.

Friction massage is performed by placing the thumb, part of the hand, or one or two fingers on the skin and moving the skin and superficial tissues over the underlying tissue in a circular fashion. No lubricant is needed and the movement is generally done fairly rapidly with moderate or increasing pressure.

Friction is valuable in loosening superficial scars or adhesions and in freeing adherent skin.

Vibration involves the transmisssion of vibratory motions of the therapist's shoulder and forearm to the body of the patient through the therapist's hand or fingers. When this type of motion is carried out on a grosser scale it is called "shaking". Vibration massage is seldom employed therapeutically.

Percussion
(Tapôtement)

Percussion refers to the technique of massage which employs percussive movements in alternation to produce stimulation. The therapist uses such movements as hacking with the outer border of the hand or relaxed fingers, clapping with the palms of the hands, beating with clenched fists, and tapping with the finger tips.

The therapeutic value of percussion massage lies in its assisting tissues to accommodate to pressure.

For the massage treatment the patient and the therapist should be as comfortable as possible. Clothing should not be worn on the body part being treated, and the involved part must be well supported.

The therapist's movements are slow and rhythmic, and she stands so that the entire stroke can be performed without undue movement or shifts in position. Maximum contact should be maintained between the patient's skin and the hands of the therapist. A lubricant, such as mineral oil, or lotion, or cream, is frequently used on the patient's skin to facilitate smooth movement of the therapist's hands.

Therapeutic massage depends upon skill rather than strength. It should rarely be painful or productive of anxiety in the patient, but, instead. should result in a general feeling of well being, pleasantness and relaxation, in addition to its specific therapeutic effects.

Indications and Contraindications

Massage is useful for relief of pain, relaxation of muscle tension, improvement of circulation, reduction of edema, and stretching of adhesions.

The clinical conditions for which massage is most valuable include fractures, dislocations, joint injuries, sprains, strains, contusions, lacerations, arthritis, fibrositis, bursitis, painful muscular contractions, low back pain, peripheral nerve lesions, scars, adhesions, circulatory disorders resulting in edema, paralytic disabilities, cerebral palsy and multiple sclerosis.

Massage is contraindicated for conditions of acute inflammation or infection, malignancies, skin lesions, and acute circulatory disorders such as thrombophlebitis. It is administered with much caution to debilitated patients and to skin areas which have been burned or are very thin.

OTHER PHYSICAL THERAPY MODALITIES

Two other methods of treatment which are often included within the broad framework of physical therapy are traction and manipulation.

Traction refers to the system of forces applied along the length of the body, or to any portion of the spine, so as to try and separate vertebral and spinal structures.

Manipulation means the sudden flexion and extension of joints in the spine or extremities to restore lost joint mobility.

Both sets of procedures are more often utilized by physicians than by physical therapists. Neither are employed as frequently as the other methods described in this chapter, and there is still some controversy within the medical profession regarding the real value of such techniques.

Chapter 8

BRACES, AMBULATION AIDS, WHEELCHAIRS AND PROSTHETICS

Because the objectives of physical rehabilitation are to make the patient as functional as possible in activities of daily living, in the use of his hands, and in ambulation, all program efforts are directed towards these goals. However, despite intensive and/or prolonged therapy, many patients are unable to achieve these aims with complete independence. That is, in order for them to return to their home and community and to function as they once did, or to approximate former functioning, certain assistive devices are necessary. This chapter will focus on those assists which are a prerequisite for satisfactory lower extremity function and which fall within the province of physical therapy.

BRACES

Introduction

Bracing is used to improve the functioning of the whole patient. If an extremity has a functional or a structural defect the entire body must be considered since it is the entire body which is affected.

Braces have a multiplicity of purposes. A brace can be used to decrease pain, to support body weight, to control involuntary movements, to aid in ambulation, and to prevent or correct deformities.

Supportive braces stabilize a body part and they are utilized with painful joints, architectural deficiencies, joints with imbalanced or paralyzed musculature, for maintenance of correct posture, and as an aid in ambulation.

Corrective braces are employed for conditions such as clubbed feet, tibial torsion, congenital hip dislocations and moderate contractures.

Protective braces are those used for emergency splinting, traction splints, weight-relieving devices and fracture bracing.

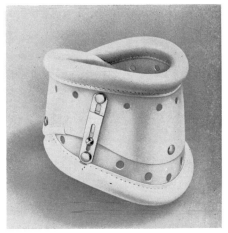

FIGURE 36. Cervical collar. (*Courtesy of Florida Brace Corp.*)

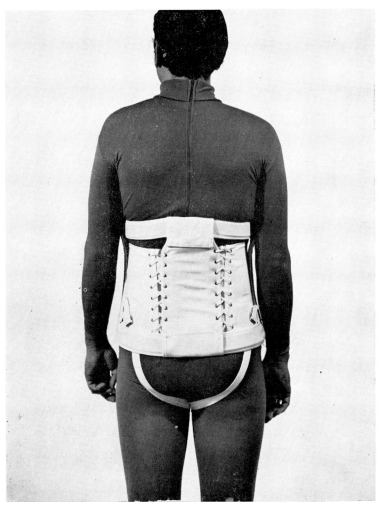

FIGURE 37. Lumbosacral corset. (*Courtesy of S. H. Camp and Co.*)

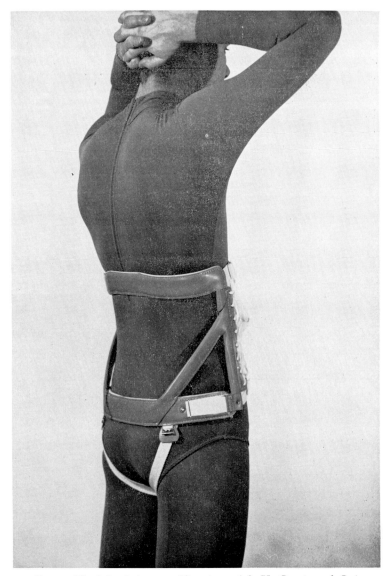

FIGURE 38. A back brace. (*Courtesy of S. H. Camp and Co.*)

Dynamic braces are seen in the form of springs, cables and elastic bands.

Preventive braces are employed to prevent deformity secondary to muscle imbalance.

Control braces eliminate involuntary movements as in athetoid cerebral palsy, thus making ambulation possible.

Prescribing A Brace

When the physician prescribes a brace for a patient he considers certain factors, namely, the purpose which the brace is to serve and the body parts which require bracing. The support of the body, motion, prevention and correction of deformities are all controlled at various joints.

The short leg brace is prescribed when the condition requiring bracing is at the ankle joint. This controls dorsal flexion, plantar flexion, pronation and supination. A stirrup, or caliper, or foot plate attaches the brace to the shoe. The use of ninety degree stops, reverse stops, or T-straps enable all ankle joint motion to be controlled.

The long leg brace is used for control of the knee joint. It is prescribed to prevent buckling of the knee due to weak quadriceps muscles, or hyperextension of the knee as a result of weak quadriceps or hamstring muscles. All long leg braces are attached to the shoe or to a foot plate. The ring lock is the best and safest of all of the various types of knee joint locks.

When the hip joint is weak attachments can be added to the long leg brace to aid in the support of body weight.

The ischial ring supports the body weight at the hip and, in addition, minimizes a limp due to gluteal weakness.

The ischial seat prevents the pelvis from tilting backward and placing too great a strain on the ligaments. It is made by extending the posterior thigh cuff of the long leg brace and molding the leather so as to form a seat.

The pelvic band controls flexion, extension, abduction, adduction, external rotation, internal rotation, and hyperextension of the hip. It is a leather band, attached to the long leg brace, which encircles the hip. When the hip locks are open, hip flexion and extension, but no other movements, are possible.

The pelvic band is used to correct the "scissors" gait of spastic paraplegia, muscle imbalance at the hip, as in cerebral palsy or poliomyelitis, pathologic spinal cord conditions below the tenth cervical vertebra, athetoid hip movements and contractures of the hip flexor muscles.

A unilateral long leg with a pelvic band can be employed to correct poor gait patterns in children, and is best used with an ischial ring or ischial seat. It has a disadvantage in that the pelvic band tends to rotate.

The Knight spinal brace is utilized for the following: to restrict motion at the lumbosacral joint and higher; to support the trunk, as in cases of fracture or tuberculosis of spinal vertebrae, scoliosis and low

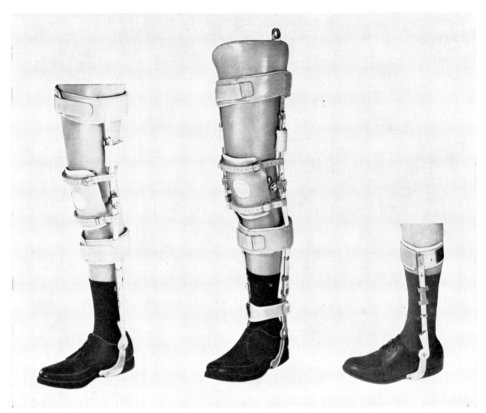

FIGURE 39. Two lower extremity braces. Left: Adjustable long leg brace, medial view; Center: The same brace, lateral view; Right: Adjustable short leg brace. (*Reprinted by permission of J. A. Preston Corp., 1971*)

back pain; for weakness or paralysis of abdominal musculature; and for continued spine immobilization.

When the patient has flaccid or spastic lower extremities with weakness or inability to control the trunk, the Knight spinal brace is attached to bilateral long leg braces. The most frequent usage of this form of bracing is with patients who have poliomyelitis, spinal cord lesions above the tenth cervical vertebra and for young children with athetoid or spastic cerebral palsy involving all four extremities.

In prescribing a brace the physician takes into consideration areas of anesthesia, problems of circulation, inflammation, progressive disease, skin lesions, general debility and acute pain. All of these variables can modify the type of brace to be prescribed and may even contraindicate bracing.

Indications for Bracing

Bracing is used in cases of lower motor neuron disorders where there is flaccid paralysis and weakness due to poliomyelitis, nerve root and nerve trunk injury, polyneuropathy, and meningomyelocele, as in spina bifida.

It is prescribed for prevention and correction of deformities resulting from muscle imbalance, fascial tightness, or prolonged, incorrect positioning.

Bracing is of value in progressive muscular dystrophy, since children so affected are prone to contractures of the heel cord, iliotibial band, and knee and hip flexor muscles.

For patients with hemophilia bracing is employed to protect against hemorrhage which results from excess motion, for stabilization of fixed deformities and traumatized joints, and for correction of deformities.

Bracing improves muscle function, corrects deformities, and eliminates involuntary motion in patients who have cerebral palsy.

In the case of a patient with a fracture, braces are utilized for support and stabilization of nonunion, for control of angular, torsional and compressive stresses, for protection of a healing fracture while simultaneously permitting movement, and to allow mobility without the need of a heavy cast.

Prevention of deformity of the involved lower extremity in spastic hemiplegia requires a brace.

Braces permit function in arthritic patients while reducing pain.

AMBULATION AIDS

There are three main classes of apparatus in addition to braces which aid the disabled in ambulation and which, in fact, often make ambulation possible. These are crutches, canes and walkers. All three come in a variety of styles, and the present section describes those which are most frequently employed in physical medicine and rehabilitation.

Crutches

Most patients who require lower extremity bracing also need crutches in order to ambulate. Prescription of crutches must consider the proper selection and correct measurement of the crutch to meet the patient's needs, the patient's muscle strength and range of motion, the need for excercises and training in crutch management, and a determination of the best crutch gaits for the particular individual in question.

Types of Crutches

There are three basic crutch types. The *underarm,* or *axillary, crutch* with double uprights and handbars is most commonly seen type. One style, the *extension crutch,* is adjustable in its total length and in the height of the handpiece, and other style, called the *permanent,*

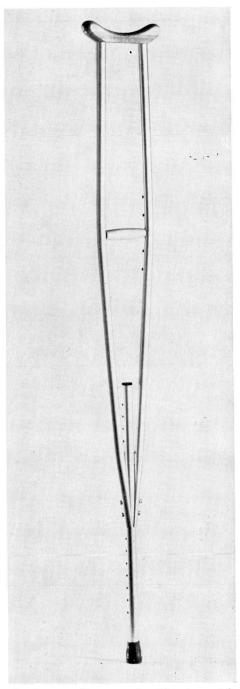

FIGURE 40. Adjustable aluminum axillary crutch. (*Courtesy of S. H. Camp and Co.*)

standard, or *plain split crutch*, is not adjustable. A variation of the latter is the *spring-top axillary crutch*, in which the underarm crosspiece is replaced by rubber or hair filling covered with leather and riveted to the uprights.

The adjustable crutch is used to meet a patient's changing needs, while the non-adjustable types are prescribed for patients whose disability is permanent, or of many years' duration, or who may have to carry some of their body weight on their shoulders as well as on their hands.

Wooden crutches are usually made of birch, ash, maple or hickory, while custom-made crutches are most often constructed of Brazilian rosewood, hard-rock maple, or lemon wood, these being more resilient and less likely to crack or splinter. Axillary crutches can also be made of tubular aluminum. The adjustable crutch is heavier than the permanent crutch.

The Lofstrand crutch is constructed of a single, adjustable, aluminum tube which is attached to a curved piece of steel having a rubber covered handbar and a metal forearm cuff. The Lofstrand can be useful as a substitute for canes. The metal forearm bar and the cuffs stabilize the wrists and make ambulation easier. In addition, because of the metal cuffs which enclose the forearm, the patient can use his hand and fingers without losing control of the crutches.

The Canadian, or *elbow extensor crutch* consists of a single aluminum tube with lateral upright attachments, a hand bar and cuffs. It has no shoulder rest. Such a crutch is used by patients who can ambulate using a four-point crutch gait and who need support for weak forearm extensor muscles. If a hand is needed to perform an activity it must be taken off the crutch, thus leaving no support for the trunk. In addition, the lack of an underarm bar on which to rest does not permit the use of the Canadian crutch for the developement of endurance.

If metal cuffs are attached to crutches of the axillary type, this provides the advantages of the Canadian crutch with the added feature of an opportunity to rest on the arm pit if necessary.

Crutch Accessories

Many accessories have been devised for crutches to make them more comfortable, safer and more functional for the user. The most important of these is probably the *rubber crutch tip*. Its purpose is to provide good ground contact regardless of the ground surface and of the angle at which the crutch is placed on the ground. Small, narrow tips do not give good ground contact and tend to wear easily. The best

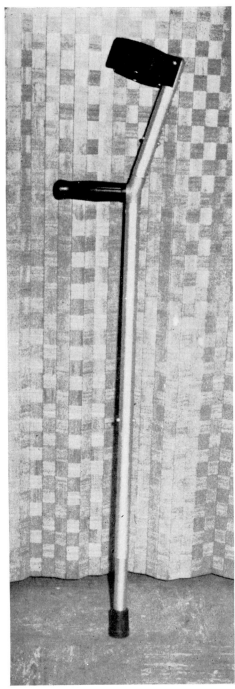

FIGURE 41. A Lofstrand crutch.   (*Courtesy of S. H. Camp and Co.*)

tip is the suction type which remains in contact with the ground regardless of the angle at which the crutch is placed.

In an effort to aid the crutch user during periods when there is ice, snow, wet leaves, etc. on the ground, the *weather tip* has been developed. Non-slip types of tips include those in which rotation of the hand bar extends a metal tip beyond the end of the rubber crutch tip, and tips made of serrated metal which are held above the rubber tip until needed.

The crab-foot tip consists of three separate tips joined as one at their base and mounted on the end of the crutch by a universal joint. Thus, at least one, and usually two tips will strike the ground at the proper angle to prevent crutch slippage.

Sometimes, when the crab-foot tip is unsatisfactory, a *disc tip,* which is a rubber-covered, metal disc about four inches in diameter, can be substituted, mounted to the crutch end by a universal joint.

The rubber axillary pad is a rubber covering, usually made of latex or sponge rubber, which fits over the underarm crosspiece. It helps to relieve underarm pressure, although its tendency to stick in the axilla can result in difficulty during certain crutch activities. It may also encourage weight-bearing on the shoulders instead of on the hands.

Rubber handgrips are also made of sponge rubber or latex and will fit all standard crutches. These are prescribed for patients who develop pain or numbness from pressure of the handpiece. However, these rubber coverings tend to rotate on the handpiece and often make it too large for comfort.

Triceps bands, forearm bands and wrist straps are added to crutches to overcome muscle weaknesses or to help maintain positions of those parts.

Preparation for Crutch Ambulation

There are primarily five muscle groups which are needed for good crutch handling. The arm flexors must be able to move the crutch forward. The forearm extensors must hold the elbows at the proper angle when body weight is on the hands or is being raised from the floor. Finger and thumb flexors have to be able to grip the crutches. Wrist dorsiflexors are needed to keep the hands correctly on the handpieces. Shoulder girdle depressors and downward rotators must support the body on the crutches when it leaves the floor.

Prior to crutch walking the patient is administered a muscle test to discover the extent and areas of muscle weakness. He is then given a program of exercises to develop the strength required in the muscle groups which are necessary for ambulation, and he is given instructions in standing and balancing on crutches.

The specific crutch gait to be taught the patient depends upon the type and severity of his disability. In determining which gait pattern can most effectively be used by the patient, the therapist evaluates him on his ability to take steps with his lower extremities, on his weight-bearing and balancing abilities on the lower and upper extremities, and on his ability to maintain his body in the erect position.

Standard Crutch Gaits

All patients who walk with the aid of crutches should learn at least two basic gaits—a fast one, which is used in the open, and a slow one, for use in crowded places where there is limited space but balance must be maintained. In addition, patients should be taught as many gaits as possible since each one requires a different combination of muscles. A disabled individual who can fatigue with one gait should be able to switch to another gait, allowing one muscle group to rest while another one works.

The Four-Point Alternate Gait. The sequence of this gait is right crutch, left foot, left crutch, right foot. This is the simplest type of gait if the patient can place one foot before the other, and it is safe because there are always three points of support on the floor. The gait is slow due to the constant shifting of weight, and it is a good one to use in crowds or in small spaces, since it does not require a large area in which to be performed.

The Two-Point Alternate Gait. This gait has the sequence of right crutch and left foot simultaneously, and left crutch and right foot simultaneously. It is actually a speeding up of four-point alternate gait, and can be taught to the patient following his mastery of the former. Since only two points are on the floor at the same time, greater body balance is required than for the four-point gait. This gait is also well suited for small areas.

The Three-Point Gait. The sequence for this gait is both crutches and the weaker lower extremity and then the stronger lower extremity. It is utilized when the patient has one leg which cannot stand full weight-bearing and one leg which can.

Tripod Crutch Gaits. Tripod gaits are taught when the patient cannot place one foot in front of the other. There are two such gaits.

The tripod alternate gait has a sequence of right crutch, left crutch, and drag the body.

When this is mastered the patient can be taught the *tripod simul-*

taneous gait, with a sequence of both crutches together and drag the body.

These gaits are both slow and laborious for severely disabled persons with spastic or flaccid lower limb paralysis. They are crutch gaits of choice in starting patients who have spinal cord injuries or residual disabilities from poliomyelitis.

Swinging Crutch Gaits. There are two swinging gaits.

The swing-to gait has a sequence of both crutches simultaneously and then lifting the body to the crutches. It is the easier of the two.

In *the swing-through gait* the patient moves both crutches in front of his body and then lifts his body and swings it forward, beyond the crutches.

Canes

Patients who have a disability which involves a lower extremity generally require some ambulation assistance. Canes are seldom prescribed for individuals who cannot bear weight on their affected leg. Patients who use one can usually do not develop a normal ambulation pattern because of the tendency to lean the body over the cane and to shorten the stride on that side. It is often found that when the cane is no longer needed this abnormal pattern tends to persist.

Determining the length of a cane for a patient is a relatively easy matter. Measurement is made so that the highest point of the cane is about at the level of the greater trochanter, including the rubber tip in the measurement.

The cane is held in the hand opposite the affected leg except in cases of a weak upper extremity on that side. In climbing a curb or steps, the patient steps up with the unaffected leg, then places the cane and the affected extremity on the step. In descending, this sequence is reversed. When there is a railing, either the railing or the cane is used, opposite the involved extremity. The patient is taught by the therapist to bear down on the cane when the unaffected extremity begins the swing phase of ambulation. This prevents tilting of the trunk over the affected leg and results in a more normal pattern of walking. If a patient is a successful cane user, pain and fatigue will not be a great hindrance, and endurance will be increased because of a more normal ambulation pattern and efficient use of muscles.

Types of Canes

Canes come in three standard sizes although any cane can be cut down to suit the user. Each type of cane has a diameter which corre-

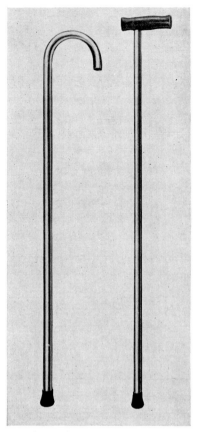

FIGURE 42. Left: Standard cane. Right: Functional grip cane. *(Courtesy of S. H. Camp and Co.)*

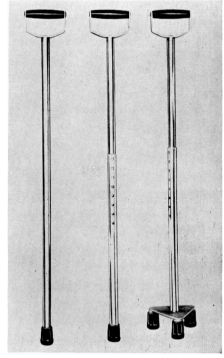

FIGURE 43. Left: Aluminum cane; Center: Adjustable aluminum cane; Right: Adjustable tripod cane. *(Courtesy of S. H. Camp and Co.)*

sponds to its length. Thus, the thirty to thirty-two-inch cane has a diameter of five-eighths of an inch, the thirty-two to thirty-eight-inch cane's diameter is seven-eighths of an inch, and the diameter of the forty to forty-two-inch cane is one inch. Canes of greater length or diameter can be specially ordered for a patient.

The *standard cane* is thirty-six inches in length, is made of wood or aluminum, and has a C-curved handle.

An aluminum *telescope cane* can be adjusted in its length from twenty-two to thirty-eight inches.

The ortho-cane has a plastic palm surface and an exclusive curved design which the manufacturer claims places the patient's weight over the center of gravity, providing better balance and control.

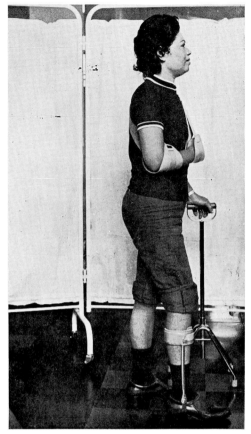

FIGURE 44. Patient with right hemiplegia ambulating with a quad cane.

The crab-cane has three prongs at the end of the shaft, attached by a flexible rubber socket, permitting movement of the shaft while the prongs remain in contact with the ground.

The quad-cane has four prongs at the end of the shaft which contact the floor. It is adjustable in length, and with four points on the ground it provides maximum support.

The four-legged cane has four points, two with rubber tips and two with small wheels, or it can be fitted with four tips. In ambulation, using the model with the wheels, the patient tilts the shaft towards the body and pushes the cane forward, maintaining contact with the floor. Using the cane without the wheels requires that the patient lift the cane and place it forward at each step. This latter type is more frequently employed since the safety of the former is questionable due to the coordination and timing which its use requires.

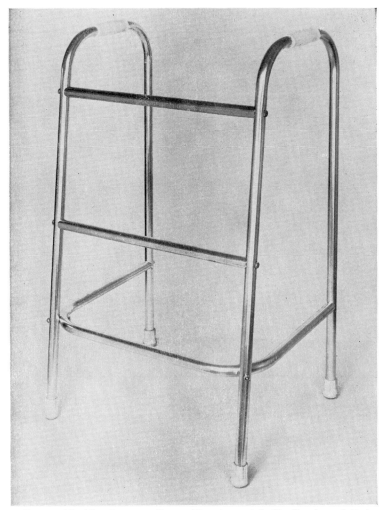

FIGURE 45. Aluminum walker. (*Courtesy of S. H. Camp and Co.*)

Walkers

Walkers also come in a variety of shapes and sizes. They are usually limited to home use and are prescribed only when a cane or crutch cannot meet the patient's ambulation needs.

Almost all standard walkers require some strength in the muscles of the wrists and hands, and strong elbow extensor and shoulder depressor muscles.

Types of Walkers

The standard walker is made of one-inch polished aluminum. Most have plastic handgrips and rubber tips on the four legs. Some models

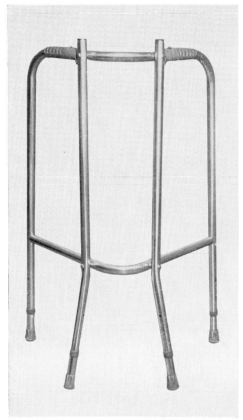

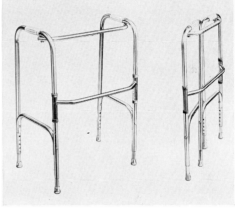

FIGURE 46. A modified aluminum walker. (*Courtesy of S. H. Camp and Co.*)

FIGURE 47. Folding walker. *(Reprinted by permission of J. A. Preston Corp., 1971)*

can be folded up for travel or storage, and the standard walker may be purchased with adjustable legs. The patient lifts the walker off the floor, places it in front of him and then walks forward between the bars.

The walkerette has runners attached to the bars and it is pushed forward along the floor, not lifted by the patient.

The Rollator®️ walker has wheels on the front legs. The patient raises the rear legs off the floor and rolls the walker forward.

The crutch walker has crutches attached to the horizontal bars to support the body weight and it also has a seat for the patient to rest on when fatigued. The crutches are adjustable and can be removed or dropped to the sides when not being used.

Walkers are most often prescribed for children with cerebral palsy who have severe involvement of the upper extremities. These walkers have a padded body ring and an adjustable saddle seat. Children who

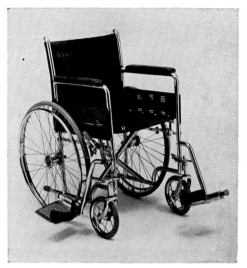

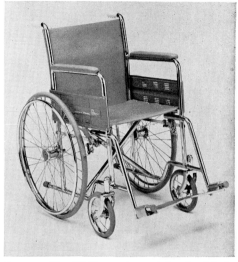

FIGURE 48. Standard universal wheelchair.   FIGURE 49. Hollywood model wheelchair.
(Courtesy of Everest and Jennings, Inc.)   *(Courtesy of Everest and Jennings, Inc.)*

cannot use crutches can usually manage well at home with a walker of this type.

WHEELCHAIRS

Despite the numerous ambulation aids which are available many patients are so severely disabled that they will never be able to walk, and thus, in order to travel about they must spend a large part of their waking lives in wheelchairs. In addition, many patients who are able to ambulate with braces and crutches find that the energy required for this is too great and prefer a wheelchair which enables them to function more efficiently. For these patients the prescription of a wheelchair is of the utmost importance.

When the physician considers prescribing a wheelchair for a patient he must take into consideration a variety of factors. These include the following: the patient's diagnosis, disability, prognosis and life expectancy; the patient's age, height and weight; transfer techniques which the patient is able to employ in getting into and out of the wheelchair; the safety of the wheelchair and its utilization; the mode of propulsion, whether mechanical or manual; the patient's style of living and the use to which the wheelchair will be put; the physical design of the patient's home, place of work and other areas where the wheelchair will be frequently used; the financial resources of the patient and the cost of the wheelchair; and whether or not the wheelchair will actually help the patient in performing the activities of daily living.

Wheelchairs and Their Components

The major wheelchair manufacturers, such as Everest and Jennings of California and Colson of Ohio, publish excellent catalogues which describe the dimensions and features of their products and the interested reader can write to them for details (please note Copyrights and Permissions section in the front part of the book). Some of the more commonly used types of wheelchairs will be described in the following pages.

Standard Universal Models. These wheelchairs have the following features: copper-nickel-chrome electroplating, durable steel tubing, a single supporting crossbrace, reinforced canvas seat and back cushion, thirty-two-ounce Naugahyde® upholstery with matching plastic arm rests, rubber tires, eight-inch casters, hand brakes, and tipping levers for getting up and down curbs and steps.

The Hollywood Style. This type of wheelchair is designed for short-term, or partially disabled patients who are ambulatory and need the wheelchair only for resting. It is a comparatively economical model but lacks versatility.

The Traveller. The Traveller is shorter than the average Universal chair but is more difficult to brake and to propel, especially at curbs and steps. It also tends to tip forward and does not lend itself to good posture. Nor can detachable arms or swinging, detachable foot rests be

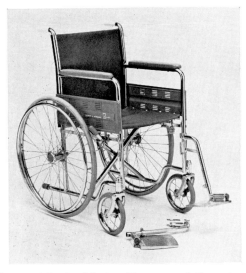

FIGURE 50. Traveller model wheelchair. (*Courtesy of Everest and Jennings, Inc.*)

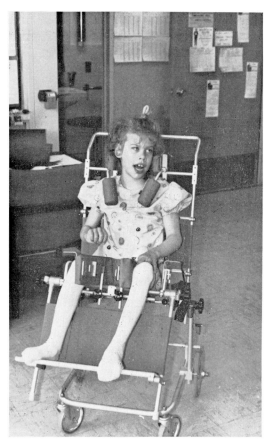

FIGURE 51. Children's wheelchair being used by a ten year old child with severe athetotic cerebral palsy. (*Courtesy of L. Mulholland and Associates*)

used with this type of chair, making close approach to work surfaces and transfers very difficult and often impossible.

All of the above wheelchair models are collapsible for travel and storage.

There are three major sizes of standard wheelchairs. The *standard adult size* is suitable for most adults, the *intermediate,* or *junior size,* is used by small adults and older children, and the *children's,* or *tiny tot size,* is ideal for children until about the age of six or seven. In addition, there is a "growing chair" which is available for children between the ages of six and twelve who are undergoing rapid physical growth. By the addition of various accessories this chair can serve the child's needs until he reaches adulthood.

Custom wheelchairs can also be purchased. The main feature which

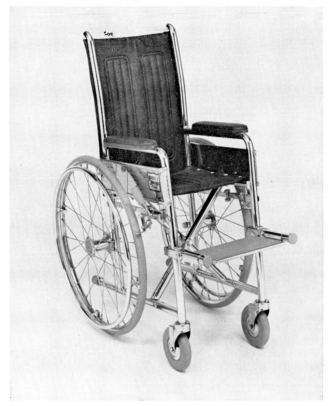

FIGURE 52. Standard tiny tot wheelchair. (*Courtesy of Everest and Jennings, Inc.*)

distinguishes them from standard chairs is detachable armrests, which the others do not have.

Accessories and Special Features

Wheels and Tires. As a general rule, if the wheelchair is to be used out of doors the large wheels are in the rear, and when the chair is intended for indoor use, the large wheels are set in front. The standard wheel size for the large wheels is twenty-four inches. A twenty-inch wheel is used by the patient who transfers sideways since it does not interfere with this act.

If the wheelchair is to be used primarily on soft, sandy, or uneven ground surfaces, pneumatic, or air-cushioned, tires increase traction and absorb shock well. These chairs are more difficult to propel, however, and are not recommended for individuals with much upper extremity weakness.

For patients with loss of grasp in their fingers, vertical projections or knobs added to the rims of the wheels transfer much of the work

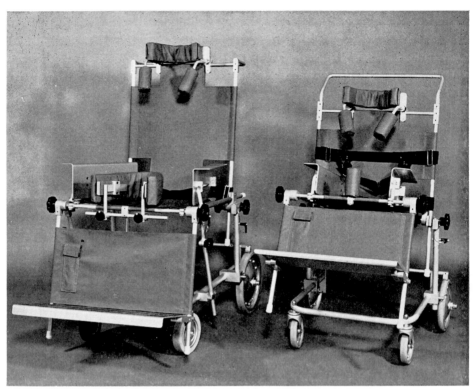

FIGURE 53. Two wheelchairs designed to be used by the growing child. At left is the Junior size model with neckrest, shoulder pads and hip abductor. This chair may be used by a child weighing between 60 and 150 pounds. On the right is a children's size model featuring neckrest, shoulder pads, trunk support belt and adduction post. It may be used by children between the ages of 18 months and 12 years. (*Courtesy of L. Mulholland and Associates*)

from the fingers to the hands, enabling a patient with such a disability to satisfactorily propel his chair.

Propulsion. For patients who have little or no power or control in their upper extremities, battery-powered wheelchairs are available. The patient can operate, by some means, such as with the side of his head or his chin, a small control stick which activates the wheels and moves the chair in any desired direction.

One-arm drive wheelchairs are often prescribed for patients who have one good upper extremity, such as hemiplegics and triplegics. With such a chair, a straight, forward or reverse direction can be maintained by pushing only one of the large wheels.

Brakes. All wheelchairs, regardless of their type, must have a good set of brakes. Brakes are required to prevent rolling down an incline

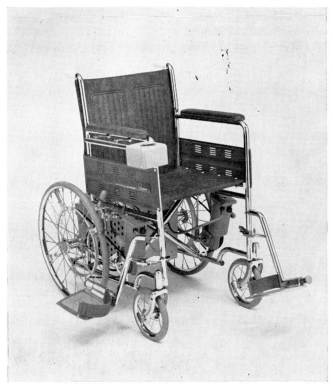

FIGURE 54. Power drive wheelchair. *(Courtesy of Everest and Jennings, Inc.)*

and to keep the chair stabile while the patient is transferring in and out of it. The brakes are hand operated.

Seats. Wheelchairs can be designed with a hydraulic seat, or a hydraulically-controlled elevating seat can be added to wheelchairs which have detachable arms. Such a device is important for the arthritic patient, or for the patient with a muscular condition who has great difficulty in rising from or sitting down into standard chairs.

Additional height can also be provided to wheelchair seats in the form of thick, foam rubber cushions which also provide relief at pressure points of the body. Cushions which are air-filled or water-filled also distribute the patient's weight evenly on the seat, thus avoiding pressure on any single body area. Some patients feel more comfortable sitting on a solid seat and this kind of bench seat is removable so that the chair can be folded for transportation and storage.

Backrests. Standard chairs have a reinforced canvas back. However, the back can also be of the type which opens and closes by means of a zipper, snaps, or buttons or small turnbuckles, for the patient who cannot transfer sideways to a bed or toilet seat, but is able to transfer backwards through the rear of the chair. This type of backrest is not adjustable to any reclining position, but other types can be made reclining or semi-reclining.

Ortho back rests are used to correct posture and reduce fatigue. Head rests can be added to standard backrests for better support of the head and neck.

Armrests. Flat, wooden or upholstered armrests are most desirable. Detachable armrests are prescribed for patients who transfer to and from the chair sideways. Desk arms, which are anteriorly scalloped, permit the patient to approach and work at desks or tables. These are not very comfortable, however, for daily use unless they are detachable and reversable so that the armrest itself is further from the patient's body. Regular adjustable armrests can be lowered for desk work and raised for comfort.

Legrests. Adjustable legrests which can be elevated and which have panels to support the legs are prescribed for patients whose lower extremities require elevation.

Footplates. Footplates can be made adjustable in length and can

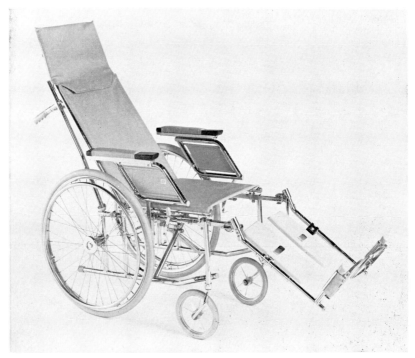

FIGURE 55. Reclining back wheelchair with back reclined and leg rests partially elevated. (*Courtesy of Institutional Industries*)

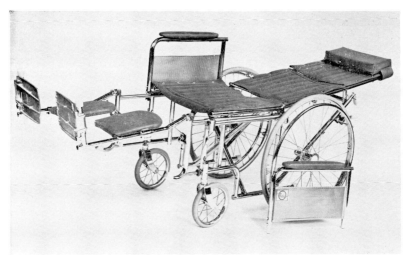

FIGURE 56. Reclining wheelchair in fully reclined position with left armrest removed. (*Courtesy of Rolls Equipment, Inc., Division of Invacare Corp.*)

be designed to swing aside or be removed if necessary. If the patient's lower extremities are spastic, toe loops, adjustable in size and usually made of canvas, are added to the footplates to hold the feet in position. Heel loops are standard on swinging, detachable foot rests and should be ordered on all wheelchairs.

Additional Accessories

Patients who use a crutch or a cane in addition to their wheelchair should have a holder, such as a leather, vinyl, canvas or cloth loop on the chair for these aids. For patients with weak upper extremities, arm slings are useful for suspending the arms in a comfortable position. They also help the patient to function more satisfactorily because they eliminate the pull of gravity. Trays which are adjustable and fit any wheelchair model enable patients to read, write, work and eat while in their chairs.

When a patient receives a new wheelchair he should follow the manufacturer's instructions for its proper care. It is encumbent upon the physical therapist to insure that he learns these instructions. She also trains the patient in proper usage of the wheelchair and in the "dos" and "don'ts" of wheelchair management.

Transfer activities which involve the wheelchair are generally the responsibility of the occupational therapist but very often both occupational therapist and physical therapist work together for the patient's welfare.

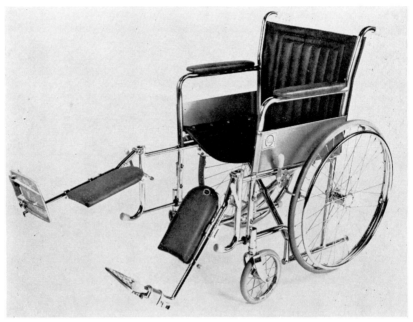

FIGURE 57. Standard wheelchair with right legrest elevated and left legrest partially elevated. (*Courtesy of Rolls Equipment, Inc., Division of Invacare Corp.*)

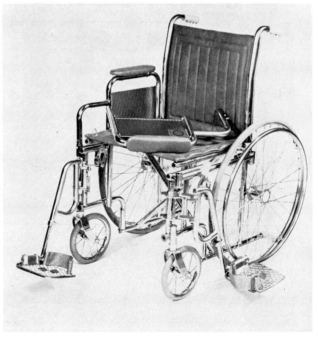

FIGURE 58. Standard wheelchair with left arm removed and left foot rest swung to the side. (*Courtesy of Institutional Industries*)

LOWER EXTREMITY PROSTHETICS

Post-Operative Physical Therapy

While much of the post-operative care of the amputee is the responsibility of the physician and the nursing staff, it is important for the physical therapist to begin an early program of exercises with the patient. For the patient who is a candidate for a prosthesis, these services are crucial since they prevent deformity, promote proper body alignment, increase range of motion, improve muscle strength, and generally prepare the patient for prosthetic training and use of an artificial limb.

The first three days following recovery from surgery are spent in performing breathing exercises which emphasize use of the diaphragm and lateral costal muscles.

By the fourth day, steps are taken to prevent contractures. These early therapeutic exercises are performed with the patient in bed and are generally done passively by the therapist although many authorities advocate gentle assisted active movement of the stump. These movements maintain the normal range of motion and aid venous return. Passive stretching is necessary when contractures have formed.

The therapist also instructs the patient as to the proper bed posture. He is cautioned against placing a pillow under his hip or knee, adbucting his stump, lying with his knees flexed, placing a pillow between his thighs, hanging his stump over the edge of the bed, and prolonged wheelchair sitting with his stump flexed. He is also told to spend at least thirty minutes, twice per day, in pronation, and to keep his pelvis level.

By the sixth to tenth day, or as the stump heals, active exercises and pressure exercises are introduced to maintain joint mobility, prevent excessive atrophy, increase circulation, and prepare the stump surface for weight-bearing. The amputee performs active exercises by freely moving his stump through the complete range of motion against gravity. Pressure exercises are done by the patient pushing against pillows and other objects of varying degrees of hardness in the directions of extension and adduction. When the stump has sufficiently healed, progressive resistance exercises are prescribed which can be conducted in the bed or in the physical therapy gymnasium.

While the main focus of attention is the amputee's stump, in order to achieve maximum rehabilitation a program of general body conditioning is instituted. Particular attention is paid to those muscle groups which are important to locomotion, such as the triceps, shoulder girdle muscles and hand flexors, which are needed for crutch walking, the abdominal muscles necessary for stability during ambulation, and the muscles of the normal leg, which is required for weight-bearing.

In addition, certain post-surgical complications may warrant treatment for pain, adherent scar tissue, slowly healing lesions, poor collateral circulation, edema, ulcerations, and other conditions. These require, besides medical care, that the therapist employ the treatment modalities prescribed by the physician, including infrared radiation, ultraviolet radiation, diathermy, whirlpool baths, contrast baths, massage, or iontophoresis.

Pre-Prosthetic Training

Preparation for the wearing and using of an artificial limb is begun as soon as it is feasible for the individual patient. (Note: Some hospitals are now fitting patients with a prosthesis immediately following recovery from surgery. The advisability of this procedure for all amputees is still under consideration). Crutch walking is initiated at this time as are hopping and balancing exercises which develop maneuverability and the sensations of walking. Lofstrand crutches are probably best suited for this because they avoid axillary pressure, discourage resting the stump on the handpiece of the crutch, and make the transition to canes easier for the patient. Hopping, balancing and proper shifting of weight are all basic to good ambulation.

Once the sutures are removed from the stump, elastic compression bandages are used to shrink and shape the stump. These are worn until the patient receives his prosthesis. The bandage can be of woven cotton or of reinforced elastic, such as an Ace® elastic bandage. The above-knee stump usually requires a six-inch bandage while the below-knee stump generally takes a four-inch bandage. Wrappings are done at least twice daily and are applied so that the pressure is greatest at the tip of the stump and decreases from the distal to the proximal end. It is the job of the nursing staff to follow the physician's instructions in performing stump bandaging, but the physical therapist is also involved in this since she views the patient's condition with regard to future prosthetic fitting.

Prostheses and Their Components

All prostheses must meet certain specific requirements. A list of such requirements includes the following: security from falling during weight-bearing, and the ability to recover from stumbling; minimum consumption of energy during normal ambulation; appearance of as normal an ambulation pattern as possible—one which compares favorably with the gait of a normal person; ability to extend the limb at any time and under any load; proper phasing of the locking action with all portions of the stance and swing phases at all joints; ability to perform incidental operations, such as stair and ramp climbing, pivoting and sitting down; proper cosmetic appearance; structural strength; durability; and proper alignment of components.

There are a great number and variety of standard prostheses for both below-knee and above-knee amputees, a large number of custom variations of these and of specialized components to suit the needs of the individual wearer, and many experimental types. The following is a description of a "standard" lower extremity above-knee prosthesis provided here as an example so that the reader may gain some knowledge of what such a device is composed of.

The *foot* is generally a solid block to which an ankle joint and a toe joint are attached. Typically, ankle joints provide only dorsal and plantar flexion but some models, notably the Habermann design, permit inversion and eversion as well.

The *axis,* or *ankle joint,* is a horizontal shaft with outer ends which rotate in plain bushings, ball bearings or needle bearings. Lateral rotation is added by using two axes at right angles or a single self-aligning ball or roller bearing, or a ball-and-socket joint. Transverse rotation is provided by using solid or hollow rubber blocks, permitting motion around the vertical axes.

The *toe joint* allows toe flexion during the latter part of the stance phase and toe extension as weight-bearing decreases approaching toe-off. The toe section is attached to the foot by simple canvas hinges or by more complex mortise-and-tenon joints. *Torsion* springs, rubber bumpers, or metal or rubber compression springs control toe joint movements. The toe is prevented from bending downward under the force of the springs by a covering or strap which joins the upper surface of the toe with the foot. Sometimes, toes made of rubber or felt are used and these do not require much springs or bumpers to restrain and restore movement.

The *SACH (Solid Ankle, Cushion Heel) foot* is currently seeing much use. Rubber is molded or laminated over a wooden or metal keel. There is no ankle joint and the foot permits eversion, inversion, plantar flexion and dorsiflexion by compression of part of the foot. The heel is made of layers of rubber of varying degrees of hardness. When the heel strikes, the rubber compresses, giving the appearance of ankle motion. The SACH foot is excellent cosmetically, but there is a gradual loss of elasticity in the material used.

In the *knee joint,* stability for weight-bearing is provided by the backward force that the stump exerts in the socket. Alignment of the

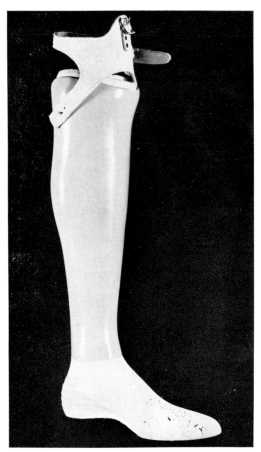

FIGURE 59. Below-knee prosthesis with SACH foot. (*Courtesy of VA Prosthetics Center, New York, N. Y.*)

prosthesis can be made so that the knee is placed in slight hyperextension during weight-bearing. In addition, manual or automatic auxilliary mechanical aids can be used to stabilize the knee by locking it.

There are several types of prosthetic knees which are commercially available. The conventional single axis knee is low in cost and simple to maintain. The friction, or breaking action does not vary during the swing phase of locomotion, and the amount of friction can be easily adjusted. A knee joint which provides constant friction with a friction lock can be used by patients with impaired stump musculature, poor balance or generalized weakness. With this knee the ends of the knee bolt are allowed to slide in a short slot. When the leg bears weight the shank comes closer to the socket and a braking surface of each segment makes contact, forming a "friction lock." During the swing phase a spring holds the two braking surfaces apart. This knee is quite stable and is often used by elderly amputees.

One other type of knee which merits mention is the hydraulic knee which permits an excellent gait. It is highly complex, very costly and not commonly used.

Limitation of knee extension is usually performed by a radial arm or projection fitted around the knee bolt and to the shank which stops the extension movements when the knee strikes it. The impact is reduced by a compressible cushion or bumper between the two parts.

A spring steel arm aids in initiating knee flexion. In addition, it can be designed to assist in bringing the leg into full extension. An elastic strap behind the knee assists in initiating knee flexion, and a similar strap in front of the knee aids in extension. It furthermore prevents excessive heel rise and helps slightly to maintain knee stability during weight-bearing.

Sockets for above-knee prostheses are usually made of willow wood. Today, the "suction socket" is the most commonly used type. It is roughly quadrilateral in shape, conforming to the contour of the upper thigh. With the "total contact socket" the stump is in complete contact with the socket, although most of the weight is borne on the ischeal tuberosities and the gluteal tissue. The socket is suspended by suction, and the valve is flush with the inner wall of the socket. Such sockets seem to provide greater proprioceptive feedback to the patient. They also reduce edema rapidly.

Suspension of the artificial limb may be provided by suction, Silesian bandage, pelvic belt, shoulder suspenders, or a combination of methods. The Silesian bandage is a light band of webbing with one end attached to the lateral aspect of the socket in the region of the greater trochanter, and the other end attached to the socket anteriorly, in the midline, at a point level with the ischeal seat. The belt rests between the crest of the ilium and the trochanter on the unaffected side. It is a valuable aid in stabilizing the prosthesis against rotation and lateral instability, and is sometimes used concurrently with suction. The pelvic belt can be used with a rigid or flexible pelvic band. It is easy to put on and permits the use of one or two stump socks, making the fit more comfortable.

Prosthetic Training

Generally, the amputee who is able to perform a swing-through gait in crutch walking, who can ambulate stairs with crutches, who is motivated for a prosthesis, and who has no medical contraindications

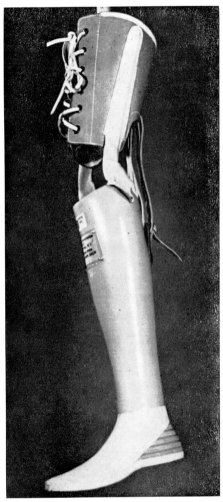

FIGURE 60. Lower extremity prosthesis with SACH foot and thigh corset. *(Courtesy of VA Prosthetics Center, New York, N. Y.)*

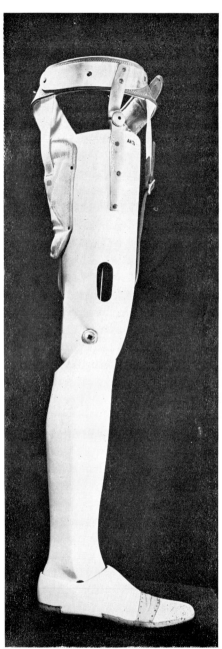

FIGURE 61. Lower extremity prosthesis with pelvic band. *(Courtesy of VA Prosthetics Center, New York, N. Y.)*

to prosthetic use, such as serious cardiac disease, obesity, greatly weakened upper extremities, or poor balance will be a satisfactory candidate for an artificial leg.

The ideal length of an above-knee stump is considered to be about ten to twelve inches from the tip of the greater trochanter. The ideal below-knee stump is felt to be approximately four and one-half to five inches from the medial condyle of the tibia, with the tip of the tibia beveled and the fibular remnant shorter, by at least one half-inch, than the tibia.

As noted previously, the prosthesis can be fitted immediately after surgery, in fact, while the patient is still on the operating table, but the more frequent case is to measure the patient for a prosthesis from eight to ten weeks following surgery. The rehabilitation team and the prosthetist, or limb-maker, decides on the limb which will best meet the requirements imposed by the patient's disability, general health, physical condition and future needs. Often, several sessions with the prosthetist are necessary before a perfect fit is achieved, since only by actually wearing and using the prosthesis can the patient and the rehabilitation staff be certain of its adequacy.

Prosthetic training often begins by fitting the patient with a pylon. A pylon is a "substitute" prosthesis. It consists of a single, or of double uprights, made of wood or aluminum, usually ending in a shoe, sometimes ending in a rubber crutch tip, attached to the patient's stump by a socket which has been measured from a plaster cast taken of the stump. Pylon walking is actually more difficult for many patients than ambulation with a prosthesis and therefore, good performance with the former is almost an assurance that the patient will do well with the latter.

With either a pylon or a prosthesis, particularly in the case of a below-knee amputee, a stump sock is of great importance. This sock is usually made of thickly knitted wool with a fleecy nap on the inside. The stump sock protects the stump against chafing, provides a cushioning effect, absorbs perspiration, and compensates for shrinkage of soft tissues.

Pylon activities begin with the patient in the parallel bars. They start with exercises involving standing balance, hip flexion and extension, and transferring weight from one side to the other, and progress to three-point ambulation, full weight-bearing, four-point ambulation, walking outside of the parallel bars with and without assistance from the therapist or canes, navigating stairs and inclines, sitting down in and rising up from a chair, walking over and around obstacles, walking in different directions, picking up objects from the floor, and turning to the left and to the right.

Training with the actual prosthesis begins with the patient being taught by the therapist how to put the limb on and take it off and how to care for it. Next, standing is initiated in the parallel bars followed by practice in balancing on one leg, shifting weight forward, backward and sideways, taking evenly paced steps, and side-stepping. The patient then performs these activities outside of the parallel bars, first with assistance, then under observation, or "spotting" by the therapist.

Following this phase, negotiation of ramps, steps, curbs, inclines and various ground surfaces is taught, as well as pivoting, rapid movements, overcoming obstacles, and falling and rising from the floor.

As a general rule of thumb, bearing in mind that there is a great deal of individual difference, it can be said that training for a below-knee amputee requires twelve sessions, while eighteen sessions are needed with the above-knee amputee. The bilateral above-knee amputee may require from six to eight weeks of in-patient training. Geriatric patients may need a longer period because of the greater amount of energy they must expend in comparison to a younger person. Each individual has an optimal rate of ambulation which requires the least energy and is most comfortable for him, and this is the rate of choice.

The type of amputation is a consideration in prosthetic training, and the reader is asked to consult the references at the end of this section for training procedures specific to disability types.

THE THERAPIST VIEWS HER WORK

It was stated at the outset of this section that physical therapy lies at the heart of rehabilitation. It might also be said that physical therapy *is* the heart of rehabilitation. Very few patients are discharged from a rehabilitation institution if the physical therapist does not feel that they are ready to be taken off the program.

To the patients physical therapy is the key to their recovery. To the rehabilitation staff it is the service to look to for knowledge of a patient's progress and prospects. To the physical therapist herself— here a quotation from a therapist of the author's acquaintance sums it up nicely: "Yes, it's hard work, tiring, both physically and mentally, and I can't say that sometimes when I'm home I don't wonder if it's all worth it. But when I see a man go from a wheelchair to ambulation, or a woman recovering function and returning to her family, or a child playing for the first time like other children, I somehow don't feel so tired and I no longer wonder about the value of my efforts. Do some other kind of work? Why, I wouldn't change jobs with anyone in the world!"

Section II

References

1. Bierman, W. and Licht, S. (Eds): *Physical Medicine in General Practice*, 3rd ed. New York, Hoeber, Harper, 1952.
2. Bloomberg, M. H.: *Orthopedic Braces: Rationale, Classification and Prescription.* Philadelphia, Lippincott, 1964.
3. Brunnstrom, Signe: *Clinical Kinesiology*, 2nd ed. Philadelphia, Davis, 1966.
4. Buchwald, Edith: *Physical Rehabilitation for Daily Living.* New York, Blakiston, McGraw-Hill, 1952.
5. Daniels, Lucille, Williams, Marian and Worthingham, Catherine: *Muscle Testing: Techniques of Manual Examination*, 2nd ed. Philadelphia, Saunders, 1956.
6. Deaver, G. G.: *Abnormal Gait Patterns. Etiology, Pathology, Diagnosis and Methods of Treatment. Crutches, Braces, Canes and Walkers* (Rehabilitation Monograph XXX). New York, Institute of Rehabilitation Medicine, 1968.
7. Gartland, J. J.: *Fundamentals of Orthopaedics.* Philadelphia, Saunders, 1965.
8. Hollinshead, W. H.: *Functional Anatomy of the Limbs and Back*, 2nd ed. Philadelphia, Saunders, 1960.
9. Humm, W.: *Rehabilitation of the Lower Limb Amputee*, 2nd ed. London, Baillière, Tindall and Cassell, 1969.
10. Kendall, H. O. and Kendall, Florence P.: *Muscles. Testing and Function.* Baltimore, Williams and Wilkins, 1964.
11. Klopsteg, P. E. and Wilson, P. D.: *Human Limbs and Their Substitutes.* New York, Hafner, 1968.
12. Knott, Margaret and Voss, Dorothy E.: *Proprioceptive Neuromuscular Facilitation. Patterns and Techniques*, 2nd ed. New York, Hoeber, Harper, 1968.
13. Krusen, F. H. (Ed): *Physical Medicine and Rehabilitation for the Clinician.* Philadelphia, Saunders, 1951.
14. Licht, S. (Ed): *Electrodiagnosis and Electromyography.* New Haven, Licht, 1956.
15. Licht, S. (Ed): *Massage, Manipulation and Traction.* New Haven, Licht, 1960.
16. Licht, S. (Ed): *Orthotics Etcetera.* New Haven, Licht, 1966.
17. Licht, S. (Ed): *Rehabilitation and Medicine.* New Haven, Licht, 1968.
18. Licht, S. (Ed): *Therapeutic Electricity and Ultraviolet Radiation.* New Haven, Licht, 1959.
19. Licht, S. (Ed): *Therapeutic Exercise*, 2nd ed. New Haven, Licht, 1961.
20. Licht, S. (Ed): *Therapeutic Heat.* New Haven, Licht, 1958.
21. Lovett, R. W.: *The Treatment of Infantile Paralysis*, 2nd ed. Philadelphia, Blakiston, 1917.
22. Lowman, E. W. and Rusk, H. A.: *Self–Help Devices* (Rehabilitation Monograph XXI). New York, Institute of Rehabilitation Medicine, 1967.
23. Moskowitz, E.: *Rehabilitation in Extremity Fractures.* Springfield, Thomas, 1967.
24. Rusk, H. A.: *Rehabilitation Medicine: A Textbook of Physical Medicine and Rehabilitation.* St. Louis, Mosby, 1964.
25. Shestack, R.: *Handbook of Physical Therapy.* New York, Springer, 1967.
26. Shestack, R. and Ditto, E. W.: *Physician's Physical Therapy Manual.* Englewood Cliffs, Prentice-Hall, 1964.
27. *Stedman's Medical Dictionary*, 21st ed. Baltimore, Williams and Wilkins, 1966.

28. Steindler, A.: *Kinesiology of the Human Body. Under Normal and Pathological Conditions.* Springfield, Thomas, 1955.
29. Turek, S. L.: *Orthopaedics. Principles and Their Application,* 2nd ed. Philadelphia, Lippincott, 1967.
30. Williams, Marian and Lissner, H. R.: *Biomechanics of Human Motion.* Philadelphia, Saunders, 1962.
31. Williams, Marian and Worthingham, Catherine: *Therapeutic Exercise for Body Alignment and Function.* Philadelphia, Saunders, 1957.

SECTION III

THE OCCUPATIONAL
THERAPY SERVICE

Chapter 9

INTRODUCTION AND METHODS
OF EVALUATION

Iᴛ ʜᴀs ʙᴇᴇɴ sᴀɪᴅ that occupational therapy is the one service where patients can work in an integrated program involving all of the aspects of rehabilitation. That is, the individual patient is not compartmentalized, but instead brings all of his abilities to bear on the therapeutic tasks prescribed for him. Occupational therapy provides activities for the treatment of the "whole" patient. Other rehabilitation services can also claim, with justification, that without their particular form of therapy or training the patient would not be restored to as complete function as possible and hence, they too are contributing to the treatment of patients *in toto*.

The obvious value of physical therapy, for example, cannot be disputed. However, while other services participate in, and contribute toward, total rehabilitation, it is in occupational therapy that the patient is most able to make use of all of his residual abilities simultaneously, or sequentially, thus transforming limitations into assets. He not only can utilize the specific strengths and skills taught in occupational therapy class, but he also is given the opportunity to employ what he has learned in other therapeutic programs. Occupational therapy is primarily remedial activity devoted to the improvement of a patient's medical, physical, psychological, economic and social conditions; yet it extends beyond the remedial sphere since many of its applications pertain to diagnosis and prevention.

The term "occupational therapy" is a misleading one. It connotes either preparing a person for vocational pursuits or engaging in hobbies, "busywork" and the like. Neither implication is correct. Activity without purpose is not true therapy. To be of therapeutic significance activities must be prescribed by a physician and carried out under the instruction and supervision of a trained professional with the definite purpose of dealing with the specific medical and physical problems of the patient.

Occupational therapy may be defined as any activity, medically prescribed and professionally administered, which assists an individual towards recovery from disabling disease or injury, or which aids an individual towards learning new methods of functioning within the confines of a disability. It is, unquestionably, one of the most crucial aspects of any physical rehabilitation program.

Occupational therapy does not provide exercises merely for exercise's sake, nor does it involve patients in tasks such as crafts for the purpose of producing a material creation or product. In occupational therapy classes, functional skills are used for retraining and re-educating specific muscle groups. It is not the exercise itself nor the end product of any activity which is important, but rather the utilization of such endeavors to increase patient independence, which is vital. When properly prescribed and carried out occupational therapy contributes to total rehabilitation by providing a set of daily activities and exercises aimed at restoring disabled individuals to as normal a level of functioning as possible.

TYPES OF OCCUPATIONAL THERAPY

Occupational therapy in a rehabilitation setting is both supportive and functional in nature and the range of activities which it encompasses is wide.

Supportive Occupational Therapy

Supportive therapy is provided primarily for psychological reasons: to overcome the depression which many rehabilitation patients experience; to provide an atmosphere within which patients can improve psychologically as well as physically; to enable patients to realize their abilities and focus their attention away from their limitations; and to give patients the opportunity to prove to themselves, through normal experiences, that they will be able to return to, and compete successfully in, their society.

Functional Occupational Therapy

The primary purpose of occupational therapy in rehabilitation medicine is to contribute to patient independence through a functional program which utilizes residual abilities following injury or disease. Functional occupational therapy may be subdivided into three main groups or categories of activity in accordance with their objectives.

The aim of *kinetic occupational therapy* is to restore or improve muscle strength, joint mobilization, coordination and posture through specific exercises and activities. Included within this category are many of the activities of daily living (ADL), arts and crafts work, the utilization of splints, braces and self-help devices, and upper extremity prosthetic training.

The goals of *metric occupational therapy* are three fold: improvement of work tolerance; measurement of improvement in work tolerance; and assessment of work tolerance potential. Prevocational tasks are also subsumed under this heading, as are homemaking activities, although both of these forms of therapy have additional kinetic aspects.

The main objective of *tonic occupational therapy* is the improvement and maintenance of genral muscle tone and psychological alertness for patients who are chronically bedridden or who must, for medical reasons, delay active rehabilitation for a period of time. It involves keeping the patient active in the normal, routine daily activities which most non-hospitalized persons engage in, such as reading, some grooming activities, etc.

THE INITIAL EVALUATION PROCEDURE

Upon a patient's admission to the rehabilitation hospital he is evaluated as to his physical function and potential by the occupational therapist. This evaluation serves the dual purpose of determining the feasibility of accepting the patient to active rehabilitation and of formulating a therapy program based upon the physician's prescription.

The following descriptions of initial occupational therapy evauations are not intended to reflect the procedures of any single institution, but are meant to provide the reader with a general picture of the kinds of assessments which are made. The Occupational Therapy Service of some hospitals may be less thorough in their examination, while others might include additional tests. The evaluation presented herein may be considered as being "typical" if the realization is borne in mind that procedures can vary widely between institutions. Furthermore, not all new patients require the same evaluation. Certain disabilities call for using specific tests and measures which are not necessary for other kinds of disorders, and, of course, each patient must be treated as a unique individual.

The first type of evaluation to be discussed will be a general one, followed by a description of the specifics involved in the assessment of some particular disabilities.

Evaluation of Range of Motion

The Upper Extremities

The therapist may begin her assessment by measuring the patient's ability to flex and extend her shoulder. She places one hand on the patient's shoulder so as to fix the scapula, the flat, triangular bone at the base of the shoulder, and one hand under the elbow to provide support, and flexes the patient's elbow to ninety degrees.

The patient is required to abduct his elbow, or lift it out from the side and away from his body. If the patient's elbow can be conducted to shoulder level, he is asked to carry his hand across his body and touch the opposite shoulder while maintaining his arm in a parallel position to the floor. With the arm remaining in the same plane, the patient must then push his elbow back as far as is possible.

(Note: As with physical therapy, there are primarily two types of range of motion activities. *Active* range of motion is that performed by the patient, unassisted. *Passive* range of motion is the excursion of a joint as performed by the therapist upon the patient. Another type is *painful range of motion,* included typically in evaluations performed by British-trained therapists. A patient may actively extend a joint a given number of degrees and, with the aid of the therapist, the joint might be extended further. However, a point may be reached between these two states at which the patient experiences pain during extension. This painful threshold is noted by the therapist.)

It should be noted at this point that range of motion is measured by the occupational therapist in terms of degrees. Anatomical position is the starting point. Canada is considered to be zero degrees and cranium is considered as ninety degrees. Rotating motions are measured from the zero degrees of the midsagittal plane, the anteroposterior postion parallel to the long axis of the body, to the 180 degrees of the lateral plane.

The simplest technique for measuring range of joint motion is with the use of an instrument known as a goniometer, or arthrometer. This consists of two shafts fastened together by a bolt, or wing-nut, permitting free movement of the shafts around a full circle. The extent of movement of an extremity is measured by a scale on the jointed end of the instrument. In examining range of motion the joint and shaft are placed on the corresponding anatomic parts of the measured extremity and the range is read directly from the attached scale. The advantage to such a device is its ease of usage, while its primary disadvantage results from the fact that it measures joint excursion in only one plane. For circular and other complex motions other kinds of instrumentation are required.

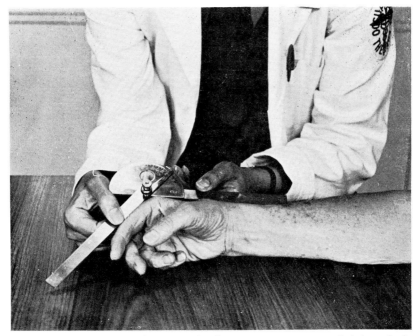

FIGURE 62. Measuring range of motion in the metacarpophaiangeal joint of the first finger with a goniometer.

Now, to continue with the evaluation procedure. Following flexion and extension of the shoulder, the patient is required to adduct his elbow, or draw it in toward the side of his body from an abducted angle of ninety degrees.

Shoulder rotation is assessed by having the patient abduct his arm to ninety degrees, turn his palm up to the side of his head as far as is possible and then turn his palm down until it is facing backwards. He next must place his elbows at the sides of his body and flex them to ninety degrees, turn his forearms out from his body and turn them in across his body. If he is able, the patient will be requested to place his hands behind his back, exhibiting medial rotation, and also down the back of his neck, providing a measure of lateral rotation.

Shoulder elevation is measured by requiring the patient to raise his arms straight up over his head through both flexion and extension.

Circumduction, or circular movement of a limb, is evaluated by having the patient place his finger tips on his shoulders and rotate his elbows. The therapist's hands may add resistance or serve only as support.

Elbow flexion is examined with the therapist holding the patient's arm above the elbow and above the wrist. The patient brings his hand to his mouth without moving his head towards the hand and straightens his elbow as fully as possible in extension.

Range of motion in the radio-ulnar joints, those formed by articulation of the two bones of the forearm, the radius and the ulna, is tested by asking the patient to turn his palms upward and downward. The therapist can provide resistance to these movements by supporting the patient's elbow and grasping his hand, splinting the wrist with her index and middle fingers.

In examining wrist motion the therapist fixes the radio-ulnar joints with her hand while the patient flexes and extends his wrists and demonstrates radial and ulnar deviations. Both sets of movements are performed against gravity and are checked by the therapist who provides resistance.

In evaluating the hand, the therapist holds the patient's wrist while he performs certain tasks, such as curling his fingers over a pencil and holding them in that position, holding a piece of paper between the thumb and each of the fingers, keeping the fingers spread and extended against resistance, and placing the hand flat on a table and extending the fingers individually.

The Lower Extremities

Although evaluation of the lower extremities is primarily the concern of the physical therapist, as has been pointed out, there are many tasks of occupational therapy which require good function in the lower limbs. Therefore, in this phase of the evaluation procedure, there is some overlapping of responsibility between the two services. This is true also of the initial assessment of trunk, neck and back function, which is discussed in the following section.

In examining the lower extremities it is best, for most tests, if the patient reclines on a plinth.

In the hip, flexion is tested by requesting the patient to draw his knees up to his chest. For the measurement of hip extension, the patient lies in a supine position and pushes his leg straight down onto the plinth with the therapist's hand placed under the heel of his foot. He then presses the heel down on the plinth and tries to prevent his leg from being raised. Following this effort he turns over to a prone position and raises his leg off the plinth.

The evaluation of hip abduction consists of the therapist placing the patient in supination, holding his ankles together and then trying to separate them. The patient also lies on his side with his legs slightly extended and tries to raise his leg from the plinth. Additionally, he is requested to stand, if possible, and ambulate for a few steps, primarily to detect the presence of a Trendelenburg symptom, a waddling gait caused by paralysis of the gluteal muscles.

The ability of the patient to adduct his hip is assessed by the therapist attempting to keep together, and then to separate the patient's ankles while the latter is in a supine position. In addition, the patient lies on the affected side with the uninvolved leg supported in abduction, and tries to raise the affected leg off the bed to touch the leg held by the therapist.

An indication of hip rotation can be obtained by having the patient roll his legs inwardly and outwardly while they are slightly abducted.

All of the above tests can be administered with the therapist supplying resistance if she feels it is required, or assistance, if instability is observed during certain movements.

Movements of the knee are evaluated in several ways. The patient lies supinely on the plinth and pulls his heel towards his trunk while keeping it on the bed. Next, he lifts his heel off the bed. Resistance may be added by the therapist. If the patient has sufficient muscle strength, he may be asked to raise his leg off the plinth while keeping it straight. These movements are repeated with the patient in pronation and also with him seated on the edge of the bed so as to obtain a good measure of knee extension.

Ankle testing begins with the therapist holding the patient's leg above the ankle and providing resistance over the dorsum and on the sole of the foot. The patient pulls his foot up toward the tibia in dorsiflexion and extends his toes downward in plantar flexion, both with the knee held in extension and also with it flexed to ninety degrees while he lies in pronation. Ankle dorsiflexion is also tested against gravity as the patient sits with his involved leg off the plinth.

In another test, the therapist holds the patient's ankles and adds resistance at the first and fifth metatarsal heads while the patient inverts his foot, or turns it inward toward the midline of his body, and then everts it, or turns it outward, away from the midline.

The evaluation of toe movements requires that the therapist firmly hold the patient's foot in order to prevent movement at the mid-tarsal joints. The patient curls his toes and holds them positioned against resistance, and then stretches his toes, again holding them against resistance.

The Trunk, Back and Neck

Abdominal muscle testing is conducted with the patient lying in supination, with his arms folded across his chest. He must first try to sit up and then attempt to lift both legs off the plinth while keeping his knees straight. Resistance can be added manually by the therapist or by having the patient change the position of the patient's arms.

In the examination of the back the patient lies prone and raises first his head and shoulders, and then both legs off the plinth. The therapist can add resistance.

Anterior neck evaluation involves the patient raising his head off the plinth while resistance is applied to his forehead. Measurement of posterior neck function requires the patient to raise his head from the prone position and lower it against resistance applied at the back of the head.

Grading of Muscle Strength

Movements involving muscular ability are measured and recorded in terms of the tasks involved, such as the length of time required for flexion and extension and the number of degrees accomplished in these activities, length of reach, position of the extremities during motions, the type or pattern of placement and manipulation of objects of various sizes, and the like.

Muscle strength may be graded in several ways. Occupational therapists who work in Great Britain, or India, or in other nations which employ the British system, use the following scale:

0   No muscle contraction noted.
1   Flicker of muscle but no actual movement.
2   Middle range movement with gravity eliminated.
3   Muscle is able to act against gravity.
4   Good; muscle can act against gravity and some resistance.
5   Full strength.

In the United States there are primarily three systems of muscle grading. Muscle power can be measured on a scale from zero to five, or from zero per cent to one hundred per cent, both of which roughly correspond to the British system, and it can also be measured by the Lovett scale, the 1916 revision of which is described in Chapter 4. Further refinement of the Lovett grades is achieved by modifying each grade with a *plus* or *minus,* as in *fair plus* or *good minus.*

Muscles which are spastic will not present an accurate picture of their true strength when measured by this method. The presence and degree of spasticity in a muscle is indicated on an evaluation report by the symbols *S* or *SS,* and the presence and degree of contractures is denoted by *C* or *CC.*

In grading the muscle power of a hemiplegic patient it is often necessary to add certain values to the Lovett scale or other systems of grading. These values are as follows: *S*—spastic; *F*—flaccid; *A*—atrophied; and *P*—painful. They are rated on a scale of from 1, indicating the least amount, to 4, meaning the most amount. Such designations are also required when reporting on the muscular status of patients with quadriplegia, paraplegia and, in fact, any neuromuscular disorder.

The main drawback of clinical muscle tests is that they test only a single performance or action of a muscles strength and, hence, do not provide information regarding endurance. For the latter evaluation repetitive testing must be conducted.

Evaluation of the Hemiplegic Patient

Prior to actual testing, the occupational therapist reads the patient's medical chart to become familiar with the history of the disability, consequences of the disability, complications, current medical and psychological problems, and other pertinent data. She particularly notes the date of onset of the cerebrovascular accident which resulted in the hemiplegia, since time is an important factor in the recovery of the stroke patient, and she will record the patient's plegic side and his naturally dominant side so as to be able to fairly judge his abilities.

The therapist determines whether or not the patient's paretic or plegic upper extremity is functional for self-care. She observes the patient's movements to detect the presence of shoulder subluxation, or partial dislocation, which would cause pain and restriction of function. The patient is asked to raise his involved hand to his mouth, raise it overhead, place it behind his neck, and place it on the contralateral knee, wrist, elbow and shoulder. Length of forward reach and degrees of flexion are also measured at this time.

The amount of time required for elbow flexion and extension, pronation and supination, and range of motion in the elbow joint are recorded.

In evaluating wrist function the therapist notes the stability of the joint, the time the patient requires to flex and extend his wrist, and any deviations which are present.

Gross hand function is assessed by having the patient pick up and release blocks of various sizes, usually ranging from one and one-half inches to three inches in diameter. The therapist particularly observes the position of the patient's wrist as he performs this task. Fine pick-up requires that the patient lift one hundred small pegs, one-eighth of an inch in diameter, and place and release them into holes in a pegboard. The therapist is concerned here with the amount of time needed by the patient to complete the task, the type of pick-up used (which fingers were used in opposition to make the pick-up, how the grasp was made, etc.), and the type of placement (directly into the hole on the board, rebounding into the hole from another peg or hole, fumbling or incoordinated placement, etc.). The length of time required at this task by the patient is measured for both the affected and unaffected upper extremities, thus enabling the therapist to judge the patient's abilities by comparative measures.

Isolated finger movements are examined by having the patient ascend and descend a finger ladder, which is, literally, a miniature ladder, with each finger and then with the fingers in sequence.

Resisted pinch is also scored. The patient grasps a three-quarter-inch theraplast ball, a synthetic, rubberlike ball used for hand exercises, and brings together his thumb and each of his fingers in a pincer-like grasp. The therapist notes the opposition, the apposition, or placement of adjacent fingers so that they can come into contact following opposition, overlap in the pinch, and hyperextension of the fingers.

In determining the neuromuscular status of the hemiplegic patient the occupational therapist is concerned primarily with the following muscles and their functions:

Sternocleidomastoid	Flexes the vertebral column and rotates the head.
Trapezius	Rotates the scapula to raise the shoulder in abduction of the arm and draws the scapula backward.
Rhomboidus major	Retracts and elevates the scapula.
Rhomboidus minor	Adducts and elevates the scapula.
Infraspinatus	Laterally rotates the humerus.
Supraspinatus	Abducts the humerus.
Latissimus dorsi	Adducts, extends and medially rotates the humerus.
Pectoralis major	Adducts, flexes and medially rotates the arm.
Pectoralis minor	Draws the shoulder forward and downward.
Serratus anterior	Draws the scapula forward and rotates the scapula to raise the shoulder in arm abduction.
Deltoids	Abduct, flex and extend the arm.

Coracobrachialis	Flexes and abducts the arm.
Brachialis	Flexes the forearm.
Brachioradialis	Flexes the forearm.
Biceps brachii	Flexes the forearm and supinates the hand.
Triceps brachii	Extends the forearm and adducts and extends the arm.
Biceps femoris	Flexes the leg and extends the thigh.
Soleus	Plantar flexes the ankle joint.
Gastrocnemius	Plantar flexes the ankle joint and flexes the knee joint.

(Note: The term *triceps surae* is used for the soleus and the gastrocnemius taken together.)

In addition, the therapist evaluates the flexor and extensor muscles of the wrist, fingers and thumb, the abductor and adductor muscles of the fingers and thumb, and the internal and external rotator muscles of the shoulder.

Facial muscles are examined for spasticity or flaccidity. This latter possibility is of importance, particularly in the case of facial nerve weakness, because many patients eventually get return of muscle power on the affected side. Knowing this, the occupational therapist will want to splint that side so as to prevent the unaffected side of the face from stretching the weak side and causing it to lose elasticity. If elasticity of the muscles is lost, when sensation and strength return to the involved side it, will remain distorted. Proper splinting procedures will prevent this from occurring.

Assessment of sensation and perception is a key phase of the initial evaluation process with hemiplegic patients since there is invariably some loss of sensation on the involved side of the body.

Tactile sensibility, or the sense of touch, is tested on the hands and fingers through the use of an instrument known as a pressure esthesiometer. This device consists of a series of plastic (or glass) rods with a nylon bristle imbedded in the end of each rod. The bristles are graded in width from 1.65 to 6.65 mm/pressure per unit cell. The therapitst holds a rod and touches the patient with the bristle, bending it so as to produce sensation. The patient keeps his eyes closed and reports whether or not he feels the touch of the bristle. Testing is carried out on the palmar and dorsal sides of both hands and all fingers, including the thumb. The thinner the bristle which the patient is able to feel, the less impaired is his tactile sense.

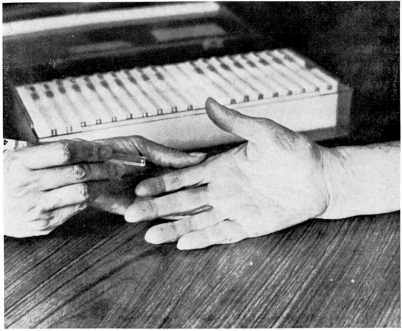

FIGURE 63. Testing pressure sense with an aesthesiometer.

In testing stereognosis, or recognition of the nature and form of objects by touch and handling, the patient is told to cover his eyes and pick up and name a set of objects and place them in a box. The objects vary, but typically include a safety pin, a coin, or coins of different denominations, a paper clip, a plastic pen, a pencil, a piece of leather, a piece of elastic, a piece of cloth, a string, a nail, a screw, a button, and a key. After the patient has completed the task with his eyes closed, he repeats it with his eyes open. The therapist notes errors which indicate loss of sensation, position sense problems and visual field defects.

A two-point discrimination test is also administered in evaluating sensory function. The measuring instrument can be a pair of pins, a compass, or a small pair of calipers. The patient is touched on various parts of his body and extremities with both points simultaneously. With his eyes closed he must state whether he felt one point or two, and where on his body the sensation occurred. The smaller the distance between the two points which the patient can distinguish as two distinct sensations, the better is his discrimination ability.

Values differ depending upon the part of the body being stimulated. In people with normal sensation two points can usually be distinguished at 0.3 to 0.5 centimeters apart on the finger tips, 0.8 to 1.2

centimeters apart on the palm, 4.0 to 5.0 centimeters apart on the back, and 4.0 to 6.0 centimeters apart on the shins. The occupational therapist can determine a patient's impairment by observing how far his responses to stimulation differ from the norm.

Graphesthesia, or the sense by which figures or numbers written on the skin is recognized, is also assessed. With the patient's eyes closed, the therapist "writes" on his skin with the blunt end of a pen or pencil, or with a stylus. She may trace letters, numbers of figures, and the patient reports what he feels or imitates to examiner by tracing on her hand. Such a test is more complex and involves a finer tactile sense than does the two-point discrimination task. It is usually conducted on the palmar surface of the hand.

Sensation in the joints is measured in two ways. One method, notably used with metacarpal joints, involves the therapist moving the joint through a wide range of motion, telling the patient whether his finger is "up" (raised), or "down" (lowered). Next, she moves the joint while the patient has his eyes covered, and he must report to her whether or not the joint has been moved and the direction of movement.

Vibration sense in the joints is assessed by striking a tuning fork and placing it against the joint. The patient reports his perception of the sensation. Both proximal and distal joints of the extremities are examined in this way.

Body part and spatial orientation is necessary for performance of many occupational therapy tasks. To evaluate this ability the therapist may ask a patient to walk between two parallel lines drawn on the floor, or to walk around obstacles which she places in his way. The patient will also be required to imitate body and limb positions modeled by the therapist. A patient will be considered more integrated in terms of his body and space if he can correctly copy the therapist's movements while facing her, than if he can only do it when facing in the same direction.

Another test requires the patient to follow a series of commands, such as placing his right hand on his left knee and vice versa, touching his left cheek with his right hand and vice versa, and so on. Many institutions additionally administer a wire-and-grommet test in which the length of time is measured which the patient requires to push an angular wire through a rubber grommet.

The most common visual field defect occurring with stroke hemiplegia is hemianopsia, usually homonymous in nature, where there is blindness for the right or left half of the visual field of each eye. Problems of this kind are detected by the therapist as the patient performs various tasks. If while picking up objects during the testing of stereognosis he only selects those which lie in the right visual field, this would tend to indicate a left homonymous hemianopsia. When the patient is engaged in activities involving fine finger dexterity, such as picking up small pegs and placing them in holes of a pegboard, if he only places them in the holes on the left side of the board, a conclusion of right homonymous hemianopsia may be warranted. Reading also provides clues to a visual field defect. The patient who begins reading in the center of a page and the patient who does not read all the way to the right-hand side of the page, both demonstrate hemianopsia. The former performance indicates a left, and the latter a right, visual field defect.

Evaluation of the Quadriplegic Patient

It must be understood that in evaluating the patient with quadriplegia or quadriparesis the occupational therapist administers many of the same tests that she does in evaluating the hemiplegic patient. That is, she is still concerned with muscle strength and range of motion, and hence, assesses these variables in the same way that she would with any patient disability. The main difference with quadriplegia is that there is more extensive involvement. While the hemiplegic patient has paralysis or weakness on one side of the body, and thus in two extremities, the quadriplegic individual is affected in all four extremities as well as in the trunk muscles of both sides of the body. Therefore, while procedures may be basically similar as those employed in testing the hemiplegic, quadriplegic patients necessarily require more extensive assessment. In addition, certain tests may have to be modified or even omitted because the patient's paralysis does not permit him to take them.

The occupational therapist assesses strength and range of motion for all extremities and the trunk. This includes the following: shoulder flexion, extension, abduction, adduction, internal rotation and external rotation; elbow flexion and extension; forearm pronation and supination; wrist flexion, extension, radial deviation and ulnar deviation; hand grasp, release and tenodesis grasp, which is comprised of wrist extension and flexion of the index and middle fingers in opposition to the thumb; finger flexion, extension, abduction and adduction; and thumb abduction, adduction, flexion, extension and opposition. In addition, she evaluates trunk balance, sitting posture, work tolerance, and the level of the spinal cord at which sensory loss begins.

The patient is also administered tests which involve grasping objects with his hand and forming a pinch grip with his thumb and fingers.

He will be asked to perform, or to attempt certain activities of daily living. Grooming includes combing the hair, washing, shaving, or putting on cosmetics in the case of a female patient, and brushing the teeth. Dressing means not only putting on a shirt and pants or a dress, but managing zippers, buttons, and snaps, tying shoelaces and tying a necktie. Eating activities are comprised of cutting meat, eating a sandwich, drinking from a cup and using a spoon. Communication assessment requires that the patient write and/or type a letter, fold it and place it in an envelope.

Evaluations are both clinical and functional in nature. That is, the therapist is interested in both the strength of muscle groups and the range of motion in the extremities, but in addition, she is concerned with how the patient uses his affected and unaffected body parts. It is not unusual to find a patient progressing well clinically but not utilizing his abilities in a functional way.

The Initial Evaluation in Activities of Daily Living

It is essential for the occupational therapist to conduct an evaluation in the activities of daily living (ADL). This assesses a patient's ability to function with respect to the tasks of everyday life, and thus provides the therapist with information regarding the number and kinds of activities which he can or cannot do at home and at work. The results obtained from ADL testing also serve the therapist as a guide in the planning of a treatment program.

The major areas of evaluation are bed activities, wheelchair and transfer activities, self-care activities, ambulation activities and elevation activities.

Testing involves requesting the patient to engage in various behaviors. The therapist does not accept the patient's statements as to whether he is able or unable to perform, but requires him to actually do, or attempt to do each activity.

The evaluation of the patient in bed activities necessitates that the patient lie down on a bed and rise himself to a sitting position. He must also roll to his right and to his left and turn over onto his abdomen. In addition, the patient is asked to demonstrate how he manages pillows, sheets and blankets, how he reaches for objects on an adjoining nightstand and whether or not he can turn a lamp on and off.

Wheelchair activities include propelling the chair forward and backward and making proper turns, opening a door, passing through the doorway and closing the door behind, and going up and down a ramp in a wheelchair.

Transfer activities in the home include the following: transferring from a wheelchair to a straight chair and back to the wheelchair; transferring from a wheelchair to an easy chair or a sofa and back; transferring from a wheelchair to a toilet and back, including adjustment and readjustment of clothing; and transferring from a wheelchair to a bathtub or a stall shower and back.

Transfer activities of travel mean that the patient must transfer from a wheelchair to a car and back to the wheelchair with and without the use of a curb, including placing the chair in the car and back again on the pavement.

Self-care activities can be subdivided into several main categories.

Hygiene, or bathroom activities involve combing and brushing the hair, brushing the teeth, shaving or applying cosmetics, turning a faucet, washing and drying the hands, face, body and extremities, taking a bath or shower, and using a urinal or bedpan.

Eating activities are assessed by having the patient actually eat with a knife, fork and spoon, demonstrating the ability to cut meat and use utensils properly, and drink from a glass or cup or use a straw.

Dressing activities are evaluated by requiring the individual to dress himself fully from undergarments to outer wear, fastening all snaps, buttons, buckles, zippers and hooks correctly. Included herein is putting on and removing braces, prostheses, orthotic devices, corsets and any other aids or appliances which the patient might require or regularly use.

Elevation activities refer to sitting and standing, and this is what the therapist instructs the patient to do: sit on and stand up from a wheelchair, bed, straight chair, easy chair, sofa, chair at a table, toilet, car seat and floor.

In addition, the patient must perform climbing and travelling activities, such as ascending and descending a flight of stairs with and without the use of a handrail; he must also be able to enter and leave a car and a taxicab, enter a bus, take a seat, rise from the seat and leave the bus, walk one block and return and step down from a curb, cross the street and step up on the other curb.

Indoor ambulation activities require the patient to operate a door, pass through the doorway and close the door behind him, walk down a hallway or corridor, leave the building and walk outside. All ambulation and elevation activities are performed unassisted or with a cane or a crutch if the patient routinely uses such aids.

(Note: Once again there is some overlap of function between the occupational therapist and the physical therapist. With the team approach to rehabilitation these disciplines can work together for the patient's benefit.)

There are several other activities which people engage in as part of their daily routines and the occupational therapist is interested in how the patient functions in these areas. They include putting on, taking off and winding a wristwatch or pocket watch, managing a pipe, cigar or cigarette and matches or a lighter, opening, reading and carrying a book and a newspaper, using a handkerchief, turning on and off lights of various types, such as a wall switch, pullchain, and button-depression type, using a public telephone, and handling a wallet or purse and their contents, such as coins, paper money, identification cards, licenses and credit cards.

ADL evaluations are important not only because they determine the individual's ability to function in daily life, but also because they provide additional information regarding range of motion in the joints and muscle strength. There are many activities which a person may perform during the day which involve different types of muscular acts than the ones which are formally assessed by the therapist. This point is best illustrated by examples.

When a patient uses his affected arm to remove a coat or jacket and to hang it on a high hook, it reveals limitations of shoulder elevation and elbow extension. The act of eating can indicate to the therapist problems of elbow flexion and forearm supination. Wrist and hand dexterity is demonstrated in managing buttons, hooks and zippers. Tucking in a shirttail at the back supplies information regarding shoulder extension and medial rotation. Shoulder flexion limitations and problems of shoulder extension in abduction and lateral rotation are exhibited when a man puts on a necktie and turns down his shirt collar. A simple act, such as placing a handkerchief in a breast pocket, demonstrates elbow flexion and forearm supination.

Irregularities in rhythm or stride are seen when the patient ambulates a short distance. Tying and removing shoes can be accomplished in several ways, such as by crouching down, sitting on a chair and lifting a knee, placing foot on a chair and bending down, or balancing on one leg. Depending upon how the act is performed it points up any stiffness in hip, knee or ankle flexion, weakness of hip and knee flexor muscles and ankle dorsiflexors, and balance problems.

In the observation of all activities the occupational therapist is looking for possible causes of difficulty, such as muscle weakness, joint stiffness, contractures, deformities, pain, anxiety or poor habits.

A final point to be made concerning the initial evaluation: while not all tests are always necessary to be administered to every patient, many, if not most rehabilitation hospitals do, in fact, conduct every measure described in this chapter. The rationale for doing so is a good one—namely, that unless all examinations are given, a disability or limitation might escape notice, thus depriving the patient of an important part of his occupational therapy program. For example, it might be thought to be unnecessary to administer all tests of sensation and perception to an amputee since there is presumably not the loss in sensation which is expected of the hemiplegic patient or the patient with a spinal cord injury. Yet, through such testing, the therapist may detect a sensory impairment secondary to diabetes, and, as a consequence of this finding, will want to include certain occupational therapy activities as part of the patient's rehabilitation program to increase sensitivity or to teach the patient to compensate for his losses.

In assessing the capabilities of patients with certain neuromuscular diseases, such as multiple sclerosis and myasthenia gravis, the therapist typically will not only give a complete evaluation but will use repeated testing techniques to ascertain work tolerance and fatigue threshold, since these are important variables in properly planning a therapy program for such patients.

As with any diagnostic procedure, which, in fact, is what an evaluation essentially is, it is wise not to omit any test which can possibly provide information useful to the therapist in helping a patient.

THE OCCUPATIONAL THERAPY RE-EVALUATION

Following the physician's prescription, the patient is placed on an occupational therapy program and a date is set, usually within six weeks, for re-evaluation of his status. At the re-evaluation conference, which was described in Chapter 5, the occupational therapist presents her observations and measurements to the other members of the rehabilitation team.

The therapist has recorded the findings obtained at the initial evaluation on a chart, and in adjoining columns of the chart has noted current muscle power, range of joint motion and ADL skills. Thus, she is able to read across the rows of the chart and compare the patient's present condition with his status at the initial evaluation upon admission to the hospital. Her report to the rehabilitation team typically begins with a brief summary of the earlier findings, followed by a detailed description of the patient's current capabilities.

The attending physical will, on the basis of the therapist's report, decide to modify his initial prescription, let it remain the same, or perhaps discontinue occupational therapy as a part of the patient's total rehabilitation program. His modifications are primarily a result of the therapist's report, but changes in the patient's home situation, psychological condition, medical status, and other factors can influence his decision.

At the conclusion of the conference a date is arranged for the next re-evaluation and in this way all rehabilitation team members are kept periodically informed of the patient's progress in occupational therapy.

———————————

Chapter 10

EXERCISES AND ACTIVITIES

THE OCCUPATIONAL THERAPY PRESCRIPTION is accorded the same considerations as that written for physical therapy. Following the therapist's report at the initial evaluation conference, the physician will prescribe a program of occupational therapy for the patient under consideration. It is important to note here that occupational therapy is never conducted in the absence of a medical prescription. The prescription includes the patient's name, age, sex, diagnosis, present physical status and general condition, and is as specific as possible in its directions so as to avoid errors in communication between the physician and the therapeutic staff.

The prescription includes the reasons for which an activity is prescribed, or its objectives, and the expected results. If, in order to achieve a desired therapeutic goal, technical modifications of tools or equipment are necessary, the physician will include this, describing in detail the changes which need to be made. Precautions which the physician feels the therapist should take are written into the prescription, including health conditions such as cardiac disease and recent suturing. The patient's work tolerance is specified, and the duration and frequency of treatments is indicated on the prescription form.

The physician states his desire for emphasis on range of motion activities, muscle strengthening, coordination activities or ADL. In prescribing ADL training he indicates whether the activities should be performed while the patient is in bed, or in an occupational therapy shop, while ambulating, or in a wheelchair, and what specific limitations will be encountered.

Any increases or decreases in work load or tempo, or changes in the nature of the occupational therapy program are medically prescribed, as are activities in a pre-vocational shop which many institutions have. Prescribing of orthotic devices, self-help aids and the like is also done by the physician, and their usage is included in the occupational therapy order.

It is very difficult, if not impossible, to describe either a "typical" occupational therapy program, or a list of all of the activities which are comprised under the rubric of occupational therapy. This is the case because the number and kinds of activities which can be prescribed for patients differ, depending upon the individual's condition, needs, and the muscles and joints which require therapy, and also because the imaginative therapist will continually devise new tasks and materials to meet the requirements of her patients. Furthermore, not all of the activities and exercises of occupational therapy are practical or feasible for all patients since the prescription for occupational therapy is dependent upon the specific disability under consideration.

This chapter will discuss, in general, the various occupational therapy exercises, activities and ADL tasks.

PRINCIPLES OF OCCUPATIONAL THERAPY

It is important for any occupational therapy activity to produce the desired objective. That is, mere action does not suffice. All activities must be designed to permit motion to be localized, primarily, in the affected joint or joints, or they must strengthen certain muscles or muscle groups. In addition, they must possess most of the following characteristics:

Provide action rather than position. If range of motion in a joint or strength of a muscle is to be increased the prescribed activity must provide for the alternate contraction and relaxation of muscles. An affected extremity should not be held in only one position, but in alternating positions of flexion and extension.

Provide repetition of motion. An activity should permit repetition of the required movement for any given number of times. The actual frequency of repetitions is theoretically unlimited, but is controlled by the therapist.

Permit gradation in range of motion of the joint. The activity should provide for a greater range of motion than that allowed by limitation of the joint. This permits an increase of motion at the involved joint as the range improves until normal movement is regained or approximated.

Permit gradation in the resistance of muscles. Muscle strengthening can only be achieved by increasing the amount of resistance given by the therapist or by the tools or materials which a patient uses in an activity.

Permit gradation in coordination. In this case, the muscle exercise required by the prescribed activity should be graded from gross to fine movements.

In the grading of treatment activities for the strengthening of muscles, the following principles are important:

If a muscle is to become stronger it must be tired by exercise. Over fatigue, however, is to be avoided. The symptoms of overfatigue include redness, pain, swelling, heat and tremor in the involved part, decrease in range of motion, restlessness, irritability, perspiration on the forehead and upper lip, and a lack of attention.

If all fibers of a muscle are to be improved, exercise should be performed against heavy resistance.

If all muscle fibers are to receive exercise, the involved body part must go through the complete range of motion.

The goal of treatment should be to help develop as much strength and endurance as existed in the involved part prior to disease or injury. Full return of function is almost always unattainable but the therapist must never set her goals short of the maximum possibility.

The priniciples of grading treatment for increasing range of joint movement are as follows:

The range of motion used in an activity must be increased in order to obtain increases in range of motion of a joint. Each time the body part is moved the joint should pass through the fullest possible range.

Once the acute phase of illness has passed, the prescribed activities should require stretching of the involved joints in the direction of their limitation.

Additional principles of grading treatment include:

In increasing muscle coordination, the amount of muscle coordination required by an activity should be increased as the condition under treatment improves.

In developing special skills the unique skills or motions normally employed by the patient is daily life should be incorporated into the treatment program as soon as he is able to do them.

In developing work tolerance the general requirements of the patient's home and work situations should be considered in his treatment.

TYPES OF EXERCISES

There are four main kinds of exercises which are prescribed for patients who are participating in an occupational therapy program.

1. *Passive* movements are performed by the therapist for the patient and require no muscle contraction by the patient.

2. *Assistive* exercises are performed by the patient to the limit of

his ability and the range is then completed by the therapist or, in some cases, by apparatus.

3. *Active* movements are those which are performed entirely by the patient and which require no more power than is used in making a movement through its complete range of motion.

4. *Resistive* exercises involve actions which are performed by the patient against resistance provided by an outside agent, such as the therapist or apparatus. Activities which make use of tools are also considered resistive.

The first form of exercise which is administered to a weakened muscle is passive motion, followed by assistive, then active, and finally, resistive movements. If early active motion is questionable

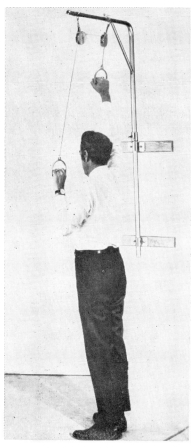 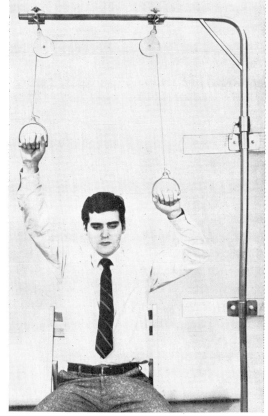

FIGURE 64. Overhead pulley system being used by an ambulatory patient on the left and a wheelchair-bound patient at right. *(Reprinted by permission of J. A. Preston Corp., 1971)*

for a patient, occupational therapy is administered in token quantities at first and is significantly increased on succeeding days in both resistance and duration. Gradual progression is always the rule.

Electrical stimulation of a muscle can influence its volume and massage may affect its suppleness, but only active exercise will increase its strength. How rapidly a muscle or group of muscles is strengthened depends upon the number, rate and duration of daily contractions and upon the amount of resistance which is overcome by the muscles during work. Muscles can accomplish the most over a long period of work when adequate rest intervals are provided. As therapy progresses, rest intervals become more closely simulated to resemble "real" work situations, in which rest is rhythmic and integrated into the activity. Occupational therapy is directed toward the strengthening of groups of muscles which operate synergistically, and activities are prescribed which require the interplay of muscles and muscle groups.

With the exception of joints which have become fixed as a consequence of irreversible osseous changes, most joints of limited range can benefit from passive or active stretching. Some joint limitations, such as those which have resulted from shortening of the flexor tendons or other deep tissue contractures, will require passive manipulation or surgery. The physical therapist may initiate passive stretching of a joint, particularly in the lower extremities, but occupational therapy provides auxilliary stretching which further increases range and maintains gains which have been achieved. If joint limitation is a result of enforced rest or disuse, as is the case in some severe disabilities, the active exercises of occupational therapy will improve the range of motion or maintain gains accomplished through stretching.

The type of exercise which is prescribed for limitation of joint motion depends upon the nature and the duration of the disability and the desired results. Only very light exercises are given for patients with recent injuries, or newly-healed infections, or arthritis. Active exercise is provided within the limits of motion. This does not actually stretch or strengthen muscles, but it does serve to prevent further limitation of joint motion and atrophy of muscles through disuse. More strenuous active motion is given initially for many patients if they have recovered sufficiently from the trauma or disease which produced the disability. This is accomplished by moving the involved joints through the greatest possible range of motion, thus stretching the contractures.

Activities which permit gradation of resistance and range of motion are given for patients who have progressed beyond the acute stage of their illness. The work is carefully graded from light to heavy, employing tools of increasing weight with longer work periods and briefer rest periods as the patient improves. Resistive exercises can be combined with stretching by increasing the weight of the tools which the patient uses and by increasing the length of reach required to perform a task. As both length of reach and tool weight are increased, the joints and muscles are stretched. Patients with contractures receive gentle stretching of the involved muscles. When the muscle is relaxed the joint may be flexed passively or extended by pressure exerted by the parts above.

There are occasions when it is important to exercise or strengthen only one muscle group and not its normal antagonists. There are two techniques of occupational therapy which can achieve such localization of exercise.

Eccentric, or *lengthening, contraction* is the gradual relaxation of a contracted muscle as it resists the pull of gravity and the weight of the body part or tool in slowly returning to the position from which it was moved. For example, when the arm is raised forward or above the head, the action which is obtained is contraction of the shoulder flexor muscles. When the arm is slowly returned to the side of the body, there is eccentric contraction of the shoulder flexors. Thus, although the shoulder has been flexed and the arm returned to the side, only the flexor muscles of the shoulder have been exercised. If, on the other hand, the am is brought down forcibly, as in the hammering of a nail, this produces *concentric contraction* of the shoulder extensor muscles. When activities are employed as exercise, eccentric contraction can be best obtained by lowering the body part slowly, resisting the pull of gravity.

Exercises without strong resistance will not strengthen a normal muscle but will only maintain its present condition. Weakened muscles can be exercised by providing resistance and allowing the body part to return to its initial position through contraction of the antagonist muscles, thus giving only minimal resistance. This is known as *return motion.* The localization of exercise in affected muscle groups can be achieved through return motion with or without some resistance. For example, an appropriate activity for strengthening a triceps muscle which is graded as *good* is sawing with a hand saw. Pulling the saw back into position for the next stroke, using the hyperextensor muscles of the shoulder and the flexor muscles of the elbow, is a return motion with only a small amount of resistance to the normal antagonists. The weakened triceps is strengthened, but the flexor muscles of the elbow which are already strong receive only enough exercise to maintain them in good condition.

Proper Positions for Exercise

When a patient is involved in a therapeutic activity it is important that he be placed in a position which permits, or provides for, the desired movements, but does not allow other motions to be substituted. Proper posture, therefore, is always essential. Compensatory movements can be eliminated by stabilizing the joint proximal to the one which is being moved or exercised. In treating both joint limitations and muscle weaknesses certain positions are more favorable than others. Since occupational therapy is primarily concerned with the upper extremities, some examples are presented of positions for upper limb movements.

For finger flexion activities the wrist should be slightly hyperextended since this relaxes the tendons of the extensor digitorum communis, the extensor muscle of the fingers which extends the wrist joint and phalanges, or finger bones, and permits greater finger flexion. For extension of the fingers, the wrist should be slightly flexes, thus relaxing the long flexor muscles and permitting greater finger extension.

In flexion and extension of the wrist, the elbow either rests on a table or is held at the side to prevent compensatory elbow motion.

During pronation and supination of the elbow the elbow should be bent to ninety degrees to prevent the substitution of internal and external rotation of the shoulder.

To obtain elbow flexion and extension the arm must be held at the side to avoid compensatory movements of the shoulder, or both arms should be used in bilateral activities. Back motion should be eliminated as much as possible.

In order to achieve flexion and lateral abduction of the shoulder, compensatory back movements can be prevented by sitting the patient in a straight-backed chair and instructing him to hold his back erect. Shoulder rotation is most easily accomplished with the arm at an angle of forty degrees of lateral abduction. Abduction is best achieved if the shoulder is at least partially rotated.

KINETIC ANALYSIS

Each tool which is used by a patient and each activity which the patient engages in can be analyzed according to the muscles and ranges of motion ordinarily involved. This is known as a kinetic analysis because its prescription is based upon a knowledge of kinesiology, or human motion, and because its execution requires motion. A kinetic analysis of occupational therapy involves a classified description of active and passive motions of the joints or body parts involved in the therapeutic activities of the program. The method of such an analysis is to execute the activity and observe another individual engaged in that behavior. That is, the analyst, usually the therapist, first performs the actions herself to determine the gross motions involved, and then observes the same motions as performed by someone else, first at normal speed and then at greatly reduced speed, so as to determine the finer movements involved. The analysis includes the cycle of motion, the type of muscle contraction, the range through which the joints move, the starting position, realism, and tool variations. These variables are discussed below.

Cycle of Motion

It is true that for every action of a tool there must be a preparatory motion. At times the preparatory motion will require greater energy than the effective action. For example, raising a two-pound hammer against gravity to a preparatory starting position, may call for more energy than that expended in striking the nail or spike, and hence, be more valuable for increasing muscle strength than the effective action. There are also cases in which preparatory motion may be contra-indicated if the muscles which perform it are too weak. An analysis of the complete cycle of motion should therefore be made by dividing it into an initial phase of preparatory motion and a second phase of effective motion.

Type of Muscle Contraction

A kinetic analysis of muscle contraction includes infomation on whether the muscle employed contract statically or intermittently, slowly or rapidly, and whether there is passive contraction, extension or stretching. While a static muscle contraction requires energy to be expended and is, therefore, related to muscle strengthening, its use is not always advisable. An example of this would be a case where muscles have been long immobilized. Static contraction will tire such muscles more readily than will intermittent contraction with periods of relaxation. A proper analysis will reveal which type of contraction is recommended for a particular patient.

Joint Range

It is important to note not only the direction of joint movement but also the range through which the joint moves. A joint may be able to flex and extend in a given activity, yet its range of motion will be so small as to render it useless for the patient engaged in the task. Thus, tasks must be analyzed in terms of joint range if an activity is to be of certain value.

Starting Position

In analyzing a tool the starting position, or stance, for its use must be indicated. Because of the nature of the disabilities which require rehabilitation, the type of work which patients perform in rehabilitation institutions, and the set-up of the workshops, most tool and craft analyses are made for seated positions. The range of motion of a joint, the energy used in performing an activity, and even the muscles which are involved, differ depending upon how a tool is held and the position of the patient during performance. Hence, the need for a kinetic analysis. As patients regain function and become ambulatory, the therapist must re-analyze the activities for the differences created by the changes in position.

Realism

Each activity of occupational therapy must be analyzed in accordance with the most effective use of body mechanics. It cannot be taken for granted that an activity results in certain muscle or joint motions. Only careful observation will reveal the actual kinetics involved. Realism requires a focus on key motions and a de-emphasis of incidental movement. The most skillful and economic way of performing a task is the desired way.

Tool Variants

Unfortunately, tools are frequently analyzed without relation to the variations in size and shape which will be used by the patient. Some tools may be too small to involve the use of joints other than the fingers, while others, because of their size and weight, will require the muscles and joints of the shoulders.

Motions can be prescribed in terms of the tools to be used rather than the exercises to be performed. The needs required by the pathology must be accurately identified and described so that the tool analysis will conform to the disability and the full value of the activity will be realized.

OCCUPATIONAL THERAPY ACTIVITIES

It must once again be stressed that activity without purpose is not therapeutic and should not be included on a rehabilitation program. The following list of therapy activities may be considered to be fairly typical of most occupational therapy programs for the physically disabled. Needless to say, programs differ from hospital to hospital, and not all activities included herein are employed with every patient within an institution. Furthermore, as pointed out earlier, the creative therapist devises exercises for the individual patient which are *unique to him* and, even as this is being written, new devices and materials are being used.

The Ankle

GOAL: Increase range of motion, dorsiflexion and plantar flexion.

ACTIVITY OR CRAFT: Operation of a treadle saw, a sewing machine, a foot-powered lathe, a bicycle jig-saw, a foot bellows, a foot-operated weaving loom, a potter's wheel, a pianola.

GOAL: Development of strength.

ACITIVTY OR CRAFT: Operating an Alexander bicycle saw, treadle sander which provides the same functions as the saw but has greater

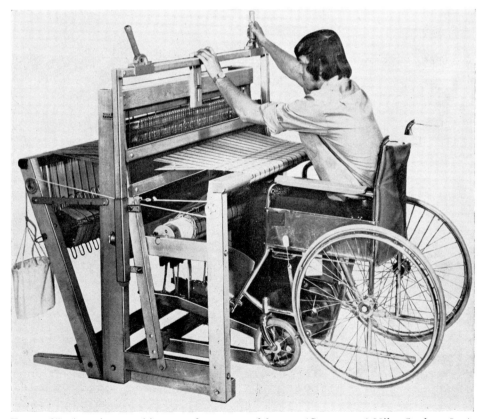

FIGURE 65. A patient working at a foot-powered loom. (*Courtesy of Nilus Leclerc, Inc.*)

resistance, a floor press, pumping with the affected leg to strengthen quadriceps muscle and provide co-contraction of ankle muscles, playing floor checkers which also strengthens the quadriceps muscle and forces ankle dorsiflexion.

GOAL: Develop standing tolerance.
ACTIVITY OR CRAFT: Any activity can be satisfactory as long as the patient stands to perform it. Some examples are as follows: assembly and use of power tools; operating a floor press, pumping with the non-involved extremity; shuffleboard; floor checkers; and similar tasks.

GOAL: Develop work tolerance for the individual's vocation.
ACTIVITY OR CRAFT: Weight lifting as performed on the job, carried out by flexing the knees and hips and keeping the back straight, climbing stairs while carrying weights, ladder climbing, kneeling, crawling.

The Knee and Hip

GOAL: Increase range of motion, flexion and extension, hip abduction and adduction, and develop strength.
ACTIVITY OR CRAFT: Operate Alexander bicycle saw, operate a floor press pumping with the affected leg, particularly to increase power in the quadriceps, use foot bellows, push treadles down on a floor loom for abduction and addiction, operate a potter's wheel for hip abduction, weave for hip and trunk flexion, play floor checkers to strengthen quadriceps and force hip and knee flexion.
GOAL: Develop standing tolerance and work tolerance.
ACTIVITY OR CRAFT: Same as for the ankle. In addition, standing provides for co-contraction of the leg muscles.

The Back

GOAL: Increase muscle tone and strength of back and abdominal muscles, improve cervical extension, general flexion and extension, and maintain correct posture during work.
ACTIVITY OR CRAFT: Operate bicycle saw to improve tone and strength of trunk muscles; use a hand-operated printing press with bilateral handles to strengthen upper back muscles; cord knotting to increase cervical extension; sanding activities for co-contraction of back muscles; operate a floor press, alternating the legs in the operation to strengthen knee, hip and back muscles; play floor checkers to maintain good posture; weave at a floor loom to strengthen trunk muscles.

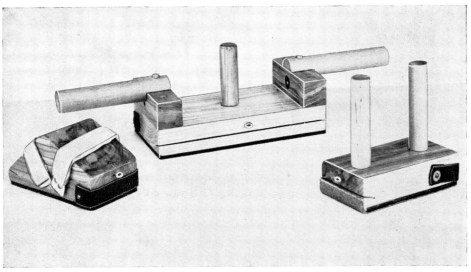

FIGURE 66. Sanding block set. Left: Metacarpophalangeal flexion sander; Center: Bilateral convertible sander, on which the dowel handles can be positioned to place the hands and forearms in mid-position, pronation or supination; Right: Bilateral sander. (*Reprinted by permission of J. A. Preston Corp., 1971*)

To increase cervical, dorsal and lumbar flexion the patient makes large willow baskets and/or pumps a printing press, threads a loom and reaches for beaters on the loom.

Improvement in cervical, dorsal and lumbar extension is accomplished through pulling cane through a chair frame in chair caning activities, pulling long cords in knotting activities, and beating material while working at a loom in weaving activities.

GOAL: Develop standing tolerance.
ACTIVITY OR CRAFT: Same as for the ankle.

GOAL: Develop work tolerance.
ACTIVITY OR CRAFT: Emphasis is placed on correct lifting procedures and on correct posture when standing or sitting.

The Shoulder

GOAL: Increase range of motion and muscle strength.
ACTIVITY OR CRAFT: Braid weaving combines flexion, abduction and external rotation and also provides for horizontal adduction and abduction. Cord knotting combines flexion, abduction, and external rotation, and provides for horizontal abduction and adduction. Operating a hand press increases flexion, extension and abduction.

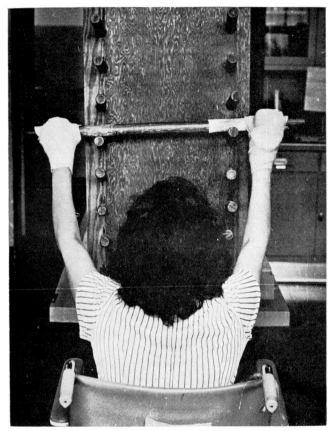

FIGURE 67. A patient increasing the strength of her shoulder extensor muscles through a wall climbing exercise. Her hands must be taped to the bar because they are too weak to grasp is voluntarily.

Weaving increases flexion and extension. Vertical or horizontal sanding activities provide for flexion, hyperextension and abduction. Hammering on metal is used to improve external and internal rotation. Suffleboard is employed for forceful flexion up to forty degrees. Tossing beanbags improves circumduction. Making baskets, notably large ones with long spokes, caning chairs in a perpendicular position, feeding and pumping a printing press, and sawing and planing wood are all employed for increasing shoulder flexion. Shoulder extension is increased through basketry work, tearing rags for braided rugs, caning chairs, pulling knots, feeding the press and typesetting in printing work, and doing woodwork. Untangling the weavers in basketry and making the warp in weaving and winding wool are good for improving shoulder circumduction.

Shoulder rotation activities include the following: basketry, where

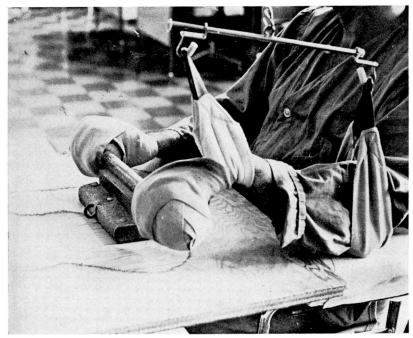

FIGURE 68. Bilateral sanding. Lack of strength in this patient's hands necessitates that they be bound to the sander.

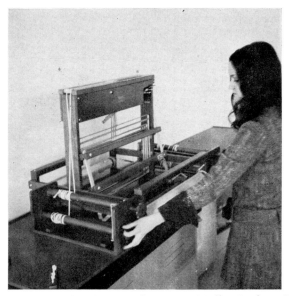

FIGURE 69. Weaving loom. (*Courtesy of Nilus Leclerc, Inc.*)

the forearm is supinated and the upper arm is extended backward and downward in using long weavers, or in sewing raffia with long threads, or in braiding rugs with long strands; chair caning, when pulling the weavers through and out with the palm held up; knotting, using long cords with the work placed high and combined with forearm supination; and weaving, when the thread is pulled out to one side with the palm of the hand up in internal rotation or with the palm down in external rotation.

GOAL: Develop work tolerance.

ACTIVITY OR CRAFT: Any activity performed at normal working level, plus weight lifting and special motions, such as reaching, which might be done on the job.

The Elbow

GOAL: Increase range of motion and muscle strength.

ACTIVITY OR CRAFT: Elbow flexion is increased by sewing, weaving, basketry, leather lacing, feeding a printing press, sawing, piercing and filing metal, typesetting, knotting, needle work, woodworking and winding yarn.

Extension exercises include hammering, unraveling and using long weavers in basketry, bookbinding, with sewing, cutting and shaping with a hammer, braiding rugs with long strips, chair caning, as in pulling out cane with long strands, pulling knots or long cords, setting type, feeding and pumping a printing press, woodworking, including use of a coping saw, plane and sander, pulling material through a frame, as in weaving, and shuffleboard.

Needle work, weaving, crocheting and braiding are valuable for elbow pronation, and the former three activities are also valuable exercises for supination.

GOAL: Develop work tolerance.

ACTIVITY OR CRAFT: Same as for the shoulder.

The Forearm

GOAL: Increase range of motion, pronation, supination and muscle strength.

ACTIVITY OR CRAFT: Playing checkers, cord knotting, using a screwdriver, hammering, weaving, and using a hand press are valuable general activities.

For increasing pronation ability active motion with strength is found in leather-lacing, filing and polishing rounded edges and sur-

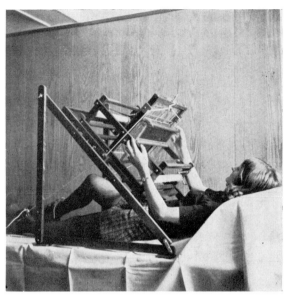

FIGURE 70. A weaving loom adapted for bed use. *(Courtesy of Nilus Leclerc, Inc.)*

faces of metal, basket weaving from right to left, braiding and wrapping braided rugs, weaving cane and driving screws. For motion and strength in supination the patient weaves baskets using an awl, wraps and sews in raffia, separates strands of braided rugs, pulls cane through a chair frame, pulls knots on long cords, laces and sews leather, files, saws and sands curved edges and polishes rounded surfaces, and engages in weaving activities.

GOAL: Develop work tolerance.
ACTIVITY OR CRAFT: Same as for the shoulder.

The Wrist

GOAL: Increase range of motion and muscle strength.
ACTIVITY OR CRAFT: Strength in the wrist can be increased by playing with weighted checkers and by braid weaving. Active flexion with strength is provided by the following: basket weaving and pressing fibers into place; bookbinding activities, such as pulling books apart for sewing, gluing and hammering; drilling holes in blocks, as in brush making; chair caning, when cane is pulled through from right to left with the right hand, and in the reverse direction with the left hand; knotting activities with the forearm maintained in pronation; leather work, such as stitching, stippling, tooling and tapping dyes; metal filing and hammering; pulling weavers tight during weaving,

with the forearm held in pronation; hammering, chiseling and sanding wood; and beating activities during loom and card weaving.

Increasing wrist extension involves basket weaving, using a needle to pull out thread in raffia work, sewing, tearing rags, brush making, especially pulling the fibers through the drilled holes, chair caning, knotting, leather lacing and weaving.

Metal tapping, stenciling and woodwork, such as curved sanding and block printing provide flexion and extension activities for the wrist.

Abduction and adduction activities include folding and creasing paper during bookbinding, knotting with the palm held up and then with the palm down, tooling curved lines in leather work, filing metal, and various weaving tasks.

Circumduction of the wrist makes use of activities such as untangling weavers in basketry, wrapping raffia over reeds, leather sewing and lacing, metal work, and winding balls and shuttles during loom weaving.

GOAL: Develop work tolerance.
ACTIVITY OR CRAFT: Same as for the shoulder.

The Fingers

GOAL: Increase range of motion and muscle strength.
ACTIVITY OR CRAFT: Finger flexion is accomplished through basketry activities, particularly when grasping and putting weavers into place and grasping tools in willow work, holding reeds in place while weaving raffia, and holding and pushing reeds into place during both reed and willow work.

In activities such as bookbinding, braiding rugs, chair caning, metal crafting and similar work it is the grasping of tools and materials which is important as well as the activities provided by their use. Any activity in which small tools are used can be employed to increase finger flexion. Some examples are drilling, sanding and bending fiber during brush making, modeling and punching leather, handling filler, cards, shuttle and thread in weaving, handling saws, planes and hammers in woodworking, and handling scissors during paper work.

Finger extension activities include braiding, frame weaving, cord knotting, finger painting, block printing and coil pottery.

GOAL: Develop work tolerance.
ACTIVITY OR CRAFT: Same as for the shoulder.

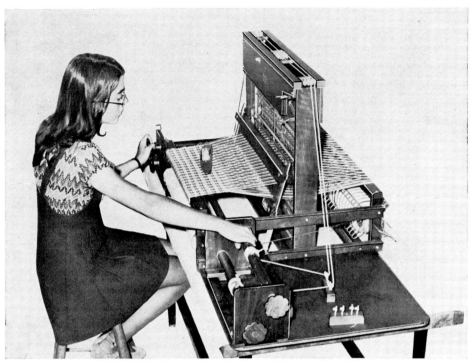

FIGURE 71. Table loom for hand exercises. (*Courtesy of Nilus Leclerc, Inc.*)

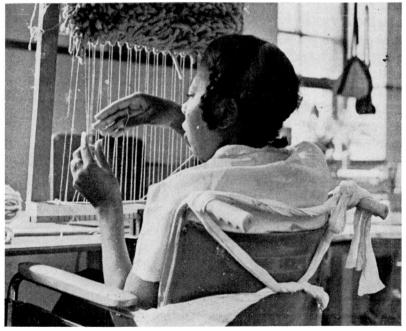

FIGURE 72. A patient doing Turkish knitting on a loom to develop fine finger coordination.

The Thumb

GOAL: Increase range of motion and muscle strength.

ACTIVITY OR CRAFT: Games, marbles, checkers, chess and Chinese checkers provide grasp and opposition tasks for the thumb and fingers. Silk screen work, woodwork, leather punching, cutting with scissors and shears, and writing are also employed.

GOAL: Develop work tolerance.

ACTIVITY OR CRAFT: Same as for the shoulder.

ACTIVITIES OF DAILY LIVING

The activities of daily living (ADL) program is an integral and highly important aspect of occupational therapy. It is on this program that the patient learns to apply what he has been taught in physical therapy and other classes to the life situation. The purpose of the ADL program is to train the patient to perform, within the limits of his disability, in the activities of his daily life at home, at work, in school and in recreational endeavors. It demonstrates to the patient the value of all that he has learned on his rehabilitation program and provides the final, practical test of how well he will manage in his daily routines.

The teaching of an activity involves breaking it down into its sim-

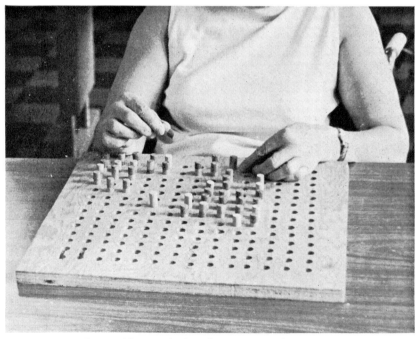

FIGURE 73. Developing fine grasp with a pegboard.

plest motions, providing exercises which will enable the patient to perform these motions, giving practice at the task and finally, having the patient actually perform in a realistic life situation.

The activities of daily living are characteristically grouped into six main areas of function. These are discussed in turn.

Transfer Activities

Transferring, in physical rehabilitation, almost invariably means to and from a wheelchair. Transfer activities are among the most important for a chronically disabled person to learn since skill in transferring often means the difference between independence and helplessness and, therefore, a considerable amount of time is usually devoted to teaching them.

Space does not permit a description of all possible transfer activities and so one activity, bed transfers, perhaps the most important of all, has been selected to serve as an example.

The transfer from bed to wheelchair and back to bed is typically the first transfer technique which a patient learns. Once he masters it he can progress to apply and modify this basic methodology to other wheelchair transfers.

The Standing or Weight-Bearing Transfer

This type of transfer can be performed if the patient has good balance, at least one stable lower extremity, the ability to maintain hip and knee in a position of voluntary muscle contraction, good shoulder depressor and adductor muscles, good elbow flexors and extensors, and preferably hand and wrist function on one side of the body. It is the preferred method of transfer for hemiplegics, unilateral lower extremity amputees and patients with unilateral hip fractures.

The bed must be stationary and of approximately the same height as the wheelchair which must be braked and possess detachable footrests. The wheelchair is slightly angled toward the foot of the bed for the transfer out of bed and angled toward the head of the bed for the return transfer. The footrest adjacent to the bed is swung aside or removed.

The patient begins transferring from the bed to the wheelchair by lying in the center of the bed. Using his uninvolved hand he places his affected arm across his abdomen. He places his good foot under the knee of the plegic leg and slides his foot down the leg to the ankle. He then partly flexes and lifts the affected leg with the normal foot and leg. Next, he grasps the side rail of the bed with the uninvolved hand, and rolling his legs to his normal side, turns onto his side. The patient then moves his legs over the edge of the bed and grasps the side rail, pulling himself to a sitting position. He then uncrosses his feet and places them firmly on the floor to provide good balance.

From his sitting position at the edge of the bed the patient checks the brakes of the wheelchair to make certain that they are in a locked position. He then leans forward and simultaneously pushes down with the noninvolved hand and foot, moving farther towards the edge of the bed. The normal knee is then flexed to an angle of ninety degrees and the normal foot is moved to slightly behind the plegic foot so that the patient's feet will be free to pivot. Next, the patient grasps the side rail of the bed, moves his trunk forward, pushes down with his good arm and, bearing most of his weight on the uninvolved leg, rises to a standing position.

He then places his hand at the center of the farther arm of the wheelchair and pivots on his feet, bringing himself into a position preparatory to sitting down. Finally, he eases himself into the wheelchair, replaces the footrest, releases the brakes and progresses on his way.

In transferring back to the bed the patient swings the footrest of the involved lower extremity out of the way and locks the brakes of the wheelchair. By leaning forward and pushing down he moves toward the edge of the chair until his feet are under him and his good foot is slightly behind the involved leg. Maintaining his hand on the armrest of the chair, the patient moves his trunk forward, and bearing weight on his normal leg, rises. After coming to an erect standing position he moves his hand to the side rail of the bed and pivots on his feet, bringing himself into a position to sit on the bed.

The Non-Weight-Bearing Lateral Transfer

The patients who are taught this method are those who have little or no function in both their lower extremities, such as quadriplegics, paraplegics, patients with neuromuscular disorders, as in multiple sclerosis, and bilateral lower extremity amputees. It requires good sitting balance and enough strength in the upper extremities so that the hips can be lifted from the bed. Strong shoulder depressor and abductor muscles and elbow and wrist extensors are also necessary. (Note: Because of the upper extremity requirements for this form of transfer, few patients with lesions higher than the seventh cervical vertebra can accomplish it.)

The bed should be at approximately the same height as the wheelchair. The chair must have swinging, detachable footrests and detachable armrests and must be braked. The most useful piece of apparatus for this type of transfer is a sliding board, which is simply a small, smooth, wooden board which serves to bridge the gap between the bed and the wheelchair. The most recent version of the sliding board is a metal one which rolls on ball bearings and slides the patient along from one surface to another.

By moving his legs with his arms the patient brings himself to a sitting position at the side of the bed. Moving towards the edge of the bed he turns so that his knees are away from the wheelchair and his hips are facing towards it. As the turn is made he must use his hands to adjust his feet so that they come directly under him. The patient then leans on his right forearm and raises his left buttock off the bed high enough to place one end of the sliding board under it. Two corners of the board must rest on the bed and two corners must rest on the seat of the wheelchair.

Using his arms for movement and maintenance of balance, the patient moves laterally across the sliding board into the wheelchair. Once he is adept at using the sliding board the patient may be able to progress to transferring without it, using his upper extremities to boost his hips for short distances instead of sliding.

The Non-Weight-Bearing Anterior-Posterior Sliding Transfer

Transferring by this technique requires loose hamstring muscles and slightly greater strength, particularly in the elbow extensors, and better balance than does the lateral transfer.

The wheelchair is braked and placed with the front of the seat directly against the bed with the footrests swung aside.

The patient keeps his head and shoulders slightly forward to maintain his balance and prevent falling backward. Using his hands he moves his legs, one at a time, to the side of the bed, away from the wheelchair. By pushing with his fists, the patient moves sideways and backwards, moving each hip and leg alternately, to bring his hips close to the wheelchair.

When he nears the edge of the bed he reaches behind himself, places his hands at the center of the wheelchair's armrests and lifts himself gently back into the chair. The procedure is reversed for return to the bed.

Other Transfer Activities

In addition to learning how to transfer between bed and wheelchair, the most frequent, and hence most important, transfers which a patient learns are as follows: transfers between wheelchair and toilet, which requires muscle strength similar to bed transfers and includes management of clothing; transfers to a straight chair; bath-tub transfers, which are perhaps the most dangerous to perform; and automobile transfers, which require strong upper extremities. Care and management of the individual's wheelchair is always included as part of any wheelchair training program.

Patients who are unable to transfer without extensive assistance have found hydraulic or mechanical lifts to be of great value. Even a small woman, if properly trained, can use such lifts to raise and transfer a man more than twice her size. Most modern rehabilitation hospitals have such apparatus for demonstration to and training of family members of patients.

Bed Activities

Included herein are all of the gross body motions which are essential in moving about in bed and in assuming the necessary positions in bed for various self-care activities.

The patient is taught to change position from supination to pronation and back to supination, to sit up and to lie down, to maintain good sitting balance while moving his trunk or arms, and he is shown how to move forward, backward and sideways while sitting and during placement of his legs.

Self-Care Activities

These may be subdivided into toilet, dressing and eating activities.

Toilet Activities

Toilet activities are primarily those which typically are performed in the bathroom, such as washing, bathing, brushing teeth, hair and nail care, use of cosmetics, shaving, and using a toilet or urinal. Use of a bedpan is also included within this category. Patients are taught the most efficient ways of turning faucets, managing toothpaste, handling razors, using bathroom tissue, and the like.

Dressing Activities

Included herein is the putting on and removing of the kinds of clothing worn by the patient, both underwear and outer garments. The utilization of snaps, buttons, hooks and zippers is usually the most difficult aspect of dressing, and often variations in the location of such fasteners are necessary, such as moving them from the back of a garment to the front. The substitution of elastic and Velcro® for fasteners, belts, laces, etc. can be an important aid to independence. More functional fashions than previously existed have recently been designed for the disabled person which make dressing an easier and more agreeable task.

Eating Activities

This set of activities requires that the patient learn to properly use his fingers and utensils to eat with and manage a cup and glass to drink from. Sitting down at, and rising from, a table are also included as part of training.

Miscellaneous Hand Activities

These are the activities which involve the use of the hands but are not included in self-care, wheelchair, ambulation or elevation training. The patient is taught to handle a telephone, elevator signal buttons, coins, eyeglasses, a watch, lights, keys and similar items which are frequently encountered or used.

Ambulation and Elevation Activities

The behaviors which are included within this group are carried out with or without the aid of canes, crutches, walkers, braces or prostheses, depending upon the patient's needs and usual mode of functioning. These activities involve ambulation on different types of ground surfaces and floor coverings, and sitting down and rising from wheelchair, bed, car, toilet seat, straight chair, etc. Climbing stairs, mounting curbs and crossing streets are all a part of this facet of the ADL program.

The relationship between occupational therapy and physical therapy is clear here. The patient is taught a safe, stable ambulation pattern in physical therapy, and the occupational therapist, in the ADL program, provides the situations and the training for the practical application of what he has learned.

Travel Activities

Traveling includes the use and maintenance of an automobile, driver education and utilization of public transportation. Today's modern rehabilitation institution provides driver education classes for patients who are taught to use specially designed hand controls when their lower extremities are nonfunctional. When retraining a disabled person to use public transportation, such as buses, trains and taxicabs, the therapist will actually accompany the patient on these vehicles after practice in the hospital has indicated that he is ready to attempt travel. Thus, the patient learns through guided experience.

Teaching An Activity: An Example

Each activity of daily living is taught differently, depending upon the motions necessary for completion of the act and the disability of the patient who is receiving the training. One activity, teaching hemiplegic to eat a meal in bed, has been selected to illustrate the complexities involved in performing an act which most people take for granted and to which they give little, if any, thought when they are so engaged.

The hemiplegic patient must first be taught to change from a lying to a sitting position. This requires rolling-over exercises and exercises for the strengthening of the arms, wrists and hands. Secondly, the patient needs to maintain his balance while sitting and engaging in various arm and hand movements. For this he is given exercises designed to improve sitting balance. Additionally, if indicated, he will receive exercises for strengthening his shoulder, back and abdominal muscles, and the muscles of the distal segments. Before the patient can take the third step, grasping and holding eating utensils, he must be given exercises in these motions, which are often preceded by activities which strengthen finger and hand muscles and improve visual-motor coordination.

Use of eating utensils may be initiated with real food, or through practice on Plasticine,® Pla-Doh,® modeling clay or similar material. Putting food into the mouth involves practicing the movements, first without food and then with food.

Many hemiplegic patients have difficulty with chewing and/or swallowing and in such a case it becomes incumbent upon the speech clinician to work together with the occupational therapist in providing specific oral exercises.

The hemiplegic must be taught to perform two-handed activities with one hand, such as cutting meat and buttering bread. It is to be remembered that during these activities good sitting balance in bed must be maintained.

There is often a long, frustrating period of time between each step of such training, particularly if preparatory exercises are necessary, or if muscle strengthening and range of motion activities must first be given, or if the patient's language impairment makes communication difficult. What is reported in a few lines here represents what may be weeks of effort on the part of the patient.

HOMEMAKING ACTIVITIES

When a patient is initially evaluated for admission to a rehabilitation program, the occupational therapist notes where the individual will be returning to upon his discharge from the hospital. It is important in the planning of rehabilitation to know the home, work and recreation environments of the patient, so that the therapy program can be meaningfully designed. A therapist would not, for example, emphasize standing tolerance with a patient who will be returning to a sedentary job. Nor, on the other hand, would driver training be omitted for the patient who is a salesman and dependent upon his automobile.

As the patient's vocation is important to know in planning a treatment program which will be of value to him upon his return to the community, so it is vital to be aware of the home to which the disabled woman will return. Not only must the physical design of the home be considered by the therapist, but also the way the existing plant can be modified, if necessary. The patient's modes of functioning at home must also be known. Training the disabled female patient to return to her home and function in it as she once did, constitutes one of the most crucial aspects of her entire rehabilitation program.

While homemaking training is primarily for women, it is not necessarily so limited. A man may be so disabled that he cannot return to work and thus, he may take over some of the household responsibilities. Disabled children who are potential homemakers can benefit from some training in this area. Furthermore, performing household tasks provides excellent practical applications in the use of prostheses, orthoses and wheelchairs.

When a patient is seen initially for homemaking training, she is evaluated as to her ability to perform routine household acts, such as making a bed, cleaning, laundry washing, sewing, kitchen activities, and often, child care as well. All areas of skill and deficiency are recorded by the therapist.

Primary considerations in the homemaking evaluation include the following: the patient's physical limitations, including type, location and extent of disability; posture and sitting balance; ability to use a wheelchair, cane, etc.; use of prosthetic or orthotic devices; fatigue threshold; visual, auditory or language defects; intellectual deficiencies; impairment of sensation in body parts, particularly in the extremities; speed of performance; and need for assistance. In addition, the therapist notes the patient's ingenuity (or lack of it) which is so important to the disabled homemaker, her concepts of work (careless or meticulous), and her attitude towards housework which, in the final analysis, can make the difference between a functioning homemaker and a person who must rely upon others to do her jobs.

As part of the evaluation process the occupational therapist is concerned with determining the type of housing the patient occupies and its location, shopping facilities in the neighborhood, other family members and their availability in the home, and any other factors which might be important in planning a treatment program for the patient.

The initial evaluation will reveal the need for retraining in home-making activities. The patient may have to be taught one-handed skills or new techniques of cooking. The home itself might require re-modeling in terms of working heights and storage arrangements.

The goals of homemaking training can be considered to be the following:

1. Retraining in basic household skills.
2. Reduction of fatigue and energy expenditure through work simplification and adaptation of household equipment.
3. Remodeling or rearranging home facilities.
4. Selection and care of clothing.
5. Child care.
6. Nutrition planning.
7. Therapeutic exercise.
8. Use of orthotic or prosthetic apparatus through functional homemaking tasks.

The Homemaking Program

Training for the disabled housewife whould be conducted in a rehabilitation facility. In such a setting the rehabilitation team can plan homemaking as an integral part of the patient's general therapeutic program. In addition, many institutions have model kitchens in which the patients can work from their wheelchairs under professional supervision.

The steps of the training program are determined by the individual's needs and rate of progress. The actual content of any home-making program varies with the patient and the disability, but there are certain aspects which are general to all patients who require help in this area. Some of these are discussed in this section. The point to remember in the planning of a treatment program is that all domestic activities involve range of reach, movement from one place to another in the home, manual activities, energy expenditure, safety precautions and communication. A therapy program is constructed around these fundamentals.

Teaching Basic Skills

Basic skills are those which are involved in activities such as cooking, washing dishes, making beds, ironing, cleaning and washing clothes. Patients are taught to perform these chores with one hand, or from a wheelchair, or with a brace, depending upon their requirements. They are taught methods of work simplification, such as how and where to place utensils and prepare work areas so that less effort is expended. This includes teaching methods of sliding items rather than lifting them, economics of work stations and equipment, proper utilization of gravity, positioning and handling of tools, appliances and controls, and many more procedures which are all designed to make the housekeeper's work easier, safer and more efficient.

Rearranging Work and Storage Areas

Selection of the proper work tools is highly important, yet it is also necessary to arrange and store these tools so that they can be of maximum value for the housewife, particularly in the kitchen.

The two factors which most frequently require alteration in the home are the heights of the work areas and the placement and type of storage units. Proper work heights improve posture and reduce fatigue. Some homes are constructed in a way that the wheelchair-bound person cannot function in the kitchen because the counter tops are too highly placed. In such cases drastic remodeling may be necessary if the patient is to continue to live there. Depths of counters must also be considered if a wheelchair is going to have to fit under them.

In addition to the heights of storage cabinets, the actual arrangement of equipment in these areas is crucial in achieving independence. Vertical filing of dishes, revolving shelves of food, pull-out bins and racks, gravity-operated or tilting cannisters and single-handle faucets are all valuable in helping the disabled housewife function in her kitchen.

The actual shape which a kitchen should be, whether *U*-shaped, *L*-shaped, or shaped like a corridor, depends upon the disability and the preferences of the person who must work in it. In most cases entire kitchens cannot be reconstructed and thus the emphasis is necessarily on teaching the housewife to function as well as possible in the existing environmental situation.

Prior to, during, and upon completion of the training program in homemaking activities, the occupational therapist, or a home economist, or a public health nurse will visit the patient's home to assess the need for training in specific areas of function. The assessment also includes determining whether changes must be made in the home, such as widening of doorways so that a wheelchair can pass through, and ascertaining how effectively the patient will be able to function in her home following hospital discharge.

It is always borne in mind that the patient must be taught to function in her own home environment. The ultimate goal of the homemaking program is the return of the patient to her home to resume her role as wife and mother. The benefits to the patient and her family are immeasurable when this objective is achieved.

THE PRE-VOCATIONAL SHOP

The well-equipped rehabilitation hospital possesses a pre-vocational shop or unit. The objectives of such a unit are to facilitate vocational rehabilitation, to provide training and experience with orthotic and self-help devices, and to help further increase and maintain muscle strength and range of motion in particularly unique ways and in ways which are not ordinarily a part of the occupational therapy program. Although the physician who is responsible for the patient's total program writes the prescriptions for pre-vocational activities, he usually acts upon the suggestion of the rehabilitation counselor.

The pre-vocational shop usually is part of the Occupational Therapy Service. Activities in the unit are conducted by an occupational therapist with special training in such work. She maintains close contact with the rehabilitation counselor who referred the patient, but the responsibility for the program is hers because of the physical exercises and movements which are involved in performing the various pre-vocational activities.

In the pre-vocational shop the patient performs simulated job tasks which represent work done in actual industry. The types of activities which are offered typically include machine operation, such as punch press, drill press, keypunch and computer technology, clerical jobs—e.g., typing, bookkeeping, filing, use of office equipment and stenography—and occupations such as printing, drafting, photography, dress designing and jewelry making. The professional staff can observe the patient at these jobs and thus gain much information which can be useful for his further rehabilitation.

The occupational therapist will measure the patient's work tolerance and note limitations in reach, grasp, manual dexterity, etc. which will lead her to modify his program accordingly. The rehabilitation counselor will be able to realistically evaluate the patient's interest in his work, his work habits, his attitudes toward work and his ability to work with others. Furthermore, verification can be made of the patient's statements concerning his work skills and experience. A patient may be given additional training in an occupation of his choice and eventually be placed in a job as a result of his performance in the pre-vocational shop.

The pre-vocational unit is not always intended as a stepping stone for the patient to vocational training and placement. Activities in the unit are often prescribed because of the type of muscle and joint action which they require. In these cases, prevocational activities are prescribed solely for therapeutic exercise.

Chapter 11

ORTHOTICS, PROSTHETICS AND PEDIATRIC OCCUPATIONAL THERAPY

ORTHOTICS

A**N ORTHOTIC DEVICE** is defined as one which pertains to, or promotes the straightening of a deformed or distorted body part. That is, it assists or corrects a nonfunctioning or malfunctioning part.

From a practical standpoint, when the occupational therapist speaks of orthotics she is most often referring to splints and braces for the upper extremities. Devices are an important adjunct to rehabilitative therapy and for many individuals with a permanent, residual disability they are an indispensable necessity for self-sufficiency.

In general, devices are prescribed for the following reasons:

1. To provide more dynamic treatment measures.
2. To permit early independence.
3. To further enable patients to actively participate in the treatment programs.
4. To provide independence in the activities of daily living.
5. To assist in restoring self-esteem.
6. To aid the patient in regaining a measure of economic independence.

Splints

A splint, or brace, is an individually prescribed device which serves to control the action of specific joints so as to prevent or to increase motion and to increase muscle strength. Splinting is both an art and a science, requiring the combined knowledge of the physician, the therapist and the orthotist, who must recognize the requirements and basic principles of how and when to splint, considering fit, comfort and cosmetic appearance as well as function.

The Classification of Splints

Splints are classed according to their basic purpose. Although the underlying pathology is a consideration, the resultant disability is the primary reason for splinting. Splints, therefore, are classified as those used for flaccidity, spasticity, incoordination, contracture, pain and trauma. Within each of these categories splints can further be divided into two types. *Static splints* are those which are designed to support the involved segment, prevent contractures, correct body alignment, provide joint stabilization, provide immobilization, prevent pain, eliminate unwanted motions, and protect the injured part. *Dynamic*, or *functional splints* are those which are designed to encourage therapeutic exercise and functional use.

There are many instances in which a splint may be designed to be useful in more than one type of disability. Prescription changes will be necessary from time to time as the condition of a patient for whom a splint was made improves or regresses.

General Objectives of Splinting

FLACCIDITY. A flaccid condition in an extremity may be due to peripheral nerve injury, poliomyelitis or other central nervous system lesion. Since the patient has been weakened by disease, he will not be able to tolerate a heavy orthosis. In the acute stage, static splinting is required for the involved parts to prevent joint laxity, contractures and, often, pain. When muscle power is sufficient to indicate activity, dynamic attachments are added to the static splints, thus providing simultaneous static and dynamic splinting functions.

SPASTICITY. Splinting for the relief of spastic conditions is typically observed in patients with spastic cerebral palsy and in hemiplegics. Static splinting is employed to prevent deformity. Dynamic splinting of the severely spastic part has limited value.

For the patient with hemiplegia, where some active flexion and extension may exist, splints are helpful in providing resistance or for preventing substitution by stabilizing some parts and providing isolated action in the retraining of motions.

INCOORDINATION. Splints which control incoordination may be required for ataxic cerebral palsy patients, patients with Parkinsonism, and patients who have multiple sclerosis. A weighted cuff, worn on the wrist, may aid the patient with athetosis. Weighted shoes and crutches may help the patient with multiple sclerosis to ambulate.

CONTRACTURES. Splints which prevent contractures are particularly important for the arthritides, burns which involve joints, cerebral palsy, poliomyelitis and quadriplegia. Static splinting aids in avoiding deformity and in the elimination of pain.

PAIN AND TRAUMA. The most appropriate form of management for fractures, dislocations, or sprains, where rigid casting is unnecessary, is immobilization of the injured part.

Splints are also employed following removal of a plaster cast as an intermediate measure prior to complete removal of support. Initially, splinting is static to promote rest and healing. When range of joint motion and hence function, can be safely increased, dynamic splinting is prescribed.

Acceptance of an orthotic device by the patient for a single upper extremity is greatly reduced by the existence of normal function on the contralateral side, since almost all activities of daily living can be performed with one hand, especially if it is the dominant one which is unaffected. The single most important factor in the prescription of an orthosis is whether it permits the patient to engage in activities which he desires, and which he could not engage in without the device. The best made orthosis is doomed to failure if it is not accepted by the patient.

While there is still some disagreement, most authorities agree that orthotics should be attempted with any patient whom they might assist towards improved function. A brace, which to some physicians may have at one time signified defeat and medical failure, has now become a symbol of progress. It enables the patient to perform new activities and to more successfully care for himself.

It must still be remembered that a splint or brace is not a permanent solution to a problem. It may be meaningfully used for months or years and then discarded when no longer needed.

Purposes of Upper Extremity Orthoses

Upper extremity splints are used to substitute in the absence of motor power, to assist weakened segments, to support segments which require positioning or immobilization, to provide traction, to enforce specific directional control, and for the attachment of devices.

A prescription for an orthosis as a substitute for absent muscle power is written when there is not enough motor strength to drive a body part through its normal range of motion with sufficient force. Power substitution methods vary from the use of rubber bands to electronically programmed carbon dioxide activators.

Many patients have some motor power but not enough amplitude or intensity. Orthotic devices can be prescribed to apply external power to assist the weakened segment through the required range with adequate strength.

When a body part has retained partial function, the question arises as to whether it is better to allow the patient to utilize his residual ability or to override the remaining, limited power completely with a device. The primary consideration is whether or not the remaining muscles will atrophy through overriding. If additional recovery is expected or even considered possible, the external power device should not override the function of the recovering muscles. If no further return of strength is anticipated, overriding by external means is indicated and is acceptable.

Adjustable power sources which assist residual muscle function without complete overriding are those which use springs, rubber bands and elastic. The tensions of these devices are adjusted to permit motion through a full range, only when the patient uses his residual strength to initiate and complete motion. There is no movement of the body part unless the patient utilizes his own remaining strength. These types of systems provide for the patient's continued employment and strengthening of his muscles and, at the least, prevent atrophy from disuse.

There are types of external power sources which provide a complete override of the remaining musculature of a segment. This is characteristic of non-elastic splints. Among these are the McKibben, the carbon-dioxide-powered, artificial muscle, and direct current torque motors. Most cable systems which make use of distant, unaffected muscles to drive weakened muscles, also override natural control. With such devices the patient is able to time, or grade his residual motor power in the involved segment to operate coordinately with external power.

Orthoses are used to support segments requiring positioning and immobilization. They are prescribed for use on either a full-time or a part-time basis.

It may be desirable for a patient to rest a group of muscles, tendon sheaths or joints for a period of time, yet require their full use at other times. For full-time immobilization a cast or removable splint may be employed.

Traction splints, or static splints which provide support or immobilization, are prescribed for the management of contractures. These are often preferred as night splints, so that while the hand may be free for action during the day, correction is provided while the patient sleeps.

If support is desired, the splint will be designed to fit the extremity exactly. If correction of a deformity is the objective, the splint will be non-conforming so that a corrective force is exerted in the desired direction.

Splinting can provide traction or tension against which a muscle can act. There are three basic principles to follow in using traction braces.

First, the amount of traction and the angle at which it is applied are crucial. Traction must be gently applied, particularly on the fingers. In general, traction must be just adequate to produce a detectable tension in the pulling device beyond that which is necessary to pull the segment to its limit of motion. The pull should be as nearly perpendicular as possible to the end position of the segment.

Second, repeated adjustments of the tension are necessary to retain efficiency.

Third, the patient must be permitted to develop tolerance to the splint. Stretching devices are not comfortable. Tolerance can be developed by first wearing the splint for a few minutes per day and gradually adding a few minutes more on each succeeding day.

Splints which permit motion must also attempt to enforce specific directional control. Most orthoses have directional control to reduce the number of planes of motion or degrees of freedom requiring control by external power sources. Certain splints are made solely to control the direction of movement, particularly when there is sufficient muscle power but abnormal directional control.

Many splints are prescribed simply because they can be used by the patient for attachment of self-help devices which enable him to perform activities which he would otherwise be unable to do.

Basic Principles of Splinting and Bracing

A fundamental principle of design which is applicable to all orthotic devices is that the splint or brace cover an adequate surface area for comfortable distribution of pressure with accurate contour. The desired function of the splint will determine the amount of surface for comfort. Accurate contouring is often achieved through the use of plastic cast models. A small adjustment in a splint can mean a great deal to the wearer. A change in position can result in a redistribution of pressure points and the splint must be adaptable for this.

Care must be taken in positioning the joints of the brace since this frequently determines how comfortable the device will be for the patient.

The part to be fitted must be examined carefully. Tender areas, areas of pain, skin erosions and bony prominences are to be avoided since pressure placed on them results in pain and frequent skin breakdown, particularly in areas which lack sensation.

The length of the lever arms of the brace is highly important. Shortness or overlengthiness of a brace may result in skin abrasions, pressure points and discomfort, all of which reduce the wearing time of the appliance.

An orthotic device must be designed to meet the functional needs of the individual. All activities which the involved part engages in should be analyzed into their components and the brace tailored to make the most desired motions possible.

Whenever possible, the wearer of the splint should be able to put it on and remove it himself. Therefore, it must be designed with ease of application in mind, and also to conserve the energy of the patient, thus encouraging activity.

The patient should be taught to put on and take off the splint. He needs also to be taught general maintenance of the device, including cleaning it, and making minor repairs. This requires that the components of the splint be simple and durable.

An orthosis must not weigh any more than is necessary to fulfill its function since even a few ounces of extra weight can significantly reduce the wearer's tolerance of the appliance.

The device should be durable and functional, but within these limits it should be cosmetically attractive. Its cost should not be high, but cost must be a secondary consideration to function and comfort.

Mechanical Principles of Orthotics

External power as a substitute for, or assist to, absent or reduced muscle strength is of four main kinds:

Elastic power includes rubber bands, springs and elasticized plastics. It is the most commonly employed type of artificial power.

Pneumatic power is the second most common source of power. The *McKibben muscle* is the basic unit in this family of appliances which is known as pneumatic actuators. These devices depend, for their power, on the transduction of expanding carbon dioxide, either through a piston or into enclosed flexible tubing which reacts by shortening. The resultant mechanical energy is used directly as tension and motion to drive orthoses. (Note: The McKibben muscle, or artificial muscle, is named for Dr. J. L. McKibben, a physicist, who began developing the device in 1955 for his daughter who was stricken with poliomyelitis.)

Electric power refers to electric motors which drive splints directly, or push or pull cables which in turn drive the orthoses.

Transmitted power is any power which activates an orthotic segment by means of a cable. It involves the transmision of force from voluntarily controlled muscles through cables.

Internal power is power supplied by the patient's muscles within the segment, whether under voluntary control or by means of electrical stimulation.

SPECIAL SPLINTS. There are primarily two major types of splints which utilize electrical stimulation for the control of muscles which are enclosed in braces. Each one depends upon an exoskeletal structure which serves to limit the motions of the braced part to a controlled number of degrees of freedom. Within this framework electrical stimulation of muscles provides movement in a single direction while return movement is managed by a spring.

The *electrophysiological splint* consists of the splint itself, an electrical stimulator, and a graded control which is actuated by mechanical movement of a distal segment under voluntary control. The control consists of a potentiometer which adjusts the stimulator output to the muscle.

The *myoelectric splint* consists of the same basic splint and a similar stimulator, but it is actuated by the electric potential output of a distant muscle which is innervated and voluntarily controlled.

Another type of internally-powered orthosis is the *tenodesis splint*. The term refers to the operation of a splint which resembles hand action following the surgical procedure of the same name. The principle involved is applied primarily to finger flexion following tenodesis. In this surgical technique the flexor tendons are attached to the radius so that dorsiflexion of the wrist produces finger flexion. The tenodesis splint produces finger flexion upon wrist action. Its function depends upon the voluntary power of the wrist extensor muscles.

A recent development in orthotics is the use of a computer to simulate central nervous system control of the upper extremity. It permits the patient with limited control of body sites because of severe paralysis to use these signal areas for the control of more degrees of freedom than would be possible through the simultaneous use of all controls. Signals can be transmitted from body control sites to the computer by mechanical, myoelectric or photoelectric methods.

A Note on Materials

The most suitable materials for the fabrication of orthoses include the following: metals, such as aluminum, steel and Monel®; Fiberglas®; Celastic®; Direkt-Form®; Nyloplex®; Royalite®; Naugalite®;

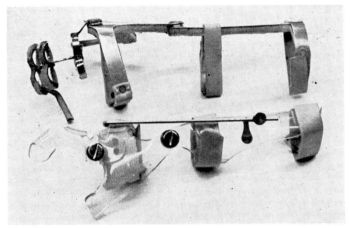

FIGURE 74. Examples of two tenodesis splints. The top splint is made of aluminum; the bottom splint is of plastic.

leather; silicone foam; paddings of foam rubber; Rubatex®; and foam laminated with jersey, latex and plastisol.

The main properties of materials to consider are weight, strength, sheer strength, elasticity, bulk, elongation, friction and life expectancy.

Self-Help Devices

A self-help device is one which assists the individual in performing various functions, or is one without which the person could not perform certain activities at all.

Aids which help the disabled person to be more self-sufficient range from very simple devices to complex electronic apparatus. Self-help equipment is designed for specific functional needs. These appliances permit the handicapped patient to perform activities which he could not otherwise do, or do only through great energy expenditure and time consumption. They provide partial or complete independence.

When a self-help device is being considered for a patient a careful analysis is made of the motions required to perform the desired activity. When it is observed that the patient does need a device for the activity in question, that he wants the device and will use it, then a self-help aid will be designed for him.

There are nine major indications for the prescription of self-help aids.

1. To provide positioning or support, as in a wheelchair, for purposes of maintaining body alignment.

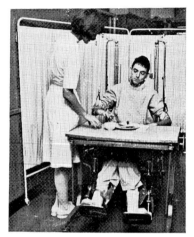

FIGURE 75. An arm counterbalance which supports a patient's upper extremity by eliminating the effects of gravity. It increases functional capacity of the forearms and hands, helps maintain range of motion, aids in relieving spasticity and edema, prevents stretching of weak muscles and helps in the maintenance of good posture. (*Courtesy of G. E. Miller, Inc.*) Shown here is the arm counterbalance being used during feeding,

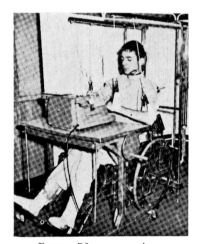

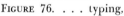

FIGURE 76. . . . typing,

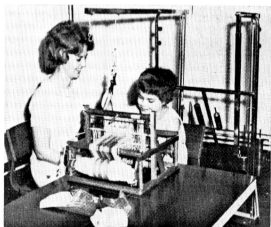

FIGURE 77. . . . weaving,

2. To provide stabilization of objects, as is seen in the use of suction cups, clamps and spikes.
3. As compensation for lost muscle power, as in the use of arm slings, or ball-bearing feeders.
4. As compensation for loss of range of motion in an extremity, an example of which is the long-handled comb.
5. As compensation for the loss of a part or loss of function of a part, as with prostheses.

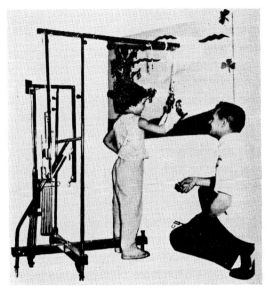

FIGURE 78. . . . and painting.

6. To reduce involuntary movements, such as with a friction feeder or weight cuff.
7. As compensation for loss of full grasp, as with a universal cuff or a built-up eating utensil.
8. As compensation for a visual deficit, as seen in the use of writing guides or reading aids, such as prismatic glasses.
9. Special self-help clothing.

It is impossible to describe or even to list the number of self-help devices which exist today. For purposes of example, however, a brief description of just some of the assists for the activity of eating is presented.

A cuff or *U*-shaped clip which fits around the palm of the hand and has a pocket into which the handles of utensils can be placed, enables patients with loss of full grasp to eat as normally as possible. Handles of utensils can be enlarged or built-up or curved for persons with weakened grasp, and pegs or rings can be placed on handles to assist grasp, as holders can be fitted onto cups and glasses. A bent knife, or rocker-knife permits food to be cut with one hand, and if the knife has a tined or serrated point it can be used as a fork as well.

Plate guards or sectional plates permit food from being pushed off the plate, and also assist in placing food on the utensil. Suction cups, or rubber mats, or damp cloths placed under dishes, or weighting of dishes, stabilizes them during eating.

Extension handles on utensils permit the patient with limited range of motion to bring the food to his mouth. Swivel spoons can substitute for lost wrist and forearm motion. Swivel cups keep the liquid level when wrist and forearm motion is absent. Weighted cuffs or heavy utensils decrease involuntary motion.

Ball-bearing feeders, suspension feeders and slings are used to support the arms at a functional level. Lapboards provide a functional eating level.

The reason for the plethora of devices is not only because of the great number which are commercially produced, but also because disabled persons all over the world are themselves, each day, devising new assists which will help them to become more independent.

UPPER EXTREMITY PROSTHETICS

As part of her therapeutic work the occupational therapist trains the upper extremity amputee in the use of whatever prosthesis he possesses. While structural replacement for a missing limb or limb segment is a relatively simple task, it is quite difficult to functionally replace an extremity through substitute mechanical or remote control techniques.

The therapist begins working with the patient shortly following surgery. All joints which are proximal to the amputation are moved through their complete range of motion at least three times per day. After the stump has healed, the patient is instructed to exercise the residual muscles of the remaining segment. The exercise program involves the muscles of both shoulders since the upper extremity amputee uses them both for prosthetic operations. Exercises progress to the resistive type as rapidly as possible.

Attention is paid to posture as well as to the specifies of prothesis utilization, since short, above-elbow and shoulder disarticulation amputees may have postural deviations resulting from loss of weight on the side of the absent extremity.

Components of the Prosthesis
The Terminal Device

In their attempts to replace hand function in the amputee, prosthetists have designed the split hook and the prosthetic hand.

THE SPLIT HOOK. The development of the split hook resulted because of the great complexity involved in designing even the simplest artificial hand. It is, therefore, a simplified substitute for a hand. There are two types of prehension control available.

In the voluntary-opening device, power remaining in a controlling member opens the finger of the appliance. When the force is released, a spring or rubber band equivalent closes the fingers on the object which is to be grasped.

In the voluntary-closing prosthesis, the device is held open by a spring when the patient is relaxed. Application of a positive control force closes the fingers against the spring's tension.

Voluntary-opening protheses are the simpler of the two forms of prehension mechanisms since they involve only a spring clamp. On the other hand, there is the disadvantage that they cannot be used to handle delicate or heavy objects. Furthermore, voluntary-opening is the opposite of normal prehension action to which the amputee was formerly accustomed with his natural hand.

The *Army Prosthetics Research Laboratory voluntary-closing hook* consists of a cam-quadrant type of clutch with an alternator-type of automatic lock operating one lyre-shaped finger against a fixed, mating, lyre-shaped finger. The operating cycle is as follows: pull

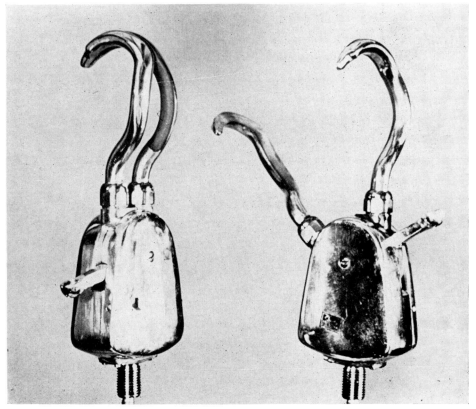

FIGURE 79. The APRL voluntary closing hook. Two views: left, closed; right, open. (*Courtesy of VA Prosthetics Center, New York, N. Y.*)

to grasp, relax to lock, pull to release, relax to open. In order for the lock to open, the cable pull must be greater than the pull that closed the hook.

THE PROSTHETIC HAND. Efforts to provide voluntary-closing devices which permit palmar prehension have resulted in the *Army Prosthetics Research Laboratory hand.* Prehension is of the three-jawed chuck type between the adjustable thumb and the movable index and middle fingers. The fingers adduct as they close. The little finger and ring finger are passive and flexible, and are positioned in a way which makes them appear natural whether the active fingers are closed or open.

This hand is very durable but it contains fine, precision mechanisms and is therefore not suggested for heavy manual labor. A plastic glove has been designed which, when fitted over the appliance, provides good cosmesis and, additionally, protects the mechanisms from dust and dirt.

Wrist Units

A wrist unit is necessary in an upper extremity prosthesis for purposes of attaching a terminal device and providing terminal device rotation for manual positioning.

The wrist unit is designed as a manual friction, manual lock, or

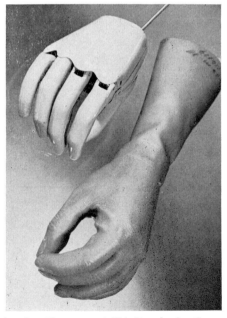

FIGURE 80. The APRL hand. (*Courtesy of VA Prosthetics Center, New York, N. Y.*)

active rotation unit. The manual friction type is the one most frequently employed. In this device a metal washer bears against a rubber one as the terminal device is screwed into place.

Wrist Flexion Units

Lost volar and dorsal flexion of the wrist can be partially replaced by the wrist flexion unit. Such an addition increases the utility of the prothesis, particularly for the bilateral amputee who must operate the terminal hook or hand close to the body.

Elbow Hinges

Flexion of a below-elbow prosthesis is permitted through the functioning of a variety of hinges. These hinges may be rigid, semi-rigid or flexible, and they can be made of leather, metal or metal cable. A stump-actuated locking hinge may be prescribed if the below-elbow stump is very short.

The Prosthetic Elbow

Elbow disarticulation, above-elbow and shoulder amputation prosthesis typically provide for forearm flexion by means of a joint which permits locking of the device at various positions. Elbow disarticulation prostheses employ external elbows. Above-elbow and shoulder appliances use internal elbows. The external elbows have five or seven locking positions while the internal elbows have eleven locking positions.

Shoulder Units

Several attempts have been made to create shoulder joints which provide flexion, abduction and elevation. These have been, in the main, relatively unsuccessful. It is possible for passive abduction to be given to the shoulder to simplify dressing activities, and a passive friction shoulder joint has been developed which allows approximately sixty degrees of angular rotation, enabling wearers to perform independent toileting.

Control Systems

Almost all upper extremity prostheses are controlled by stranded, steel cables that glide inside a cable housing which is frequently lined with nylon.

CINEPLASTY. Cineplasty is the surgical procedure whereby a skin-lined tube is constructed through a muscle in which, after healing has taken place, a pin can be inserted and linked to a terminal de-

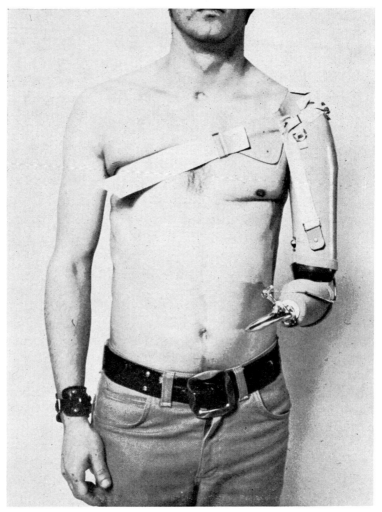

FIGURE 81. Upper extremity prosthesis with split-hook terminal device. It is secured with an above elbow chest strap harness with a leather shoulder saddle. (*Courtesy of VA Prosthetics Center, New York, N. Y.*)

vice. The use of cineplasty is still somewhat controversial but the current general consensus among authorities in the field is that it is a successful procedure and can be recommended for selected patients.

Recent Prosthetic Developments

Prostheses which derive control information from bioelectric sources in the body eliminate the gross body movements and direct use of body power of cable prostheses. When cybernetically coupled

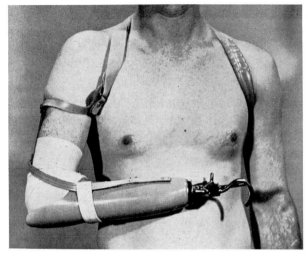

FIGURE 82. The same prosthesis fitted with an above elbow figure-eight harness. (*Courtesy of VA Prosthetics Center, New York, N. Y.*)

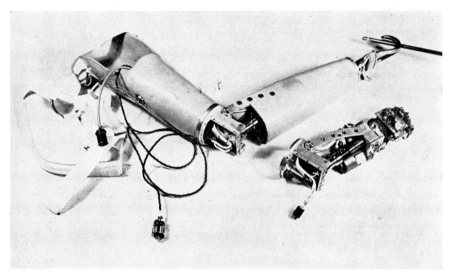

FIGURE 83. The "Boston Arm". (*Courtesy of VA Prosthetics Center, New York, N. Y.*)

to the human central and peripheral nervous systems, as when electromyographic (EMG) signals from muscles that previously controlled the amputated joint are utilized, training is virtually eliminated and amputees achieve volitional efferent control immediately after fitting. Proprioceptive-force sensing has been achieved in the EMG limb known as the "Boston Arm" by electronically sensing force and feeding this information back to the limb servo-mechanism in opposition to the body-generated EMG signal. The resulting demand for additional muscular output from the patient stimulates force-sensing organs in the residual muscles and at the interface between the limb socket and stump. Basically, then, the "Boston Arm" is a prosthesis which is powered by the EMG signals of the patient's own remaining muscles.

A modification and improvement of the EMG arm has been developed which uses a sensory-aids display system to transmit information to the user through the location of a vibratory sensation on the skin. Thus, kinesthetic feedback from the prosthesis is provided. When this sensory feedback is added to the EMG arm the resultant prosthesis achieves all of the volitional, efferent control and conveniences of EMG activation and external power in combination with the positioning sense of the traditional mechanical prosthesis.

Prosthetic Training

Training procedures are designed to be congruent with the type of amputation which the patient has had. The general objective of training is to enable the patient to become as self-reliant as possible in all of the activities of daily living. (Note: It is considered practical to teach the unilateral amputee to use his prosthesis as an assist to his natural hand while performing two-handed activities.)

The patient is taught initially how to care for his prosthesis, including putting it on and taking it off, cleaning it and maintaining its proper function, and adjusting the harness.

A stump sock of cotton, nylon or wool may or may not be worn, depending upon the individual patient's preference.

The patient is taught correct prosthetic terminology and the characteristics of his prosthesis' components. Then he is trained in the use of the controls.

Training in utilization involves prepositioning, and drills in approach, grasp and release. The final phase of instruction involves the application of these basic procedures to ADL and vocational activities.

PEDIATRIC OCCUPATIONAL THERAPY

Occupational therapy for children does not differ in its basic objectives from that which is prescribed for adults. Increasing range of motion, improving muscle strength, learning self-care activities and ADL training are the primary goals of any rehabilitation program. What is unique about dealing with disabled children is the approach used by the therapist to the patient and the modifications which are made in methodology and in the materials that are used.

Basic Qualifications in Work with Children

The occupational therapist who works with children must have a thorough knowledge of normal human development in order to be able to evaluate a child's performance. She must be familiar with the evolution of motor behavior so as to appropriately select therapeutic toys, games and activities. The mere simplification of adult crafts is not adequate for the treatment of a child. Imagination and creativity are required if activities are to be meaningful and valuable for the young patient.

The therapist must know how to grade activities for certain disorders and thus, she requires knowledge of pediatric illnesses. She needs to be able to organize and plan activities for both individuals and groups in such a way that the children in her care will be interested and anxious to participate. She must have the necessary skills in providing outlets for a child's dramatic, constructive and creative play and energy, with sufficient direction and control. She must be able to provide an atmosphere which is friendly, reassuring and understanding to the child who has become hospitalized due to a disability, and who has been separated from his parents and family because of the hospitalization. Much of the success of a kinetic occupational therapy program depends upon the cooperation of the patient which, in turn, is a result of the kind of rapport which the therapist establishes from the initiation of training.

There are certain specifies which the pediatric occupational therapist must consider in the planning and course of her work. These include the following: the child's age and his relevant maturity; his powers of concentration; his attention span; his comprehension of time; his level of interests; his lateral dominance; his susceptibility to fatigue; and his habits.

When selecting toys to be used in a therapy program it must be remembered that in addition to the loss of strength and function produced by the disability, a child's strength is normally less than that of an adult. Thus, the proper size and weight of the toy, and the power required to operate it has to be carefully considered.

The child's adjustment to his handicap and his reactions to the hospital play a large role in how well he will do on a rehabilitation program. Above all, the therapist must remember that she is dealing with a child, not just a small adult, but a child with all of the concomitant variables associated with that status. Kindness, patience, good humor and love are all needed in very large doses.

As anyone who has worked with children knows, one rarely works only with the child, but rather with the child and his parents. This is true also of occupational therapy in physical rehabilitation. Once the patient is considered to be ready for discharge to the home, if further therapeutic activity is indicated, the parents will be instructed on a home treatment routine. They will be informed as to the purposes of the home therapy program, and will be given a list of necessary restrictions, each one of which will be interpreted to them.

If the child uses any supportive devices, such as splints, braces or slings, their purpose and uses are carefully explained to the parents. Recommended activities, including time allowances and probable areas for increasing activity are listed for the parents, as well as suggestions for handling activity readily in the home environment. Parents are cautioned regarding the activities to be avoided and are, of course, informed of the reasons for these contraindications. Finally, a list of supply sources for equipment and a list of sources of home assistance are provided.

In addition, the therapist holds discussion sessions with the parents, provides demonstrations of therapeutic games and techniques whenever possible, and supplies brief notes which can act as a reference and guide for the family during the first few weeks the child is at home.

Space does not permit a complete description of occupational therapy programs for each of the childhood disorders discussed in Chapter 3 of this book. As stated previously, the objectives of improving muscle strength, range of motion in the joints, coordination and management of daily activities do not markedly differ from the goals for adults. Materials and procedures must be modified, not only for disabilities involved, many of which are not found in older persons, but also because of the reduced size, weight and strength of the patients involved. And, of course, the therapist's manner and approach in working with children differs from what is employed with adults.

It is possible, however, within the confines of this section to examine in some detail occupational therapy for one disability. Cerebral palsy has been selected for purposes of illustration because of its prevalence in rehabilitation institutions, and because of the wide variety of systems, theories and approaches to treatment regarding the kinds of exercises which should be employed with patients suffering from this disorder. The methods referred to below pertain to exercises of the upper extremities.

Occupational Therapy for Cerebral Palsy

The Method of Phelps

Phelps' work was the first truly concerted effort to apply technics specifically to cerebral palsy and a great deal of his methodology has become incorporated into basic treatment approaches. He employs classical conditioning in compliance with Sherrington's law of reciprocal innervation and Jacobson's principles of relaxation and motion from a relaxed state. Phelps uses bracing extensively to prevent and correct deformities and to maintain the body in an erect position. Self-help skills are taught as muscle groups achieve a desired condition of efficiency, and these skills are then utilized to further develop the action of the muscles.

With the very young, and with the uncooperative child, conditioned motion is employed. This consists of passive range of motion activities, each of which is carried out in time to a song, a different song being used for each movement. In time, a conditioned response develops to these stimuli, initiating active motion and preparing the child for the next step in the progression of exercises. Reciprocal movement is employed at the proximal joints, with treatment beginning at these sites and progressing distally.

Exercises for the spastic type of cerebral palsy are directed at overcoming the stretch reflex and increasing the contractility of those muscles which act antagonistically to the spastic ones. For the latter, massage is used, which also builds strength and improves the tone of non-spastic but weak muscles. Active-assistive, active, and finally, resistive motions are used as indicated.

The athetoid type is treated primarily by training in techniques of conscious relaxation and in motion from the relaxed position. Awareness of muscle tension is taught through resistive motion by palpation or by verbal instruction. Once the patient learns conscious relaxation, movement is initiated, progressing through stages of passive, active-assistive and active motion, avoiding tension and involuntary movement as much as possible. The least involved segment is the first to be treated, and therapy progresses from there.

Ataxic children are treated by teaching them combined motions. Two unidirectional movements are taught separately and then in combination.

Development of balance and position sense is important in the training process for the recovery of sitting or standing balance. Phelps employs special apparatus extensively, including mirrors, weights on the wrists, shoes and crutches, shoes with extended soles, standing tables, relaxation chairs, stabilizers and reciprocal skis.

The Method of Fay

Fay's technique involves exercises in which normal and pathological reflexes are used as forces for movement. His theory is based upon the phylogenetic evolution of homo sapiens. The midbrain and spinal cord, when released from cortical control, function in a manner which produces the primitive movement patterns seen in amphibian and reptile stages. The tonic neck reflex, for example, is described as the initiator of a caudally-directed flow of impulses which unlock muscles and consequently produce a projectional response.

Exercises are carried out by producing a number of reflex responses, such as the Babinski sign. "Unlocking" reflexes and positions are used to establish movements which are later brought under the patient's voluntary control. These are considered by Fay to be precursors of movement patterns. Continuation of these exercises through deep tendon and skin stimulation results in improved function, improved volume and strength of the spastic muscles, and diminution of muscle tone and postural disturbances.

The Method of Kabat

Kabat bases his system of exercises on six principles. They are as follows:

1. The therapeutic effect of voluntary motion is based on repeated activation of the nervous pathway.
2. Continued activity is essential for maintaining power, endurance and coordination.
3. Voluntary motion of the agonist muscle results in relaxation of the antagonist.
4. Training of new patterns of motion depends upon the formation of new functional pathways.
5. Performance is facilitated by repetition of motion.
6. The amount of muscle activity is contingent upon the percentage of excited motor units.

Mass patterns of motion are treated as being spiral and diagonal in character, that is, as a pattern of voluntary motion which includes in the one motion, at a number of joints simultaneously, three components—flexion or extension, abduction or adduction, and external rotation or internal rotation. The two diagonals of motion for each of the major body segments are comprised of flexion and extension components and are always combined with lateral motion and rotation. Movement is initiated and terminated with rotation and progresses through extension into flexion.

Exercises employ combinations of isometric and isotonic contractions using maximum resistance. The movement begins in the position of extreme stretch and ends in extreme shortening. Reinforcement is added through the therapist's stimulation of skin receptors and by verbal instruction. In the general treatment plan, proximal defects are corrected first, but in individual exercises timing of movement progresses from distal to proximal.

Kabat employs pulleys, weights and manual techniques to provide heavy resistance. Work is performed against gravity and friction to increase awareness of contractions, first in elementary motions and then in combinations of motions and in skilled activity.

The Method of Knott

Knott's technique of proprioceptive neuromuscular facilitation to stimulate and strengthen the response of the neuromuscular mechanism is based upon Kabat's original efforts. She employs reinforcement and repetition of motion to develop endurance, and changes in activity to overcome fatigue.

Stimulation proceeds from the proximal to the distal, and strong muscles are utilized to reinforce weaker ones. Resistance is provided to the isotonic contractions of agonist and antagonist muscles.

Knott, like Kabat, focuses on patterns of motion, particularly the spiral and diagonal, in order to accelerate learning and to improve strength and balance.

The Method of Bobath and Bobath

Bobath and Bobath focus on the inhibition rather than the utilization of reflexes. It is their belief that abnormal muscle tone and primitive reflex patterns of movement are common to all cerebral palsied children. Incoordination in the ataxic patient is considered to be a consequence of lack of muscle tone. Movements and postures are felt to basically consist of the combined action of the muscles which belong to either the flexor or extensor groups, and lack of function is held to be a result of lack of control over this mass action.

The initial treatment step involves teaching the patient to inhibit the primitive and exaggerated reflex activity by holding the various joints in the position opposite to that which they tend to assume. Movements are not taught but many different postures must be learned before the patient can move correctly from one to another. If a gap is observed between postures where there is a lapse into spasticity, a reflex-inhibiting posture must be devised which will bridge the movement defect.

The Bobaths feel that deformity results from encouraging movement appropriate to later stages of development *before* the child is able to control the motor activities of earlier stages. Thus, a young child is prevented from standing or walking until treatment has prepared him for these activities.

The Method of Rood

Rood's system is based upon stimulation of cutaneous and musculotendinous receptors in the activation of muscle responses for either contraction or relaxation. Motor responses are facilitated by bombarding the sensory-motor system with more efferent impulses than normal to cause the contraction of a muscle and the inhibition of its antagonist to produce motion, or the contraction of a muscle and the simultaneous contraction of its antagonist for holding a part.

Rood stimulates cutaneous receptors by light stroking or brushing, or by the application of ice, which promotes reciprocal inhibition between agonist and antagonist muscles. Proprioceptive nerve endings in muscles and tendons are stimulated by stretching, manual pressure, and pounding on bony prominences.

Treatment proceeds developmentally. Functional activities are not attempted until results of the treatment of body parts indicate their readiness and advisability.

The Method of Deaver

Deaver finds that the greatest success occurs when all but two movements of an extremity are restricted during the performance of a functional activity. He employs extensive bracing to achieve this objective.

Emphasis is placed by Deaver upon training in activities of daily living. He feels that most children will benefit from a period of inpatient care and he utilizes this time to compile an accurate inventory of skills so that training may be given in deficient areas of performance.

Bed and wheelchair activities are considered to be of primary concern. Various techniques are taught to the child, often employing assistive devices as aids in performing ADL tasks such as transferring, propelling a wheelchair, rising from a chair, and bathroom care.

Hand activities are also taught by the method of eliminating all but two movements, in this case movements of the arm. Feeding is taught with the use of splints and adapted utensils which are gradually removed as control is established.

The Method of Pohl

Pohl's treatment of cerebral palsied children is founded upon three principles—conscious muscle relaxation, voluntary muscle control, and building of developmental patterns. All forms of the disorder are managed by the same methods although variations are introduced depending upon the specific needs of the individual case. Since the emphasis is on voluntary control, braces are not employed.

Each treatment session includes relaxation, active motion and functional activity. Relaxation is continually stressed. Mild stretching of contractures is used to aid in the development of control of antagonistic muscle groups.

General relaxation is first induced by instructing the child in the feeling of tensed muscles. Each muscle group of the body is relaxed through passive movement or palpation. Attention is then directed towards individual muscle groups where voluntary contraction is to be taught, usually progressing from proximal to distal joints. Isolated relaxation is taught simultaneously with active contraction of the prime mover or of the antagonist.

Training of voluntary muscle control involves three principles—muscle consciousness, function and coordination. Muscle education is conducted through isolated contraction with the body segment aligned so as to eliminate substitutions and mass movements. Training in functional activities is developmentally ordered and begins with passive motion and total relaxation, followed by an active pattern where there is active motion of prime movers and inhibition of antagonist muscles.

The Method of Schwartz

It is Schwartz's belief that psychological abnormalities are the most important causative variables in retardation of physical development. He maintains that progress in treatment depends upon successful emotional, intellectual and physical self-expression, and in the child with cerebral palsy this is best accomplished through simplification of the environment and the providing of motivation.

Putting these ideas into practice, Schwartz uses an apparatus known as a Hartwell Carrier.® This consists of a ceiling track extending around a large room, from which are suspended numerous slings, tricycles and dollies. The motor-driven machine is under selective control and has different speeds of operation. A child placed in a sling or on a tricycle receives the stimulation of pressure of his feet on the floor, develops reciprocation, and can progress without fear of falling. Group activity and successful performance of play activities provide motivation.

Bracing is not employed since it is felt that neuromuscular training must be accomplished according to natural patterns.

Basic Principles of Occupational Therapy for Cerebral Palsy

Therapy for Spasticity

Spasticity represents muscle imbalance. Thus, the fundamental objective of treatment is muscle re-education to correct that imbalance. This is accomplished through strengthening of weak muscles, reducing the power of strong muscles and protecting and/or re-educating the zero cerebral. (Note: Damage to a cortical area will deprive a muscle of its upper motor neuron while leaving the lower motor neuron and thus, the reflex arc, intact. The flaccid muscle is termed zero cerebral or OC. Spastic patients generally have some OC muscles.)

No muscles are treated until the relative strength of the antagonist has been assessed. The function of the spastic muscle can be improved by repeated exercise without elicitation of the stretch reflex to teach gradual control through the complete range of joint motion. Speed of contraction is also used to improve function. Once the slowest speed has been noted, rhythmic exercises are employed at that speed until the child works consistently well. Then the speed is increased while the rhythm is maintained. Muscles which are antagonistic to a spastic muscle are also exercised without constant stimulation of the spastic muscle, since they often become weak through disuse. Exercise through a controlled range of motion will strengthen them.

There are two types of deformity which the occupational therapist works to correct. A *primary* deformity is one caused by the imbalance of spastic versus OC muscles. *Secondary* deformities arise indirectly from abnormal muscle pathology. Exercise, bracing, splinting, proper seating, and muscle re-education are employed to prevent and correct such conditions.

Therapy for Athetosis

Treatment for the athetoid type of cerebral palsy is based upon the child's ability to develop conscious relaxation and control over the relaxation so that he can increase or decrease it in accordance with the state of his athetosis. With the very young child, braces, proper seating and repetitive exercises are required to encourage relaxation. In all cases, braces and splints are employed to control movement in certain joints while the patient learns to control others voluntarily.

Once relaxation is achieved, specific motion from the relaxed position is initiated. Movements are carried through to completion, as in the follow-through of a baseball pitcher when he throws the ball. First, single motions are taught, then combinations of motions. The smaller the muscle group, the slower is the desired pace since athetotic patients often lose accuracy with increased speed. Steady progress is made when the patient learns to pause between motions in combination activities, since this avoids a build-up of tension.

Therapy for Tremor

Tremors are dealt with by teaching the patient to relax the involved extremities. Weights are used to reduce the amplitude of the tremors and progression of treatment is from gross to fine motions.

Therapy for Ataxia

Treatment is aimed at developing compensatory mechanisms to substitute for cerebellar dysfunction. In the case of loss of balance, increased use of the kinesthetic sense is taught through developing an awareness of weight distribution. When the kinesthetic sense is absent, emphasis is placed on the development of balance sense and exaggeration of kinesthetic sensation, since motivation can be a contributing factor.

Basic motions such as grasp, release, clutch and return can frequently be performed, if inaccurately. Conditioning helps to establish the correct pattern if it is done in the position from which the skill is naturally performed.

Because of flabby musculature of the patient, strengthening exercises are usually conducted. Both gross and specific exercises are beneficial to the child and are carried out repetitively and with increasing resistance.

Therapy for Rigidity

For rigidity alone the basic treatment principle involves the development of speed of muscle contraction and release. This is performed through repetitive motion, beginning with passive motion, followed by assistive and, finally, active movement.

The patient is generally forced to work at a rate which is slightly faster than he wishes. Exercise proceeds from one joint to another and from one speed to another prior to the development of combined motions or skills.

Naturally, cerebral palsied children are taught ADL skills aided by built-up eating utensils, self-help aids, special clothing, modified tools and implements, wheelchairs, bracing and splinting.

CONCLUDING REMARKS ON OCCUPATIONAL THERAPY

The great number and variety of activities which comprise an occupational therapy program make it an indispensable service to any rehabilitation institution. It is an integral part of every patient's total rehabilitation program, for without the essentials taught by the occupational therapist complete rehabilitation or habilitation is not possible. For many patients, even the most basic and minimal activities of daily life cannot be performed, and they would be unable to leave the hospital and return home were it not for the training they receive in occupational therapy. It may conclusively be said that without occupational therapy there is no rehabilitation.

Section III
References

1. Alles, D. S.: Information transmission by phantom sensations. *IEEE Transactions on Man-Machine Systems, MMS–11:* 85, 1970.
2. Anderson, M. H.: *Functional Bracing of the Upper Extremities.* Springfield, Thomas, 1958.
3. Anderson, M. H.: *Upper Extremities Orthotics.* Springfield, Thomas, 1965.
4. Bierman, W. and Licht, S. (Eds) : *Physical Medicine in General Practice,* 3rd ed. New York, Hoeber, Harper, 1952.
5. Cromwell, F. S.: *Occupational Therapists Manual for Basic Skills Assessment.* Los Angeles, United Cerebral Palsy Association, 1960.
6. *Dorland's Illustrated Medical Dictionary,* 24th ed. Philadelphia, Saunders, 1965.
7. Dunton, W. R. and Licht, S. (Eds) : *Occupational Therapy: Principles and Practice,* 2nd ed. Springfield, Thomas, 1957.
8. Grinker, R. R. and Sahs, A. L.: *Neurology,* 6th ed. Springfield, Thomas, 1966.
9. Hirschberg, G. G., Lewis, L. and Thomas, Dorothy: *Rehabilitation: A Manual for the Care of the Disabled and Elderly.* Philadelphia, Lippincott, 1964.
10. Jones, Mary S.: *An Approach to Occupational Therapy,* 2nd ed. London, Butterworth, 1964.
11. Jones, Mona (Ed) : *Work Adjustment as a Function of Occupational Therapy.* Dubuque, Brown, 1962.
12. Krusen, F. H., Kottke, F. J. and Ellwood, P. M. (Eds) : *Handbook of Physical Medicine and Rehabilitation.* Philadelphia, Saunders, 1966.
13. Lawton, Edith B.: *A.D.L. Activities of Daily Living. Testing, Training and Equipment* (Rehabilitation Monograph X). New York, Institute of Rehabilitation Medicine, 1956.
14. Lawton, Edith B.: *Activities of Daily Living for Physical Rehabilitation.* New York, McGraw–Hill, 1963.
15. Licht, S. (Ed) : *Orthotics Etecetera.* New Haven, Licht, 1966.
16. Licht, S. (Ed) : *Rehabilitation and Medicine.* New Haven, Licht, 1968.
17. Licht, S. (Ed) : *Therapeutic Exercise,* 2nd ed. New Haven, Licht, 1961.
18. Lovett, R. W.: *The Treatment of Infantile Paralysis.* Philadelphia, Blakiston, 1916.
19. Lowman, E. W.: *Self-Help Devices for the Arthritic* (Rehabilitation Monograph VI). New York, Institute of Rehabilitation Medicine, 1962.
20. Lowman, E. W. and Rusk, H. A.: *Self–Help Devices* (Rehabilitation Monograph XXI). New York, Institute of Rehabilitation Medicine, 1967.
21. MacDonald, E. M. (Ed) : *Occupational Therapy in Rehabilitation.* London, Baillière, Tindall and Cox, 1961.
22. Mann, R. W. and Reimers, S. D.: Kinesthetic sensing for the EMG controlled "Boston Arm." *IEEE Transactions on Man-Machine Systems, MMS–11:* 110, 1970.
23. Meldman, M. J., Wellhausen, Marilyn and Jacobson, Joanne: *Occupational Therapy Manual.* Springfield, Thomas, 1969.
24. *Rehabilitation Equipment and Devices Constructed in Wood. Instructions for Making Exercise Equipment, ADL Devices and Occupational Therapy Progress*

Kits (Rehabilitation Monograph XXXVI) . New York, Institute of Rehabilitation Medicine, 1968.

25. Rusk, H. A.: *Rehabilitation Medicine. A Textbook of Physical Medicine and Rehabilitation.* St. Louis, Mosby, 1964.

26. Rusk, H. A., Kristeller, Edith L., Judson, Julia S., Hunt, Gladys M. and Zimmerman, Muriel E.: *A Manual for Training the Disabled Homemaker* (Rehabilitation Monograph VIII) 3rd ed. New York, Institute of Rehabilitation Medicine, 1967.

27. Rusk, H. A. and Taylor, E. J.: *Living With a Disability.* Garden City, Blakiston, 1953.

28. Schad, Carol and Dally, A. T.: *Occupational Therapy in Pediatrics: A Student Manual.* Dubuque, Brown, 1959.

29. Steindler, A.: *Kinesiology of the Human Body.* Springfield, Thomas, 1955.

30. Wagner, Elizabeth and Zimmerman, Muriel (Eds): *Approaches to Independent Living.* Dubuque, Brown, 1962.

31. Willard, Helen S. and Spackman, Clare S. (Eds): *Occupational Therapy,* 3rd ed. Philadelphia, Lippincott, 1963.

THE SPEECH AND HEARING SERVICE

Chapter 12

ADULT SPEECH AND LANGUAGE DISORDERS

LANGUAGE IS MAN'S most important communication medium and when the ability to verbally express one's thoughts, feelings, needs, desires and emotions is lost or impaired, the consequences are dire both for the affected person and for the society in which he lives.

INTRODUCTION

It has been estimated that there are more than one million aphasic individuals in the United States. There are over two million school-age children with a speech disorder, which means that ten per cent of this total age group is afflicted by some form of language handicap, one-half being seriously affected. Six per cent of the total United States population has some speech or language problem, and when a special group, such as the cerebral palsied, is considered, it is known that approximately sixty-five to seventy per cent of such persons are speech and/or language impaired. In addition, it has been reported that, among children of elementary school age, the incidence of hearing loss varies from two to four per cent, while in the cerebral palsy group it is somewhat higher, at about five per cent or greater. When it is realized that the deaf individual is also likely to have a consequent speech defect, the problem is compounded.

While these statistics are important they most probably do not accurately reflect the actual incidence of speech and hearing disorders in the population. They have been obtained from studies of hospitalized patients, clinic patients and selected school children, and there are undoubtedly many more individuals with such problems who never come to the attention of a speech clinician, an audiologist or a physician.

In a rehabilitation setting the incidence of persons who are in need of, or who can benefit from speech therapy is naturally higher than

297

in the general population. Estimates of the number or rehabilitation patients who are seen by a speech and hearing service, range from twenty to sixty per cent of the total in-patient population, depending upon the type of institution concerned and the population being considered. These are primarily individuals who have lost their language or have had their speech and/or language impaired as a result of brain injury, such as a cerebrovascular accident, and these consist mainly of patients with aphasia, apraxia and dysarthria. As these facts are understood, the crucial role played by the speech therapist on a rehabilitation program becomes clearer.

While in some respects the speech and language problems seen in a rehabilitation institution resemble those met with in university clinics, general hospitals and out-patient speech centers, there are certain distinct differences. In the non-rehabilitation speech clinic the defects which are treated are primarily stuttering, functional articulation problems, voice impairments and defects resulting from oral deformities, such as cleft palate cases, and these are likely to exist in isolation from other medical problems. In a rehabilitation hospital, however, the speech or language disorder is usually secondary to neurological disorder or vascular disease and as such is encountered in patients who are multihandicapped. In these cases speech therapy becomes more complicated since gestures, which are often an important part of language, may also be difficult or impossible for a patient because of a paralytic condition. In the individual with only a communication disorder this is generally not a problem.

While the terms "speech" and "language" have been used more or less interchangeably thus far, such usage is technically incorrect. *Speech* may be thought of as referring to the non-content aspects of verbal behavior, such as volume, rate, pitch, inflection, rhythm, phonation, and the functions of the peripheral speech mechanisms. *Language* may be considered in terms of the content facet of verbal behavior, the verbal expression of ideas which permits functional communication between individuals. The speech therapist, or speech clinician—which is the preferred title in many institutions—deals with both of these components of communication and hence, the term speech and language therapy is most appropriate.

There are several services which the speech clinician performs in a rehabilitation hospital. These include the initial evaluation and continuous re-evaluation of speech, language and hearing functions, therapy for patients with communication impairments, and auditory rehabilitation with patients who have a hearing loss. In addition, recommendations are made by the clinician for the prescription of orthotic devices, such as hearing aids, prosthetics, which may be indicated for a patient with a palatal defect, and even dentures, if their absence or poor fit is interfering with adequate speech production. Many speech clinicians also engage in research and in the education and training of students who are preparing to enter the profession. The speech clinician frequently maintains close contact with the psychologist and the physician since problems in the behavorial and medical spheres are most likely to interfere with progress on a therapy program.

The majority of persons speak "normally" and therefore give little or no thought to the complexities involved in producing oral communication. Yet the act of speaking involves some of the most complex motor coordinations which humans make. It has been written that a German scholar once devoted a lengthy monograph entirely to the muscular acts involved in uttering the single syllable "pop," and concluded his treatise with an apology for its incompleteness. In diagnosing a speech or language disorder the speech clinician must be aware of the phenomena she is dealing with, in order to properly determine the existence and extent of deviations from normal speech.

The term "speech" can be either a noun or a verb. In its noun form it may be defined as an established system of communication of both conventional and arbitrary acoustic symbols, primarily produced by the muscular movements of the respiratory and upper alimentary tracts. When used as a verb, speech means the communicative behavior of humans through the use of such symbols. Speech, then, is *a system of verbal abstractions and the use of this system as a type of communicative behavior.*

Communication is based upon words, which are themselves symbols representing objects and thoughts, and, as such, are substitutes for the meanings the words convey. In addition, words have an arbitrary significance in that their meaning is unique for the individual or group employing them and, in fact, may bear only slight resemblance to their represented concepts. It is this arbitrary and self-inspired symbolism which distinguishes verbal communication from other kinds of human behavior and which is so essential to language.

Speech is considered to be normal when the listener attends more to the content of the speaker's utterances than to the way in which these utterances are produced. Conversely, speech is defective when attention is distracted from the communication and drawn to the communicative effort. Thus, the evaluation of a speech defect is highly dependent upon the listener. It is generally assumed that the listener's perception and language familiarity are unimpaired and thus, if he is unable to respond properly to what he hears, the judgement is made that the problem resides with the speaker.

There are certain characteristics which, if present in an individual's speech, are considered representative of a defect. Speech is defective if it is:

1. Not easily audible;
2. Vocally or visibly unpleasant;
3. Not readily intelligible;
4. Deviant with respect to specific sound production;
5. Effortful in production;
6. Lacking in conventional stress, or rhythm, or tonality or pitch change;
7. Linguistically impaired;
8. Inappropriate to the speaker when the variables of age, sex, or physical development are considered;
9. Productive of a psychological maladjustment or behavior problem in its possessor.

Briefly then, a speech defect focuses attention on the speaker because of one or more of its characteristics, interferes with communication, or causes a psychological problem in the individual possessing it. It is often the case that all three of these areas of difficulty are found within an individual and it is the function of the speech clinician to evaluate their presence and extent, provide therapy where indicated, and make appropriate referrals to other professional services.

COMMUNICATION DISORDERS OF ADULTS
Aphasia and Related Disorders
Aphasia

Aphasia, broadly speaking, is a loss or impairment of language as a result of brain injury. It is a general language deficit crossing all language modalities and may or may not be complicated by other consequences of the brain damage which produced it. It is characterized primarily by a reduced vocabulary, difficulty in utilizing the remaining vocabulary, impaired auditory verbal retention span, and impaired perception and production of communicative sounds.

Shortened attention span, reduced concentration ability, and losses in the visual-motor, auditory and sensory spheres may be associated with the language impairment. Behavioral changes such as lability, hostility, depression and anxiety are also possible sequelae to the brain injury which results in aphasia.

Linguistically, aphasia is an impairment of the patient's ability to deal with symbols, and thus represents a disturbance in both symbolic formation and expression. The aphasic typically has difficulty in formulating, comprehending and/or expressing meanings.

Aphasic patients may have problems in comprehension of written symbols and thus, with silent reading, or *alexia*; in writing, such as use of faulty grammar, omission of words, notably connectives such as conjuctions and prepositions, or *agraphia*; in performing arithmetic computations, or *acalculia*; in remembering or finding specific words to use, or *anomia*; and in maintaining a proper melodic or rhythmic pattern in speech, or *dysprosody*. The tendency to substitute words, to make grammatical errors, to use letter transpositions, and to omit words and letters in written and oral communication may be considered together under the term *paraphasia*.

These aphasic disturbances are considered to be on a high symbolic linguistic level of production. There are disturbances which are frequently observed in aphasic patients which are known as subsymbolic disturbances. These are the agnosias and the apraxias. Dysarthria may also be considered as subsymbolic but this disorder will be discussed separately.

Agnosia

Agnosia is a receptive disorder manifested as a disability in the recognition of configurations through the sensory channels when the disturbances are not produced by specific sensory losses.

Visual agnosia refers to the inability to recognize configurations such as objects, colors, patterns, letters or words through the visual sense. The involved individual is aware of seeing, but does not recognize what it is that he sees.

Auditory agnosia means a disturbance in the recognition of sounds. This impairment can be for nonsymbolic sounds, such as those made by machinery, animals and the like, for human nonsymbolic sounds, as in sneezing or handclapping, or for spoken symbols, i.e. words, phonetic units, phrases and sentences. In the patient who cannot recognize sounds which he hears, the ability to evaluate auditory sensation is lost. The person with auditory verbal agnosia cannot cannot understand what he hears.

A less important disturbance of this kind is *amusia*, or an impairment in the ability to recognize previously familiar music. This can present a more serious problem if it also interfers with the individual's ability to detect tonal and inflectional changes in speech.

Tactile agnosia, or *astereognosis*, is a disturbance in the ability to recognize objects through the sense of touch. This disorder is more thoroughly discussed in the section on occupational therapy.

Apraxia

Apraxia is a motor disturbance, sometimes referred to as "motor aphasia," which is frequently seen in aphasic patients. While not all aphasics are apractic, most apractics are aphasic. Apraxia is an impairment in ideation. A patient so affected lacks the ability to recall the motor patterns of speech. He may remember the appropriate words but not the oral movements required to produce these words.

Nonverbal apraxia is a disability involving the use of tools such as writing implements, eating utensils and mechanical devices, so that these tools are not employed in the purposeful way for which they were intended and designed.

Verbal, or *oral apraxia* is a defect in the motor aspects of speech production. Inner symbolic formation may be intact, yet the patient can remain inarticulate because of an inability to transfer the ideas into speech. The peripheral speech mechanisms and the neurological transmissions involved in speech production are unimpaired but the affected individual cannot form the words necessary for communication. At times, the apractic patient who cannot on command protrude his tongue, purse his lips, or smile, may perform these movements spontaneously when they are not related to language.

A final characteristic of aphasia which is of interest is the so-called "automatic speech" which some patients exhibit. Sometimes, the aphasic who cannot say words meaningfully, will be able to sing a simple song which contains those words. In response to a greeting he might be able to reply "Hello," or "I'm fine," and often he may use profanity when other words are lost to him. This kind of verbal behavior involves well-learned, automatic language which is almost reflexive in nature and it is not an adequate measure of language function, not a satisfactory prognostic indicator.

It should be realized that the verbal behavior of aphasic patients fluctuates markedly during the first few days, and even the first few weeks after the initial brain injury. This is because of the various neurophysiological changes which take place during this period such as recovery of brain tissue from shock, healing following surgery, decreases in edemic pressures on the brain, and stabilization of blood pressure, pulse rate and temperature. During this time, which is known as the period of spontaneous recovery, the patient's performance is variable and may show considerable improvement from day to day. How much he will improve or how rapidly improvement will progress cannot be predicted.

The period of spontaneous recovery is generally estimated to be of approximately three months' duration, although this is an arbitrary figure which varies widely between patients. It is also possible that an adverse condition such as intracranial hemorrhaging, infection, or a chronic disease process can inhibit recovery of speech and language and even cause a regression in the patient. If the condition is arrested recovery may begin again. Diagnostic tests which are administered during these times will, obviously, be unreliable, and results obtained from the same patient on two different occasions can have a very low correlation. Eventually, however, most patients become neurologically stable and further changes in their performance can be expected to be slow, gradual ones which result from the practice and exercise given in therapy, and the stimulation and practice received in everyday living situations. At this time performance becomes more regular and predictable, evaluation measures are more reliable, and therapy becomes more meaningful.

THE EVALUATION OF ADULT COMMUNICATION DISORDERS
The Screening Procedure

All patients admitted to a rehabilitation hospital are, as a rule, given a general screening by the speech pathology service. This screening differs from a complete speech and hearing evaluation in its thoroughness. It is aimed primarily at determining whether a problem exists and identifying the nature and extent of such a problem. The screening is conducted upon the initial admission of a patient and, since time is usually limited during this period, it is designed towards making a recommendation regarding the patient's need for speech therapy. Once a patient has been accepted to a rehabilitation program, the problem areas which were detected during the initial screening session are more intensively evaluated.

The main questions which the speech clinician attempts to answer during the screening session are these: Can the patient communicate adequately? Can he "get across" what he wants to say? Does he comprehend what he hears? Is there a hearing loss?

The speech clinician frequently begins by asking the patient questions of general information, such as his name, occupation and interests, and by having him describe his present physical status and its antecedents. By doing this she may begin to draw conclusions regarding the patient's audition, ability to understand what he hears, and verbal intelligibility. In an additional test of auditory comprehension the patient will be asked to follow simple, and then more complex, instructions. These can range from having the patient point to and name objects in the room to requiring him to select a particular object from a group of several, name it, place it in a receptacle and hand the receptacle to the clinician, all of which requests are given as a single command. The patient with impaired auditory comprehension will make errors in performing these tasks and, if severely impaired, may not be able to do them at all.

In her examination of the functioning of the patient's peripheral speech mechanisms, the tongue, lips, palate and facial muscles, the clinician is concerned with whether the movements of these organs and muscles are adequate for speech. She looks for weaknesses of the muscles which are involved in speech production.

The patient is asked to protrude his tongue and push against the restraining force of a tongue depressor. His cheeks are pressed inward while he is requested to keep his lips in retraction. He is told to say "Ah" as the clinician notes palatal movements. Diadochokinesis is tested. This involves performance of repetitive movements such as lowering and raising the mandible, occluding and opening the lips, and the rapid, repetitive production of sounds, as in "pa-pa-pa-pa-pa," "ta-ta-ta-ta-ta," and "ka-ka-ka-ka-ka." The patient's ability to imitate vocal and nonvocal movements of lips and tongue are tested by having him first observe, and then mimic the clinician.

In the initial assessment of hearing, the speech clinician notes whether the patient speaks significantly loudly or softly, if he asks to have questions or instructions repeated, or if his answers to questions or responses to directions are inappropriate, or irrelevant.

At this time the speech clinician makes an initial diagnosis of existing problems. If the patient demonstrated an inability to express himself, and difficultly in producing words, could not name objects correctly, showed impairments in counting, writing, telling time, spoke in jargon, could not understand what the clinician said to him, or revealed a reading deficit, the diagnosis may be of a form of aphasia. The patient who demonstrated an inability to utilize his speech musculature in a coordinated way so as to communicate effectively, who showed weakness or paralysis of the peripheral speech mechanisms, and exhibited impairments in phonation, volume, rate and other noncontent verbal behaviors, may be judged to be dysarthric. If there was no neuromuscular involvement of speech mechanisms, but the patient could not voluntarily move the appropriate muscles of his face, tongue and lips, could not imitate the therapist's vocal actions, and showed phoneme dysfunction, a tentative conclusion of apraxia may be warranted. In the case of the individual who frequently requested that questions be repeated, who responded inappropriately to queries and directions, or who showed marked deviations from the norm in volume, a hearing loss would be suspected.

It is on the basis of these preliminary diagnoses that a patient is recommended for a program of speech or language therapy and he is then given a further evaluation in the problem areas uncovered by the initial screening procedure before therapy is actually begun.

The Evaluation of Aphasic Disorders

The speech clinician employs the evaluation session to more thoroughly test the patient in all verbal and nonverbal communication spheres and to focus upon the areas of difficulty which the patient exhibited during the initial screening procedure. The evaluation, furthermore, provides information for the initiation of language retraining and, on the basis of the findings of this session, the starting point for therapy is determined.

There are several areas of communication which the clinician is interested in evaluating. These include the following:

Auditory and visual perception and comprehension of language.
Ability to understand and use symbols in reading, writing and arithmetic computations.
Oral and written formulation and comprehension of propositional language, or general expressive ability.
Auditory retention.
Performance of motor functions required for speaking and writing language.

The attempt is made to determine the extent to which drain damage has interfered with these functions.

To test the patient's visual recognition and comprehension capacity the clinician may have him name letters of the alphabet by showing him single letters on cards and asking him to identify them. The same procedure can be used for the recognition of individual words and numbers. The patient may be given the task of reading and then carrying out written directions, such as "Give me the pencil," or "Close your eyes."

In the evaluation of auditory comprehension, commands are given verbally to the patient without any hint by gesture or glance on the part of the clinician. While, in the initial screening procedure, commands were also given, they were primarily simple and concrete in nature. In a thorough evaluation there will be two- and three-step commands as well as more abstract ones, such as "Point to what you call people on," rather than "Point to the telephone," and "Give me what you write with," instead of "Give me the pencil."

The patient will be asked to imitate the clinician's verbal behavior, first with his eyes open and then with his eyes closed.

Auditory retention span can be tested by giving the patient a picture and having him point to the items he sees and names, and then removing the picture from sight and asking him to recall what he had just named. It is quite possible for an aphasic person to understand what he sees and hears but not be able to retain the memory of it for any length of time.

Reading comprehension may be evaluated by presenting the patient with several names or addresses printed on cards, his task being to locate his own. Words are presented to him which he must match to the appropriate pictures described by the words. The patient is directed to read short sentences to himself and is then asked written questions based on the reading material which can be answered by a simple negative or affirmative response. Simple arithmetic problems are given to the patient to solve to determine his ability to handle basic mathematical processes. He is also requested to spell common, familiar words, such as *house, cup, dog, Sunday, mother,* and the like.

General language functions are assessed by asking the patient to name objects which are pointed out to him by the clinician, by having him write a sentence or two without assistance, and by an appraisal of his spontaneous language production in which his use of grammar, syntax and vocabulary is evaluated. The patient is required to name objects and their functions, and is asked differences between objects and pictures—e.g. an airplane and a train, a telephone and a typewriter, a shoe and a dress. He may be shown a picture and be requested to describe what is happening in the scene. He is given words to define. The basic question to be resolved by these procedures is this: *Are the patient's language functions adequate for daily communication?*

The motor functions which are involved in speaking and writing are examined by having the patient imitate the speech clinician in pronunciation of words and in oral movements, with and without phonation. The patient is also asked to write or print spontaneously. If he is unable to do this, he is given the task of copying from material provided by the speech clinician. If even this is too difficult, he is permitted to trace over the material. While motor functions such as those involved in communication have naturally been involved during other phases of the evaluation process, it is here that the clinician views them with certain, specific aims in mind, such as the possibility of diagnosing an apractic disorder, and hence, she is evaluating them more specifically and intensively.

An audiometric evaluation is also an integral part of the total evaluation procedure and this will be dealt with in Chapter 14.

LANGUAGE THERAPY

Basic Principles

The primary goal in the treatment of aphasic disorders is increased communication. This objective can mean many things depending upon the individual patient who is undergoing therapy. Some patients will be content if they can express their daily needs with a rudimentary vocabulary and understand what their family says to them. Others feel that, while their speech and language may be adequate for daily functional usage, they might err while speaking to a business patron and thus not perform at their jobs in a satisfactory manner. Still others expect to achieve the level of language skill which they possessed prior to their disability.

The speech clinician must decide how realistic each patient's goals are, contingent upon her knowledge of their past history and present disability. It is a general working principle that whenever they are realistic, a patient's objectives should be accepted. On the other hand, it is known that few aphasics whose language impairments persist for months following brain injury, ever recover their former communication level. Thus, the speech clinician must work both within the framework of the patient's goals and the realities which can be expected.

For this reason it is usually felt to be advisable to inform the patient at the beginning of treatment that therapy will probably require a fairly lengthy period of time and will proceed slowly, one step at a time, requiring much patience on his part. This tends to prevent over-optimism on the part of the patient, which would lead to unrealistic expectations from speech therapy; yet it also tells him that he is expected to make progress. Once gains are seen by the patient, therapy becomes a positively reinforcing situation.

There are several guiding principles which the speech clinician heeds in her treatment of aphasia and related disorders.

Since the object of therapy is the retraining of the brain to deal with communicative processes, a "natural" technique to employ is sensory stimulation. This refers mainly to auditory and visual stimulation and, thus, one principle which is followed states that *intensive stimulation through the auditory and visual modes of perception is effective in eliciting language.* This stimulation is maintained until the patient can function through each modality on any given level of complexity which is appropriate for him.

The second principle involves insuring that *the appropriate stimuli are utilized.* Since aphasics are often auditorily impaired, it is encumbent upon the speech clinician to manipulate and modify stimuli so that the patient perceives them, interprets them correctly, and is able to make use of them. By combining visual stimulation with auditory stimulation, greater results may be obtained than if one modality alone were employed. Once the patient correctly perceives the stimulus, then progress can be made with a shift in emphasis to a single modality. In addition, it is helpful to employ stimuli which are meaningful to the patient rather than those to which he has few associations. Thus, for most patients, words such as *car, eat* and *home* are preferable to *diesel, masticate* and *domicile*. This is because both short-term and long-term memory are better for familiar words, and because auditory retention span is greater for words of one syllable than for polysyllabic words.

It may also be an aid to the patient's perception if the stimuli are presented slightly louder and/or more slowly than they would be in ordinary conversation.

All of these techniques are attempts at enabling the patient to properly perceive presented stimuli which, in the case of aphasia therapy, are words. This is a difficult task for the therapist but one which obviously must be performed correctly if learning is to take place.

Another basic guideline followed by the speech clinician is that *successive repetitions of a stimulus are important for recognition*. Many patients who do not perceive a word correctly upon first hearing it will come to recognize it if it is spoken repeatedly. What may appear monotonous to an observer is essential to the patient.

As important as presentation of material is the requirement that *each stimulus should elicit a response*. Stimuli are not merely presented in sequence. The patient is required to respond to each one before the next is given to him. By following this principle the speech clinician can determine the adequacy of the stimulus she is using, and the patient is able to receive feedback regarding his performance. If the stimulus which was presented is an appropriate one, it should elicit a response. If it does not, either the stimulus was not an adequate one or more stimulation may be required. The response may first be gestural in nature, as in pointing to an object, but as stimulation is increased or repeated, gesture language becomes replaced by verbal behavior.

The feedback involved in seeing one's own performance, or in hearing one's own speech is highly important in providing the patient with information which he can use for self-correction. Many patients are unaware of errors they make until these errors are demonstrated to them via their own behavior.

Speech clinicians also adhere to a principle of *stimulation rather than teaching and correction,* the underlying belief being that as language improves incorrect responding decreases. Patients are therefore stimulated to emit correct responses which will replace defective ones.

The speech clinician must work *within the boundaries imposed by the patient's general condition,* the irreversible brain damage which produced the aphasia, and the patient's needs and motivation to enable him to achieve maximal recovery of communicative functions.

Factors Affecting Prognosis

There are certain rules of thumb which a speech clinician uses to determine the prognosis of an aphasic patient. While it may generally be claimed that improvement from aphasia is highly correlated with overall physical recovery, this is not always the case since some patients do improve almost completely physically, with little or no corresponding improvement in language ability. The clinician then looks at other variables in attempting to predict recovery.

One factor is age. The younger the patient, the more optimistic the outlook. Another factor relates to the etiology of the condition. Patients who have had their aphasia caused by head trauma have a better prognosis than those whose disability resulted from cerebrovascular disturbance or disease. Premorbid personality is also a variable to be considered. Patients who were previously sociable people show more rapid recovery than those who were of a withdrawn nature. The patient who demonstrates flexibility in thinking is considered to be a more hopeful therapy candidate than one who exhibits rigidity of thought processes.

General behavior characteristics play a prognostic role. Extreme lability, depression, apathy, disorientation, confusion, serious memory disturbances, marked neurotic symptoms and psychotic behavior are negative factors when working with a patient to bring about improvement.

Finally, the patient's awareness of his language dysfunction is considered. The individual who realizes that he is making errors while speaking, or knows when he is emitting jargon, who receives some feedback of his performance through his own sensory modalities is a better therapeutic risk than the person who lacks this kind of awareness. The patient who is not cognizant of his deficiencies is probably more seriously brain-damaged and, as a consequence of absent or impaired feedback, is probably less motivated for therapy. This is not to be interpreted as a hard and fast rule, however, since many patients who reveal such impairment in the early stages of recovery from their disability, do gain an awareness of self-behavior and become better therapeutic candidates as time goes on.

Therapeutic Techniques

Therapy is begun as soon as the patient's medical condition permits him to attend. The earlier therapy is initated, the greater the probability of recovery of language functions. While early language retraining need not be intensive, it is important to begin with at least brief sessions of stimulation. This shows concern for the patient, prevents nonverbal communicative methods from becoming in-grained, and aids the patient's morale.

There are two main schools of thought regarding the starting point for therapy. One maintains that therapy should begin at the level of language breakdown and proceed from easier to more difficult tasks. The other point of view holds that training ought to be initiated with the patient's most immediate needs serving as a guide. There is certainly room for both approaches and both can be incorporated into a therapist's procedure.

Aphasia Therapy

With patients who have little or no functional speech, the therapist can begin by showing them cards on which are pictured objects or scenes of action and corresponding descriptive words. These cards are either purchased commercially or are made up by the therapist and are appropriate to the patient's age, education and background. Thus, childish pictures are not shown to an adult, nor are yachts shown a poor man who has never seen one. A few cards are selected at a time, and, as therapy progresses, one subset is re-placed by another with the earlier ones kept for periodic review.

The patient is instructed to look at a card and its corresponding word, to think about the word, and when he feels he knows it, to say it aloud. The clinician first points to the card and then to the word, saying it clearly. This is done for many repetitions with intervals between repetitions so that the patient can think of the word and re-peat it. Should the patient be unable to repeat the word the therapist stops after a few words, spreads these cards on the table before the patient, and has the patient point to the card she names. The cards are then named, first in sequence, then in random order until the patient has mastered them. This procedure is repeated with all of the cards.

If the patient is able to point correctly, the therapist may become more abstract in her requests by asking the patient such questions as, "What do you drink from?" or "What do you drive?" And the patient must indicate the picture of the glass or the automobile. Pointing is then gradually replaced by oral production.

When the patient errs, he is told to listen to the therapist who then pronounces the word correctly for him. Patients often want to say the word spontaneously, or before the therapist does, but they are encouraged to wait, listen, and think before speaking.

Once the patient is able to fluently say single words, he is advanced to short phrases, such as "in the cup," or "drive a car." Note that the phrases revolve around the previously learned words. Following this phrasing the single words are reviewed by showing the patient the cards and asking him, "What is this?" Patients are given time to respond, which can be up to one minute in length. As therapy progresses, patients typically have increasingly shorter latencies of responding. This technique is continued until the patient experiences no difficulty in naming items and using them in short phrases.

The same words are employed for the improvement of writing skills. The patient is given a few words each day and he practices copying them. When he performs correctly, he is advanced to writing the words without looking at the copy. Then he is asked to write the words from only looking at the pictures they were derived from, and finally, to write them without the pictures being present. With each writing the word is spelled and pronounced aloud by the therapist and the patient.

Once the patient has become adept with single words and phrases, he is started on short sentences. These are placed singly on cards and read aloud several times in unison by the patient and the therapist. Then the patient is directed to read the sentences alone and, finally, to write them.

Words, phrases and sentences can be written on Language Master® cards and the patient can work solitarily with the Language Master, an apparatus which presents the cards visually while also stimulating the user aurally. He sees the word or group of words, hears the correct response and then repeats it aloud.

There are several techniques employed in therapy which elicit responses from the patient. The simplest of these provides a frame for a word which is missing and must be supplied by the patient. He may be asked to complete phrases or short sentences such as, *a cup of* _____, *bread and* _____, *comb your* _____, and *wind a* _____. This exercise can provide both needed stimulation and early success. Later, once the correct word is supplied, the therapist asks the patient to say more about it, to use it in a sentence, or to respond to a question, using the word as part of his response.

As the patient's abilities become more advanced, short paragraphs are read in unison by patient and therapist, with the latter leading strongly at first and gradually dropping out as the former improves. The therapist asks the patient questions about the reading matter to test his comprehension of what he has read.

It will be noted that with all procedures therapy is begun at a simple level and increased to greater complexity as the patient improves. It is often difficult to determine precisely when to advance from one level of complexity to another and exactly how large the step of advancement should be. Such decisions are dependent upon the subjective judgement of the speech clinician.

There are primarily three techniques which are employed with the higher level aphasic. The first involves the syllable writing of a word by the therapist who then pronounces it and has the patient repeat it after her. Next, patient and therapist say the word together, with the therapist leading at first and then gradually fading out as the patient becomes able to say the word alone. The therapist then uses the word in a series of sentences, having the patient first listen and then repeat them. Finally, the patient is requested to define the word. This last task is usually a difficult one for aphasics, and the therapist asists the patient until a functional definition is achieved.

Patients who are at this language level are given sentences which illustrate the uses of these words as "homework", to practice reading and writing them when they are away from the therapy situation. These individuals can also be instructed to read a newspaper and report back to the therapist on articles which interested them, or to listen to a radio or television program and describe to the therapist what they heard and saw. Aphasic patients will, at first, understand little of these programs but, as progress continues, they are able to report more and more information.

The majority of aphasics exhibit impairment in recognizing letters of the alphabet. While we do not normally learn to speak by first memorizing the alphabet, to some patients not knowing it is frustrating and anxiety-producing. The patient who requests training in this area is given practice in saying and writing the letters in serial order until they can be reproduced correctly in this manner. Next, the patient is stimulated by a group of letters simultaneously. Severely impaired aphasics are presented with the letters in triads, such as *abc, def, ghi,* and so on, while less impaired individuals are presented with them in larger groups, as in *abcd, efgh, ijkl,* and the like. The letter is sounded by the therapist several times and the patient repeats it afterward.

Letters may be paired with words beginning with them such as *a-ate, b-big, c-car,* etc. The letters are placed on cards with the words on the backs of the cards. There can also be an assisting card with the entire alphabet printed on it in the order grouping which the patient learned. At first the patient merely points to the letter named by the therapist, then he is required to say the word when the letter is named. Next, letters are dictated randomly by the therapist to the patient who must write them as they are spoken. Then the patient names a letter, produces its sound, and gives examples of its usage in words. Finally, the words are sounded and the patient spells them orally, unassisted.

As the patient becomes fluent in alphabet usage new phonemes and diphthongs are gradually introduced, and in the last stages of alphabet training several words are used for each sound, placing the sounds in various positions within the words.

There are patients whose aphasic disturbances are so mild that therapy is often believed to be unnecessary for them. However, these persons may have a greater potential than their present level of functioning indicates and can benefit from treatment. Such individuals typically do not require lengthy periods of language retraining and can carry out many procedures on their own. These patients receive intensive stimulation aimed at retrieving lost vocabulary and increasing verbal retention span. The materials which are employed in therapy are commensurate with the patient's age, education and occupation, and special tools which are needed by the patient to function maximally at his work are often required.

Patients practice sentence and paragraph repetition, as well as repeating names, addresses and telephone numbers. They are given specific questions to answer based upon their reading materials and work in arithmetic processes.

It is obvious that the mildly involved aphasic is less hampered by loss of language skills in many areas than is the severely or moderately impaired patient. However, since he must function in the community his need for treatment may be as important for his success and happiness as that of the hospitalized patient with the more serious disorder.

Apraxia Therapy

Since the patient with apraxia cannot recall the motor patterns necessary for speech, the early stages of therapy revolve around imitation of the speech clinician. This is done either in a face-to-face position or with the clinician and the patient seated before a large mirror, so that the patient can see the oral movements of the clinician as well as his own, thus receiving feedback which is important for self-correction.

Initial steps in retraining apractic patients are concerned with control of the speech musculature. Either by direct command, or an imitation of the therapist, the patient is given a series of exercises to perform. These include protruding the tongue, placing the tongue alternately at both corners of the mouth, touching the inner cheeks with the tongue, touching the back teeth and extending the tongue to the roof of the mouth, pursing the lips and blowing out air as if to extinguish a match, and smiling. Each exercise is demonstrated by the therapist and performed by the patient until done correctly.

The second step is designed to produce or increase phonation. Beginning with simple sounds, such as *ah* and *ooh,* the patient is aided physically by the therapist. She may place her hand firmly over the patient's larynx and say "Push hard," or "Press here and say *ah* together with me." Phonation may not immediately result and so this exercise is repeated until the patient is successful. When he does perform the exercise properly, he is reinforced and encouraged by being told that he will find the tasks easier each time he does it.

Following this, the patient is required to produce the sound without assistance. Several attempts are made, followed by a rest period, followed by more attempts, and so on. Once this sound reproduction is achieved, manipulation of the sound is attempted by having the patient vocalize louder and for a greater duration so that more control is gained over phonation.

The third step involves the use of consonant sounds. This is done by using the visible (lip motions clearly seen) consonants, such as *m* and *p,* first, then moving on to the semi-visibles—e.g., *t* and *l,* and, finally, to the invisible consonant sounds, such as *k* and the hard *g.* For each consonant, a card with the letter printed on it is shown simultaneously with the patient's pronunciation.

To produce the consonant sound *m,* the patient is asked to place his lips tightly together and hum, either monotonically or in a tune. To produce *p,* the patient's lips are placed together and opened with a slight expulsion of air, as in saying "pah". Holding a match or a tissue in front of his mouth can be an aid in showing him the proper pronunciation through its effects. For the sound of *f,* the patient is told to bring his lower lip up to his upper teeth and blow. The voiced counterpart of *f* is *v,* and this is produced by adding sound to the previous task. The *l* is made by the patient touching the roof of his mouth with his tongue and adding sound. The most difficult consonants are those which are not orally visible. For production of *k,* the patient's hand is placed over the therapist's throat while she coughs and makes the *k* sound. She presses upward on the patient's throat as he tries to imitate her phonation. The hard *g* sound is made by adding sound to the *k.*

For each consonant, should the patient be unable voluntarily to place his lips or tongue correctly, it is done for him by the therapist using a tongue depressor, or an orange stick, or her hands until the positions are learned. Tongue movements are aided by exercises, such as having the patient protrude and retract his tongue repetitively, and by singing a song utilizing the syllable *la* as a substitute for the words. As sound production increases, vowels are added to the consonants and the patient practices saying "ma", "pa", "la", "ta", "ga", "ka" and the like.

In the fourth step, vowel sounds, diphthongs, and vowel and diphthong combinations are added and practiced in much the same step-by-step manner. Simple arithmetic is performed orally to provide the patient with practice in placement of speech musculature. Thus, for example, for the *f* sound, he can be asked to add two plus two, three plus one, nine minus five, seven multiplied by two, and so on for each consonant and vowel sound.

Reading exercises can be given from the beginning of treatment. Apractic patients may understand what they read but cannot make the correct sounds in reading aloud. In reading training the vowels and consonants retained by the patient are employed predominantly at the start. Reading of cursive writing is generally preferred to reading of printed words.

Finally, work is begun with individual words as drill practice, such as *me, mine, money, mat, more* and *may.* Sentences are then introduced which primarily incorporate the known or learned consonants, as for example, "*My money is here*," and I *miss my hat.*" Next, meaningful sentences are incorporated into the training, such as "I want to eat," "Pass the salt," and "Open the door." Familiar phrases, like "How are you," and "Good morning," are also included in the practice. Rote tasks, including counting from one to ten, or reciting the alphabet, or naming the days of the week, are also helpful. In this way more and more material of increasing difficulty and of greater importance to the patient become incorporated into his speech.

Agnosia Therapy

Agnosia, as previously mentioned, is a loss of recognition through a sensory modality. Since this loss generally involves only one of the senses (although this is not necessarily true), the therapist utilizes another sense as a substitute for purposes of stimulus identification. Thus, the patient with visual agnosia who, upon seeing a pencil, does not recognize it, may be brought to recognition by having him hold the pencil, running his fingers around its contours, feeling the point and the eraser, and come to identify it through the tactile sense. The auditory sense can also be employed, as in dialing a telephone or in turning the pages of a magazine or newspaper, for the patient who does not recognize these objects visually. Even taste can be employed by a patient to identify foods and beverages when his visual sense is impaired.

In addition to the above, there are several techniques which are regularly utilized by speech clinicians in treating visual agnosia. Pairing items is one method. Several identical items are placed before the patient in random order, such as pencils, matches, pins, combs and books. The therapist demonstrates the pairing task and then directs the patient to pick up the items which are the same. A more advanced pairing task requires the patient to pair pictures of like objects in dissimilar scenes or poses, such as pictures of Chevrolet automobiles, of cocker spaniels, of Presidents, or of baseball players.

A second procedure is matching. The patient is asked to match identical pictures, or colors, or in a more difficult variation of this procedure, to match pictures with actual objects, or to match geometric designs.

Discrimination tasks are also employed. From a series of geometric forms the patient must select the one which is different from the group, or choose the letter of the alphabet which is unlike others in a series.

Finally, the therapist can draw a stick figure of a man or a dog and ask the patient to select the corresponding picture from a group which he has already worked with. She may draw a pencil or a glass and the patient then selects the matching object. The act of drinking or writing may be performed by the therapist in pantomime, and the patient chooses the item used in, or implied by the act.

In treating the patient with auditory verbal agnosia, lip reading or phonetic instruction in which the patient can learn to follow the observable movements of the oral musculature has been found to be helpful. The patient is instructed to touch the therapist's laryngeal musculature and facial muscles as she speaks, so as to gain a tactual picture of speech production. Therapist and patient can also sit before a mirror while the therapist vocalizes simple sounds and sound combinations with clear, visible movements. These movements are imitated by the patient and eventually are performed by the patient after only hearing the sounds without observation and imitation of the therapist.

Sounds or musical selections are played on a tape recorder or record player, and the therapist points to pictures of the object, animal or person which produces such sounds so as to gain and strengthen associations between sound and sound source.

The tactile sense may be employed by having the patient actually strike a wooden board with a hammer, thus associating sound and object.

The basic principle which underlies all techniques is that *the use of non-affected senses can help a patient to recognize sounds, and constant, intense stimulation is important in retraining sound distinction.*

DYSARTHRIA

Dysarthria is a defect of articulation occurring on a neurological basis. The lesion can be peripheral, with nerve involvement of the face, lips, tongue or palate, or it may be central, as is most likely the case with aphasic patients who are also dysarthric.

Dysarthria is most basically described as an inability to produce or articulate correctly because of lack of muscular control. It is manifested as distortions and omissions of the sounds of speech. The dysarthric patient typically speaks in a slow, laborious manner with slurred sounds because his articulatory mechanisms have become cumbersome to him. Difficulty in swallowing and hence drooling and choking on foods and liquids are other characteristics often associated with dysarthric speech.

The Evaluation of Dysarthria

In evaluating a patient for a suspected or possible dysarthric defect the clinician is listening, not to the content of speech or language functions, but rather to the non-content aspects of verbal behavior. She observes the patient's speech for deviations in rate, pitch, volume, voice quality, phonation, articulation and general intelligibility. The observation is done both in a face-to-face manner and also with the speech clinician's head turned away from the patient

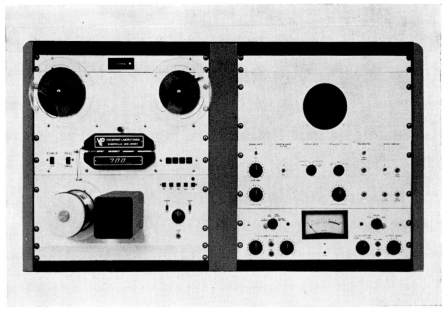

FIGURE 84. A sound spectrograph which can be employed for speech research and diagnostics, speech analysis and speaker identification. (*Courtesy of Voiceprint Laboratories Corp.*)

so that omissions, sound substitutions, and distortions may be detected without visual cues. The patient is asked if he experiences difficulty in swallowing, chewing or sucking. Facial asymmetry is examined, the gag reflex is tested, and signs of drooling are noted.

Labial (lip) and lingual (tongue) movements are tested by having the patient open his mouth, smile, purse his lips and protrude his tongue. He is asked to push his tongue against the resistance of a tongue depressor. His palate is viewed during pronunciation of consonants and vowels to determine its efficiency of operation. The existence of difficulty in facial mobility is determined by having the patient smile, frown and wrinkle his brow, since weakness or paralysis of facial musculature will hamper speech production.

Nonverbal and verbal diadochokinetic movements are tested, first by asking the patient to open and close his mouth and to lateralize his tongue repetitively within ten second periods, and then by requiring him to rapidly repeat syllabic sounds, such as *pa, ta* and *ka,* many times in succession.

Problems of respiratory insufficiency may be assessed by requesting the patient to count digits in a single breath.

If a patient's speech reveals faults which indicate impairment of vocal musculature to the extent that intelligible language is interfered with, a diagnosis of a dysarthric defect is made and therapeutic steps are taken to correct it.

Dysarthria Therapy

There are primarily two spheres of speech therapy in the treatment of dysarthric patients. These are exercises for improvement of muscular movements and phonetic training.

Exercises are given to the patient for the purpose of increasing the range of motion and strength of muscles which are essential for correct speech. Repetition of syllables such as *la* and *ma,* and upward, downward and lateral movements of the tongue are helpful, and these are practiced rapidly and regularly. As the muscles required for these acts are strengthened and brought under control by the patient, articulation becomes clearer.

There are several techniques for improving phoneme production. Generally, specific defective sounds are treated first in isolation, then in the context of words, and finally, in connected speech. The defective phonemes are often found to be *s, sh, ch, j, r, l* and consonant blends. One method involves practicing the consonant or consonant blend as it precedes first long vowel sounds and then short vowels. A list of words containing each combination, and of phrases which use these words, is compiled by the therapist and pronounced by the patient. This provides rhythmic practice, forcing the patient to make many repetitions within a short period of time. A second procedure consists of having the patient read a list of phonetically-edited sentences aloud and then repeat these sentences without looking at the list. With each defective sound emitted by the patient, the therapist interrupts and requires the patient to repeat it. Still another technique requires that the patient read a list of words which contain the problem sound or sounds. The therapist asks him to repeat each incorrectly pronounced word.

There are procedures which are employed to aid patients who have a problem of slow rate of speech. With one method, polysyllabic words are listed on a card and these are divided into syllables with the accented one being underscored. The patient repeats each word after the therapist, who proceeds slowly at first and then with increasing rapidity until normal rate is achieved. When the patient can pronounce a word correctly, he is asked to use it in a sentence.

A procedure which is designed to increase ease of natural inflection and fluency, and to make connectional units of speech more automatic, is repetition of short phrases, with emphasis placed on the important word in the phrase—e.g., in the *house,* at the *store,* a big *book.*

When a patient's vocal volume is too low to permit good intelligibility, the therapist first ascertains that he is able to achieve and maintain an adequate tone. The patient is then given a simple task, such as counting or reciting the alphabet, and each time his volume

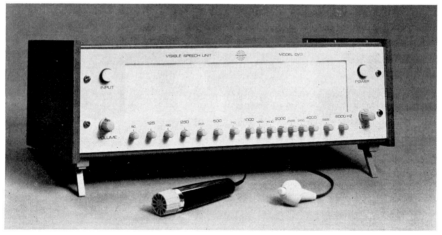

Figure 85. Visible speech and articulation trainer. (*Courtesy of Precision Acoustics Industries, Inc.*)

decreases, he is stopped by the therapist and told to continue at a louder volume. A second technique involves requiring the patient to speak against a background masking noise so that he must speak loudly in order to be heard. Each time his voice fades the therapist stops him, has him repeat what she did not hear, and then directs him to continue. Thus, by these methods, both loudness and duration of phonation are improved.

While dysarthria is typically a less complex disorder than aphasia and is more readily amenable to therapy than the more serious language disabilities, it nonetheless requires the expert attention of a speech clinician, particularly in severe cases where intelligibility may be quite poor. As is true of aphasics, the sooner the dysarthric patient is treated following initial onset of the problem, the greater the chances for improvement of articulation.

Chapter 13

DISORDERS OF SPEECH AND LANGUAGE IN CHILDREN

Aᔆ ɪꜱ ᴛʀᴜᴇ ᴏꜰ ᴀᴅᴜʟᴛꜱ, the majority of children who are seen by a speech pathology service in rehabilitation medicine have problems which are additional to any speech, language or hearing deficit they may possess. While children may be seen on an out-patient basis for a communication disorder alone, it is more typically the case that a physical disability, such as cerebral palsy, for example, has resulted in the child's hospitalization and has produced a speech handicap.

The speech clinician who treats such children must be aware not only of the primary disability and how it affects communication, but also of the fact that children present unique problems which result from such variables as a more plastic and growing nervous system, and a younger chronological age which permits speech patterns that would be unacceptable in an adult. In addition, children are usually less well able to express their needs and wants than are adults, exhibit different modes of thinking and ideation and engage in different behaviors than do older people. And, of course, the family, especially the parents, plays a greater role in the total life of a child than is the case with an adult patient.

For these and other reasons, which will become more apparent as this chapter progresses, a special kind of skill and understanding is required by the speech clinician who treats the communication disorders of children.

AN INTRODUCTION TO THE DEVELOPMENT OF LANGUAGE

In order to determine whether the speech and language of a child is defective, or inappropriate, it is necessary to know what normal speech and language are for different chronological age levels. There are two main categories, or levels, of verbal behavior, which can be referred to as the *pre*linguistic and the linguistic.

The *prelinguistic level* roughly describes the patterns of vocalization during the first year of life. It is marked initially by reflexive sounds which are associated with physiological states. Vocalization during this period occurs as a result of physiological changes within the child or as a consequence of changes in the environment; yet it is not differentiated for the nature of the stimuli which elicit the vocalizations. At this time, the majority of the vowel-like sounds which are uttered by the child resemble adult front vowels. The average infant under two months of age has approximately seven phonemes and a few consonants. Following this period the back vowels become more frequent and the number of consonants increases.

During the third month of life babbling appears and increases in frequency during the following months. By the sixth month a noticeable rhythm can be detected in the babbling and certain similar sounds become repetitious. During this period another person's speech will interrupt the vocal play if the speaker is an effective stimulus for the infant. If not, babbling continues or even increases. After the sixth month, the babbling, or vocal play, shows greater variety and more inflections. Near the end of the eighth month or beyond, the child begins to repeat familiar syllables of his parents, such as *mama, dada* and *bye-bye,* although these are said more as part of the babbling than as purposeful responses to specific individuals and situations.

In the last trimester of the first year the child begins to respond to the speech of others by emitting similar sounds. This period marks the transition from prelinguistic to linguistic levels, and it is here that the adult becomes important in the learning process. Echoic responses increase following adult interruption of infant vocalizations, or adult voicing of a sound which is familiar to the infant. Some children attain their first true words at the end of the first year.

At one year, the *linguistic level* of vocalization replaces the prelinguistic. At this point the child's environment becomes important with regard to the rapidity with which language is learned. Between twelve and eighteen months of age the average child has said a few words. These words, while similar to those of an adult, may have different meanings for the child. They may be used inappropriately by adult standards and may be used as one-word sentences, usually being general in their reference. Echoic responses continue at a high rate for as many as twelve to sixteen months longer.

By eighteen months the front vowels and back consonants become mastered and the child has a vocabulary of between ten and twenty meaningful words. There is jargon and echoic behavior but the child is learning to respond to, and control, his environment through the use of language. Jargon reaches its maximum usage at about eighteen months and then declines until by the end of the second year it occurs very infrequently.

By the time the child is two years old he has advanced to phrases. He is talking as we consider "talking", although speech is often awkward, grammatically incorrect, and confused in meaning. At two and one-half years of age he has mastered about twenty-seven phonemes, and now decelerates in the acquisition of new sounds but accelerates in the frequency with which he uses his vocabulary. Prior to this, vowel acquisition, which marked initial learning, has yielded to increased consonant acquisition. By the age of three the child is using simple sentences, and by three and one-half, the great majority of his responses are comprehensible. His vocabulary contains nine hundred to twelve hundred words and he speaks in well formed sentences, using plurals.

At four years of age the child is using conjunctions and understands prepositions. He has a vocabulary of approximately fifteen hundred words. By the age of five or slightly beyond, his speech should be relatively free of infantile articulation.

It must be stressed at this point that the "time-table" of language development which has just been described refers to the *average* child and not to all children. Some children possess several clear words by their eighth month while others do not have true words until their eighteenth. These developmental steps of language learning merely serve as norms, and some deviations from the mean are expected and are not considered abnormal. It is only when the manner or content of a child's language usage is *significantly* below the norm for his age that he is considered to have defective speech.

COMMUNICATION DISORDERS OF CHILDREN IN REHABILITATION
Aphasia

Aphasia is a language disorder which results from damage to the brain. Thus, an aphasic child is a child who has either failed to develop normal language or who has suffered a loss of language as a consequence of brain injury.

There are many possible causes of such injury in children, including complications of delivery, premature birth, birth injuries, congenital anomalies, incompatible blood factors, tumors, trauma, altered blood chemistry, vascular disorders, glandular disturbances, central nervous system infections and convulsive disorders.

Asphasia in children is most easily diagnosed when there are no other accompanying handicaps, such as auditory or visual defects, or intellectual retardation. The child with an auditory receptive language loss, for example, may appear initially to have a hearing impairment. A brain-damaged child may exhibit behavior similar to that of an emotionally disturbed child. Such complications tend to make an accurate differential diagnosis difficult, and therefore, a team approach to the problem in which a psychologist, a speech clinician, an audiologist and a physician combine services in a diagnostic evaluation is often necessary.

One important distinction to be made is between congenital and acquired aphasia. The congenitally aphasic child has failed to develop language ability because of brain damage which occurred prior to, or shortly after, birth. The child with acquired aphasia sustained the brain injury considerably after birth as a result of one or more of the causes listed above.

Since aphasia is a disturbance of language function, an accurate diagnosis must wait until the child is of an age where language appears. The child who does not speak "normally" at age six months, for example, could not be termed aphasic since speech at that age primarily consists of babbling. If at age three, however, language is markedly retarded in development, or is inappropriate, a diagnosis of aphasia is more likely to be correct. In congenital aphasia then, we are dealing with a child of two and one-half to three years of age who exhibits lack of adequate language development. There are usually no clear neurological sings of brain damage or disease, and the presenting problem is one of a speech and/or language defect. There is a marked discrepancy between the child's language skills and his development in motor activities, and while problems may be present these are simply concomitant with the communication deficits.

There are several characteristics which serve to help identify the aphasic child. Linguistically, the child exhibits marked retardation in the comprehension, evaluation and production of language. There is also a wide discrepancy between language comprehension and production. On a developmental level, the child does not show the expected regular increments by which most children increase their communicative skills. There may also be agnosias, articulation defects, poor name associations and an inability to acquire symbolic language. Behaviorally, the aphasic child may be hyperactive or hypoactive, aggressive, fearful, withdrawn, uncooperative, compulsive, hostile, perseverative, labile and inconsistent in responding.

He may demonstrate a brief attention span, lack of concentration ability, impaired judgement, depressive reactions and other emotional problems. In the learning sphere there may be sensory perceptual difficulties, sensory-motor coordination defects, undetermined handedness and intellectual deficiency. These problems may exist in isolation, but more typically occur in combination, adding to the difficulties ordinarily encountered in the therapeutic treatment of aphasia.

Articulation Disorders

Articulation has been defined as a series of overlapping ballistic movements which place varying degrees of obstruction in the way of the outgoing air stream and simultaneously modify the size, shape and coupling of resonating cavities. The phonemes produced by these series of movements are highly variable and their characteristics are influenced by the phonetic contexts in which they appear. Any factors which interfere with the development of these series of movements will result in defective articulation.

Articulatory defects are most frequently grouped into two major categories, dyslalias and dysarthrias. While the symptoms for both may appear identical if only the acoustical features of speech are considered, there are important distinctions.

Dyslalia

Dyslalia refers to an articulatory disorder due to faulty learning, or to abnormality of the speech organs and not to any central nervous system impairment.

Dysarthria

Dysarthria refers to disorders of articulation resulting from lesions within the cerebral centers, pathways and nuclei of the nerves which are involved in speech production. It is not a problem of an isolated paralysis of a particular cranial nerve, but rather of a central lesion in a certain brain area. Depending upon the location and extent of the lesion or lesions, all phonetic functions which are involved in speaking are affected. Dysarthria disrupts the total motorics of speaking, including articulation, phonation and phonic respiration. Often, dysarthric syndromes occur in combination with other verbal defects, such as aphasia. In children undergoing rehabilitation, the dysarthrias represent the most frequently encountered articulation disorders.

Dysarthria can be caused by tumors, hematomas, toxic and metabolic disorders, degenerative processes, brain abscess, vascular disorders, inflammations or central nervous system infections such as encephalitis and meningitis, congenital malformations of the skull or of brain tissue, and head trauma, as in a skull fracture when cortical tissue has been damaged. In children, it is the last four which most commonly produce the motoric defects responsible for the dysarthria.

Visible signs of dysarthria include paralytic conditions of the lips, tongue, jaw, palate, pharynx or larynx which result from lesions involving the fifth, seventh, tenth or twelfth cranial nerves. There may be slight disorders of motility of the tongue, lips or palate. Coordinated disorders of motility might be manifest while isolated movements of articulatory structures remain normal. Sometimes, higher functions of speaking are lost, such as rate, clear enunciation, and rhythm, as in the case of epilepsy. The dysarthria can be minimal and involve sound selection, fluent articulation, word finding and sentence structure. Auditorily, dysarthrias resulting from paralytic lesions involving the articulatory mechanisms can produce open nasality, closed rhinolalia and vocal disorders of pitch, loudness, modulation, registers and clarity. When slight disorders of motility affect speech musculature, the sounds are often slurred, distorted or irregularly pronounced.

Coordinated disorders of motility result in slurring, inexact and fatigued articulation, stumbling over syllables, cluttering, repetitions of syllables and words, and a disturbed relationship between voiced and unvoiced consonants. Disorders of higher functions of speaking are heard in alterations of voice timbre, distorted or slurred speech patterns and rate deviations. Minimal dysarthric defects exhibit disabilities in speaking, reading, writing and arithmetic.

THE EVALUATION OF COMMUNICATION DISORDERS IN CHILDREN

In attempting to determine whether a child has a speech or language disorder, the speech clinician must always ask herself if the phenomena she observes are comparable to the child's age. Certain errors of language are considered normal for certain age levels and it is only when the errors made by the child are those which should have dropped out by his age that the clinician will be concerned about a possible problem.

With a language-impaired child there are often a host of problems other than the specific communication disorder, including medical and psychological difficulties, which the speech clinician needs to be aware of. She therefore relies upon information from parents, which includes the child's medical, behavioral and educational histories, from the obstetrician, pediatrician, neurologist and other physicians who have had contact with the child for detailed medical reports, and from the psychologist specifically, for data on the child's behavior, intellectual capacity and present level of functioning, perceptual and perceptual-motor abilities, and social maturity.

The clinician's task is the evaluation of language and speech. This includes testing visual and auditory recognition, naming, oral formulation, conceptualization and articulation, recognition of symbols and receptive language ability.

In assessing a child's language capacity, the clinician must determine the reliability of the sensory modality which she is utilizing. Thus, oral instructions would not be used extensively with the child who is receptively impaired, nor would tasks involving motor performance be given a child who has a paralytic or marked paretic motor disability.

Visual Recognition

To test visual recognition the child's reactions to people in his environment are observed. The focus of attention is placed on whether or not he recognizes familiar persons, such as his parents. Toys are placed before the child so that observation can be made of his handling of them. Should he not respond, the clinician encourages him to play with the toys, even placing them in his hands. Proper handling of these objects indicates recognition.

The child is asked to imitate the therapist in the touching of parts of his face and body. He is given a blank cardboard or flannel face and asked to place cut-out features in their proper position. He is given the task of drawing a person by telling him to "Draw Daddy," or "Draw a girl."

Figure-ground perception is examined through having the child point out a picture which has been superimposed on a diffuse background, or by requiring him to draw around the outline of the figure with a crayon.

Several differently colored blocks are presented to the child whose task is to place blocks of the same color together. He is given cards having vertical and horizontal dots printed on them which he must connect with a pencil or crayon. In such a manner, an assessment is made of the child's ability to correctly perceive spatial relationships.

The child's recognition of basic shapes is tested by presenting him with different geometric shapes for identification. Pictures of familiar items, such as a ball, a doll, a cup, a hat or a crayon are shown to the child who can either name them or match them with actual objects on the therapist's desk. Action scenes in pictures can also be shown to him for identification of parts of the pictures. Alphabet letters, numbers and words which are printed on cards are presented to the child to test his visual verbal recognition skills.

Auditory Recognition

There are several ways in which auditory recognition can be evaluated. At first, the clinican observes the child's reaction to her voice or to a parent's voice so as to determine the child's awareness of the sound. She observes the child's perception and recognition of other sounds in the environment, such as the ringing of a telephone, the closing of a door, and an automobile's horn.

Next, the clinician tests recognition of specific sounds. This is done by concealing a sound-producing object behind a screen or under her desk, demonstrating the sound and having the child select the object which makes the sound from an array of several items which are placed before him. These may include a bell, a rattle, a squeeze toy and the like.

Auditory verbal recognition is evaluated by placing familiar items, such as a doll, a cup, a ball and a block, in front of the child and requesting him to select the one named by the clinician, by asking him to point to parts of his head and body, by giving him simple commands to follow, as in "Give me the doll" and "Throw the ball", and by giving more complex directions, such as "Put the pencil in the cup and give the cup to me."

Naming Ability

The child's ability to name is examined by handing him objects and requiring that he identify them, by asking him to name people and objects in the environment, and by requesting him to name items in pictures, geometric figures on a formboard, colors, letters and numerals. The clinician determines the correctness of the child's identifications and his pronunciation of the names. Such tasks provide information regarding the child's expressive vocabulary and articulation abilities.

In evaluating articulation, the clinician notes the recognizability of the words used by the child or, if no words are recognizable, the consistency of neologisms and specific vowel and consonant sounds. If there is no true speech the quality and quantity of babbling is recorded. A formal articulation test can be administered. The Templin-Darley Screening and Diagnostic Tests of Articulation or the Laradon Articulation Scale are frequently employed and are commercially available.

The clinician is alert to spontaneous speech production, requests and questions asked by the child. She may perform certain acts, such as drawing, throwing a ball or drinking, and ask the child to describe what she is doing. Pictures are exhibited and the child's task is to describe what is taking place in the picture or in a series of related pictures. The clinician may ask the child a question, such as "What did you do this morning?". Thus, the child's ability to formulate ideas into proper speech is evaluated.

Basic Academic Skills

When a child is of school age it is important to determine if defects are present in reading, writing or arithmetic.

In the assessment of reading skills pairs of words are presented to the child such as *see-see, house-comb, take-take* and *dog-cat,* and he must draw a line through, or circle the pairs which are alike (or dissimilar). The child is presented with a series of simple words or sentences and he is directed to encircle the ones which the therapist pronounces. A frame of a sentence is shown to the child and he has to complete the sentence by adding the correct word from a choice of several, only one of which makes the sentence meaningful. He is asked to read a brief passage aloud and the therapist then queries him regarding what he has just read.

To assess writing and spelling abilities the therapist directs the child to copy single letters, to write or print his own name, to write or print specific letters, to copy sentences, to write sentences spontaneously, and to write words as they are dictated to him.

Arithmetic skills are evaluated by having the child count blocks, sticks or marbles placed before him, by requiring him to copy numbers and to match the correct number of objects to the written numerals, by asking him to add numbers mentally when given marbles or sticks, and by requiring him to compute simple arithmetic problems which are written on paper or on cards.

In addition to testing language and speech functions the clinician observes the child's perception and sensory-motor behavior. She notes delays in responding and discrepancies between verbal and nonverbal levels of performance. Behaviors, such as hyperactivity, lability and withdrawal, are recorded and the extent to which emotional problems seem to be interfering with language is estimated. Finally, an audiometric examination is administered to the child.

At the conclusion of the evaluation all data are reviewed and the speech clinician, on the basis of positive findings and of ruling out certain possibilities for lack of sufficient evidence, makes her diagnosis. The diagnosis includes whether or not there exists a speech, language or hearing impairment, the extent and severity of an existing deficit, the probabilities that therapy will alleviate the problem, and a tentative prognosis for improvement and length of therapeutic time which may be required to bring about such improvement. It is important that an evaluation report provide this information since merely specifying a speech defect is not sufficient. The evaluation must yield clues which can aid the clinician is selecting an appropriate starting point for therapy and for determining a level of expectation for improvement. It is upon the information obtained during the evaluation that therapeutic treatment is initiated.

THERAPY

Aphasia Therapy

General Principles

It is generally believed that the room in which treatment takes place should be a small one which is relatively free of distracting stimuli. A small room is preferred because an important aspect of language training is the proximity of the therapist to the child. It is often found that aphasic children perform more successfully when they remain near the therapist. This aids is providing structure to the situation and in sustaining concentration on the given tasks. The therapist may begin by sitting side by side with the child and, as treatment continues, gradually lengthen the distance between them.

The therapy room itself is quiet and free of distracting influences since the aphasic child's attention is easily commanded by stimuli external to treatment. Therefore, a room which is painted in a solid, subdued color and is without decorations is preferred. All toys and other materials are kept out of sight when not in use. A certain amount of soundproofing is desirable since excessive background noises become distracting, but total soundproofing is not advocated. This would not provide opportunity for the child to increase his perception skills, to learn to differentiate signal from ground and to learn to reduce and control his distractibility.

Language therapy for aphasic children parallels that given to adults in many ways. There are certain distinctions, however, and there are differentiations made depending upon whether the child is congenitally aphasic or has become aphasic because of trauma or other brain pathology.

It is important to instill in the congenitally aphasic child the desire to speak. Since this child has not had language from birth, he has probably developed other methods of obtaining his needs. It is incumbent upon the speech therapist to impress upon the child the need to talk, both to gain satisfaction of wants and to use as a social tool. This is often accomplished by having the child play with toys and games with a few other children, including normally-speaking ones, with speech coming from within the group and the therapist acting as a guide. The aphasic child learns to see the value of speech in communication, and motivation is thereby increased.

The activities which are provided for the child are those which make verbal behavior pleasant. Therefore, although language is the eventual goal, early treatment can involve making animal or mechanical sounds as part of games. The child is gradually "weaned" to verbal representations of the sounds and, finally, to language.

It is helpful if, in the use of recordings or stories, the child's name is interjected periodically as an attention-holding device which also tends to personalize his therapy.

Continual positive reinforcement of behavior is important in that it both rewards the child for correct performance and demonatrates to him that his language can command services and control his environment. Thus, when a child learns to say "I want water," the therapist gives him a glass of water. For language which is not demanding in its implication, candy corn, M & M's®, Hersheyettes,® gumdrops, small marshmallows, peanuts and the like are employed as reinforcers.

As with all aphasics, the speech clinician must determine what sensory approach to initiate treatment with. For some children, who look closely and directly at the therapist when she speaks, the visual modality may be deemed best for approaching therapy. If the child listens intently but becomes confused by watching the therapist's oral movements, the chosen approach would be via the auditory sense. Some children may learn best through tactile stimulation and hence, touch would play the dominant role in therapeutically reaching them.

The congenitally aphasic child may learn best when speech volume is of a greater intensity than in ordinary conversation, and he most probably requires many repetitions of stimuli. Furthermore, the rate of presentation of materials should be slower than for the normal child and the units of material employed at each step of training must be small. Thus, a short unit, presented at increased volume and repeated often for the appropriate sensory modality, represents the most satisfactory method for training the congenitally aphasic child.

Materials which are employed in working with the child are associated with a real object or person as often as is possible. When learning has been established the concrete item is replaced by a picture. Items employed in therapy are demonstrated by the clinician so that their several functions are seen. A doll, for example, is for hugging, and for rocking, and for dressing, and for spanking and for feeding. These functions are taught gradually to the child so that full knowledge of them, at least as they are present in his life, is gained. Items are also presented in their different forms. A doll can be large or small, blonde or brunette, rubber or cloth, male or female. By doing this the clinician is aiding the child in gaining flexibility of thought concepts and language.

The first words which are taught to the child are usually those which he needs to satisfy his wants, such as "Mommy," "Daddy," "eat," "water," "potty" and "toy." At first, a liberal attitude is assumed by the clinician with regard to pronunciation. Speech must be encouraged and too strict a view of how a word should sound can inhibit a child's expression and, perhaps, even extinguish the speech he already possesses. Once the habit of oral speech is clearly established, accuracy may be considered a goal to work towards.

The training of the child with acquired aphasia who has had normal speech but is now language-impaired, proceeds along lines similar to those used with the child who is congenitally aphasic. There are, however, some special problems of importance to consider. Such a child is greatly handicapped by his disability. He may withdraw or act out in response to frustrations which he feels from his inability to express himself. To reduce this frustration, gesture language is immediately introduced. Beyond this, the child must be reoriented towards using and understanding conventional language.

The prognosis for a child with acquired aphasia is relatively good and, in fact, many such children spontaneously recover language function. There are, however, a number of cases where the brain damage is so extensive that only limited goals can be aimed for. Original objectives must be continually reassessed as therapy progresses.

Distractibility, lability and hyperactivity are some of the other problems which the speech clinician must face and control if therapy is to be successful. As with the congenitally aphasic child, therapy

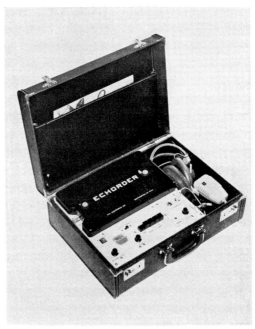

FIGURE 86. The Echorder® speech and language training unit which provides auditory reinforcement of speech by automatic speech playback through preselected time delays. (*Courtesy of RIL Electronics, Inc.*)

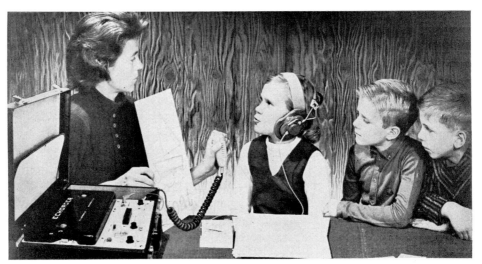

FIGURE 87. The Echorder® in use with a group of children. (*Courtesy of RIL Electronics, Inc.*)

usually begins with prelingual activities, advancing to echoic behavior, gestures accompanying monosyllabic or disyllabic words and
finally, to emphasizing conventional words only.

Specific Techniques

The materials which are employed in the treatment of children
must, of necessity, differ from those used with adults. What is appropriate for an adult may well be meaningless for a child. The items
used with children generally include simple household objects and
furniture—either actual—or doll-sized; food and clothing—either
real or of toy status; dolls and puppets; toys; items with raised numerals and letters; phonograph records; noisemakers; play houses and
towns; games; picture books; possibly live animals; and the like.
Materials such as cardboard boxes, chalk boards, colored paper, felt
cloth and musical instruments are also employed.

NAMING. Naming is one aspect of language. Common objects, such
as a ball, a doll or a shoe, are presented to the child and he is asked to
name them as they are handed to him by the therapist. If he cannot
name them, the child's attention is directed to the therapist who
names them, and the child then imitates her. As he progresses, more
complex stimulus units are used, such as a doll house, and the child
names the items in the house as he places them in the correct rooms
in response to the therapist's directions. The child may be taken for
a walk about the building and grounds and asked to name what he
sees. Here too, failure by the child results in the clinician's supplying
the correct name until it is learned.

The therapist also presents pictures to the child for identification
of the objects in the picture. He is also required to match pictures
with real objects. Naming of important or familiar people, either
in person or from photographs, is included in this practice. In addition,
the child is taught to match common geometric forms and colors
which are produced on paper for him by the therapist. The concept
of identifying numbers is introduced at a later stage through drawings,
actual objects or counting on the fingers.

VISUAL VERBAL RECOGNITION. In this sphere of training the child
is first shown an easily identified letter of the alphabet, either as a
raised block letter, or as felt flannel board or as a cut-out. After the
child sees the letter he is permitted to feel its shape and is shown the
shape of the mouth in pronouncing it. He is given the task of tracing
the letter, then copying it, and finally, writing it upon command.
Letters are then shown to him in groups, all of the members of each
group having similar contours, and he is taught to distinguish be-

tween them. Words which are of interest to him are presented in large print with colored letters for easy identification. The child is requested to match the words with real objects, to match like words and unlike words when they are presented in pairs, and to match upper and lower case letters. He may be given a "family" such as *at* and be asked to place consonants like *f, c, p,* and *h* before the *at*. Following this, the child is told which word he has made and is taught to say the word himself.

AUDITORY VERBAL RECOGNITION. This type of recognition may be initiated by having the child give physical responses to stimuli until language is more fully developed. Thus, with a doll, for example, it can be shown to the child, its name told to him by the therapist, and the child can then be asked to lift the doll. If he is able to imitate the word *doll,* he is encouraged to do so. Procedures are repeated as frequently as is necessary for learning to take place.

Objects and pictures are associated by first giving the child an object such as a ball, by having him play with it, and then by showing him a picture of a ball, all the while repeating the word *ball* to him. This technique is repeated with many objects and their matching pictures. Then the child is permitted to choose an item from several upon hearing the therapist say its name. He is taught how to choose by pointing to its picture and naming it. He is shown simple action scenes and asked to describe them in a sentence.

Simple commands are given to the child, such as "Get the doll," "Bounce the ball," "Shake the rattle," "Hold up your hand," and "Open your mouth." At first, the therapist demonstrates these acts and, each time the child is unable to follow her instructions, she repeats the demonstration. Then more complex commands are given, such as "Bring me two marbles from the table over there," or "Take the rattle and put it in the box." It must be emphasized that each new step in therapy is repeated many, many times and it is rare if one-trial learning occurs on any given level.

FORMULATION IN SPEECH. Following reception and assimilation of language, formulation in speech is taught. Some aids which are employed include simple conversation between therapist and child, puppets and pictures, and the acting out of familiar stories. These encourage spontaneous speech and expand upon what the child has already learned.

Stimulating pictures may prompt questions from the child and therefore the therapist employs these early in training. The therapist pantomimes acts such as combing the hair and drinking water, and the child is asked to describe her behaviors. Using puppets the child is able to dramatize an event which he has seen or has participated in, and to verbally describe the event and its participants. A series of related pictures can be helpful in teaching sequence and timing. The therapist may begin telling a story and have the child continue it at some point.

In teaching prepositions, objects are placed in, under and behind tables, boxes and the like, with the child first watching the therapist and then carrying out the tasks alone. He may also be required to sit on the chair or under the table, and thus learn prepositions through actually engaging in their prescribed behaviors.

Defective non-language visual recognition and lack of auditory recognition of nonverbal sounds are rarely observed in children, and when they do occur they are treated in much the same way as with adults, the main exception being the materials which are employed. Reading, writing and arithmetic are similarly taught to children as they are to adults who have losses in these areas.

Articulation Therapy

This section is devoted to the treatment of children with dysarthric impairments.

The aim of articulation therapy is often thought of as teaching the child to make new sounds. For those children who are able to pronounce sounds correctly in one or more phonetic contexts, the goal of therapy is considered to be one of helping the child to increase the number of phonetic contexts in which the sound is produced correctly.

A primary objective of articulation therapy is to heighten the child's awareness of the auditory, proprioceptive and tactile sensations that are associated with speech. This can be accomplished by providing auditory stimuli which the child must imitate. This type of exercise provides opportunities for the movements of the peripheral speech mechanisms necessary for clear articulation. It may be initiated through activities which increase the flexibility of the articulators, and specific exercises can be provided for each one individually. These can be performed by the patient in face-to-face contact with the therapist or before a mirror, depending upon the child's wishes and the judgement of the clinician as to which method is preferable for the individual case.

It is important to sharpen the movements of the lips since labial mobility has a salutary effect on the tongue, palate and mandible as well as being crucial in itself. It can be achieved by having the child look at pictures of clowns' faces and imitate them, exaggerating the expressions. The vowel sounds which correspond to the lip features may be simultaneously emitted.

The sounds of mechanical devices, such as a squeaking door or an exploding balloon, are also emitted by the child. These can be produced upon command of the therapist, or modeled by the therapist and imitated by the child, or played on a phonograph with the child first listening and then imitating what he has heard.

Whistling, blowing plastic autos across a table, blowing ping-pong balls up an incline, and imitating the sound of the wind are other types of lip exercises used in therapy. Diadochokinetic movements, as in uttering *pa-pa-pa-pa* and *ba-ba-ba-ba* are practiced, with emphasis on the plosive nature of the breath stream in the consonants.

Exercises of the tongue include babbling, first with the tongue tip on the lips, then on the teeth, then on the alveolar ridge and finally, on the hard palate. Licking the lips, in imitation of removing candy, imitating a cat licking milk from a saucer, running the tongue around the inside of the mouth touching the inner cheeks, teeth and palate with the tongue tip, and alternately pushing against and retracting the tongue from the lower incisors are other tongue movements which are practiced regularly. Sound is added as the child is told to imitate a train's wheels, a chicken's clucking, or other non-human noise.

The movements of the jaw are given training as the child imitates the sound of a steeple bell, a dog's bark, or a siren, dropping the jaw as far as possible with each sound. Jaw movements are exaggerated in the prolongation of vowels, in hearty laughing and in make-believe exclamations of pain and surprise.

Velar-pharyngeal muscles are more difficult to control because their action is not as precise as the other articulators and because it is not visible for ready imitation. Therefore, the speaker must rely upon kinesthethic feedback for knowledge of the correctness of the movements of these muscles. This feedback is corroborated by the auditory evaluation of the sounds. It is well known that if the other articulators are functioning properly the velar-pharyngeal muscles will also be more agile in their action.

Exercises are begun by the patient yawning before a mirror and noting how the posterior part of the tongue drops, the velum rises and the pillars of the fauces widen. This is repeated until the child has developed a strong feeling of the rising velum and open pharynx.

Practice at feeling velar action is provided by having the child say "Ah" and switching to a *p* sound, by holding the air in the mouth under pressure before exploding the consonant, and by opening the mouth widely and panting, much like a dog in hot weather. Changes from velar relaxation to contraction are made when the child says "m-pah" repeatedly, puffing out his cheeks between syllables. Sounding different vowels in succession provides kinesthetic feedback of velar tension, as does holding the nose and releasing it as "mm" is voiced. Velar control is checked by the therapist placing a small mirror under the child's nose. Since the velar-pharyngeal muscles close the nasal port, there should be no clouding of the mirror with correct pronunciation. Clouding indicates the need for further practice.

The child is also given practice in imitating the therapist's production of bisyllables, such as *bibi, baba, bubu, babu* and *biba*. Bisyllabic exercises include those which require shifting of articulation, as in *taka* and *kata,* in which the former requires a shift from the tip to the back of the tongue, while the latter requires just the reverse.

Training the child in auditory stimulation and discrimination of speech sounds is achieved in several ways. The child may link new sounds with familiar ones in his environment, or with sounds of nature as heard on phonograph records, or with the speech of others. The therapist can intensively stimulate him by repetition of the sound.

Certain exercises for auditory discrimination may be utilized, such as showing the child several pictures and asking him to select the one which makes a particular sound. The clinician can read a story which contains new sounds and the child's task is to raise his hand each time he hears them. These types of "game" exercises can be varied in many ways and it is up to the ingenious therapist to do so in a manner which provides the necessary training and maintains the child's interest.

Following successful completion of these basic exercises, the child is ready to produce new sounds, first in isolation, then in systematically varied phonetic contexts and, finally, in structured, formalized speech.

COMMUNICATION PROBLEMS IN CEREBRAL PALSY

It is safe to say that there is no single pattern of speech which may be labelled as typical of cerebral palsy. While "cerebral palsy speech" is often described as being slow, jerky, labored and distorted, there are actually a myriad of different speech disorders associated with the disability which vary, not only between the types of cerebral palsy, but from child to child within each type.

The problems of the cerebral palsied individual can usually

be placed within several large categories, including delayed language, articulatory disorders and intelligibility, disorders of rhythm and disorders of breathing.

Language Development

Studies of the language development of cerebral palsied children have reported that from fifty to seventy-four per cent of such children are delayed in language abilities. Some investigators have learned that among persons so affected, even individuals past their teen years may have only one year of oral language development. Other researchers have found vocabulary development to be from three to four years behind that of normal children.

Language retardation may be broken down in terms of developmental levels. It has been demonstrated that children with cerebral palsy are three months delayed in the appearance of first words, twelve months delayed in the use of two-word sentences, and forty-eight months delayed in the use of three-word sentences. Some other involved children do not use single words until from nine to twelve months after normal children do, but lag only six months behind in the use of two-word sentences.

These discrepancies serve to point out the differences between the means of the groups studied, and show the variety of delays which occur within the total cerebral palsy picture. The important conclusion to be drawn is that cerebral palsied children are considerably retarded in language development.

Articulation Disorders

Articulation disorders with their consequent problems of intelligibility are frequently found in the cerebral palsy population. Between seventy and eighty per cent of all affected children have some articulation defect. In many, the disorder is of a magnitude which renders speech unintelligible. The athetotic type of cerebral palsy generally suffers greatest from this defect.

The most common articulation problem is dysarthria, which is found in all cases of cerebral palsy when there is neuromuscular involvement of the speech mechanisms.

In the spastic child the involvement can be hypertonic speech musculature resulting in slow, labored movements, oversusceptibility to the stretch reflex, or flaccidity, in which case the muscles of the tongue and jaw are too weak for adequate movement. Furthermore, there may be an overtonicity of opposing muscles making synergistic movements difficult or, in some cases, impossible. In the athetotic type, speech problems result from involuntary movements of the involved muscles. When the muscles of respiration, voice and articulation are involved, speech may be arhythmic and accompanied by clicks and other extra noises resulting from involuntary movements being superimposed upon those which are required for correct speech. Dysarthria is more frequently encountered in the athetotic than in the spastic type of cerebral palsy.

Characteristically, cerebral palsied children have the greatest difficulty with tongue-tip sounds and with sounds which require fine coordination. Their speech is typified by omissions rather than primarily by substitutions. Tongue movements are the most difficult of all to make. Diadochokinetic rates are slow. The difficulty of movement patterns in producing a speech sound is influenced by the sound patterns immediately preceding and immediately following the sound. Final sound positions are more difficult than initial or medial ones. Articulation is inefficient since cerebral palsied children tend to use sounds which are easily produced and, even if they are inexact, will continue to use them if their purpose is served.

Rhythm Patterns

Abnormal patterns of rhythm, such as stuttering or stuttering-like symptoms, have been reported for cerebral palsy in general, as well as jerky, arthythmic speech in athetotic children in particular. This may be a consequence of extreme tension which produces contacts hard enough to result in stuttering, or to lesions in the extrapyramidal tracts of the brain which disrupt rhythmic speech.

Problems of Respiration

The involvement of cerebral palsy can include those muscles which are responsible for respiration if there is damage to the respiratory regulation centers in the brain. Since respiration produces the air currents necessary for phonation, speech-sound production, and phrasing, difficulties of respiration result in impairment of speech.

The hypothalamus influences respiratory centers in the medulla through the pneumotaxic center and hence, is important for the regulation of respiration. As it is contiguous to the basal ganglia it can be affected in children with predominantly athetotic cerebral palsy. Those children with spastic cerebral palsy are less likely to have respiratory system involvement since their brain damage is mainly cortical.

Respiratory Anomalies

Included among respiratory anomalies are the following:

Irregular cycling, in which there are gross deviations from normally predictable time and amplitude of breathing movements.

Rib flaring, where there is thoracic expansion in the region of the ninth and twelfth ribs with little abdominal expansion.

Thoracic-abdominal opposition (reversed breathing), which occurs when the thorax or abdomen makes either inspiratory or expiratory excursions while the other is doing the reverse.

Shallow breathing, which is a rapid series of low amplitude excursions coupled with low vital capacity.

Breathing interfered with by athetosis, or involuntary movements of the respiratory muscles.

Respiratory-laryngeal incoordination, the asynchronous timing of expiratory movements and valving of the larynx.

Stertorous breathing, as a result of the halting or impeding of either inspiratory or expiratory movements by spasmodic or tonic occlusions of the airway.

Thoracic breathing, which is respiration performed mainly by the intercostal and other thoracic muscles.

Abdominal breathing, where respiration is primarily performed by the muscles of the abdomen or diaphragm.

Mouth breathing, as when respiration is carried on through the oral cavity.

Non-volitional breathing, in which survival oxygen exchange patterns cannot be voluntarily altered.

Deformed thoracic cage.

Laryngeal Anomalies

In addition to problems of breathing which impede normal voice production, cerebral palsied children can have abnormalities involving the larynx which also impair speech. Among these are the following:

Spasmodic anomalies of glottis constriction, in which constrictors of the vocal folds tend to hold them closed by opposing action of the dilators during phonation.

Dilator spasm, or slow valving.

Spasmodic anomalies of extrinsic muscles, where there are abnormal pulls of the extrinsic laryngeal musculature.

Ventricular fold spasm, in which the ventricular folds serve a sphincter function.

Breathy valving, or asynchronous timing of the expiratory muscles and valving of the larynx.

Obtuse thyroid angle, which is a deformity of thyroid cartilage as the result of abnormal muscle pulls.

Athetosis of the vocal folds, which occurs when laryngeal muscles function in an irregular, arhythmic pattern.

Monotones.

EVALUATION OF SPEECH AND LANGUAGE DISORDERS
IN CEREBRAL PALSY

Speech

Evaluation of the speech mechanism comprises the functioning of the lips, tongue and mandible.

Tongue movement is examined by having the child protrude his tongue, touch the corners of his mouth with his tongue, place his tongue behind the upper incisors, and rapidly lateralize his tongue from one side of his mouth to the other.

Diadochokinetic rates for tongue-tip alveolar and tongue back-palatal movements are measured in five-second periods, both with the mandible kept stable and with it unstabilized. If it is observed that voluntary tongue control is impaired, the child can be given a piece of candy or a cracker to determine function during vegetative motion. The cracker is given while the lips are held in retraction, and specific movements are elicited by placing bits of cracker in different parts of the mouth and on the lips and teeth. Then pressure is applied in opposition to tongue elevation and lateralization at the tip and posterior part of the dorsum and also to tongue protrusion to determine whether increasing sensation elicits improved function.

Other procedures involve having the child open and close his mouth rapidly, and compress, retract and pucker his lips repeatedly. These movements are often measured with a criterion of ten times in ten seconds. Rate of repetition of syllables such as *ka, pa* and *ba* are also evaluated by this standard.

Certain criteria have been suggested for minimum requisites of function of speech mechanisms for normal speech production. They are as follows: prolongation of a steady tone for ten seconds; extension and protrusion of the tongue five times within ten seconds; touching the tip of the tongue to the rugae ten times within ten seconds with the mandible stabilized; opening and closing the lips ten times within ten seconds with the mandible stabilized; opening and closing the mouth ten times within ten seconds; and propelling food and liquid from the front of the mouth to the back and swallowing them without drooling. These tasks can all be incorporated into the evaluation procedure.

Breathing

Respiration is evaluated by the clinician first noting the presence of any of the respiratory anomalies which have been previously described. Respiratory function is measured in terms of rate and amount of air intake of the lungs. It can be assessed by observation or through the use of pneumographic apparatus.

The rate of breathing is usually much more rapid in children with cerebral palsy than in normal children of the same age. With the child in a prone position he can be timed as to the number of respiratory cycles that occur per minute during quiet breathing.

The vital capacity, or amount of air the lungs can hold during inspiration, is reduced in cerebral palsy to varying degrees. Kymographic recordings can be made of breathing irregularities which occur during speech.

Voice

The diagnosis of voice problems depends upon the ability of the speech clinician to recognize patterns which are deviant from the age norms of the child in question. She listens to the child's speech to determine if intensity and intensity change are adequate, if pitch is flexible, or if the child occasionally breaks into falsetto, if voice quality is clear and resonant and pleasant, or harsh, metallic, nasal, or hoarse, if voice is coordinated with articulation, and if prosodic aspects of speech are normal in sound.

By listening to the child's speech the clinician can also obtain a judgement of intelligibility, depending upon her percent of correct reception of what he says.

Oral Language Development

The language development of the child is diagnosed by making a comparison between his present language and language norms which are appropriate for his chronological age.

SPEECH AND LANGUAGE THERAPY
WITH CEREBRAL PALSIED CHILDREN

It is believed that either prior to, or in conjunction with, speech and language therapy, the child with cerebral palsy should be given training in improving his general neuromuscular control. This means exercises in proper breathing, relaxation of involved muscle groups, training in chewing, swallowing and sucking, and in control of drooling, reflex inhibition, and postural correction.

Although these variables are highly important for correct speech and language production, the exercises are most frequently conducted by a physical therapist or by a physical therapist with assistance from the speech clinician. There are a number of excellent books which describe these procedures and the interested reader is referred to the references at the end of this section. The present section will discuss only those techniques which are directly related to the training of speech and language, and which are considered to be within the province of the speech clinician.

Relaxation

For cerebral palsied children undergoing speech and/or language training, relaxation is highly important. This is particularly true for athetotic types since in their case relaxation precedes other forms of treatment. There are many methods of teaching relaxation, including Jacobson's progressive relaxation which is applicable to some patients, Korzybski's semantic relaxation, hypnotic suggestion and drugs, all of which can be utilized by the speech clinician, either alone, or in conjunction with a physical therapist, psychologist or physician.

Breath Control

Some techniques of breath control can be employed by the speech clinician. One involves the eliciting of steady prolongation of expelled breath by having the child try to keep the flame of a candle bent without blowing it out. A more difficult variation of this technique requires the child to keep a small piece of tissue paper against a wall by blowing on it. Other blowing activities include blowing a ping-pong ball up an inclined plane, blowing a balloon about, blowing plastic bubbles and blowing toy musical instruments.

Directional control may be achieved through prolongation exercises and by the therapist holding the child's nose or stroking his throat, tongue and lips gently to suggest the avenue along which the breath should be expelled.

Improvement in rate of breathing can be accomplished through exercises which involve voluntary breathing in rhythm, such as to a metronome's ticking or to the singing of simple rhymes by the therapist.

Phonation and Articulation

In order to increase phonation and articulation skills the therapist might begin by reviewing techniques of relaxation. She then may produce the sound *ah* softly, slightly depressing her mandible with her tongue placed slightly forward in her mouth, and with a minimum of breath pressure. After she demonstrates this the child is requested to imitate her. Once this is learned by the child the same procedures are employed for other sounds.

Length and steadiness of tone are encouraged by having the child phonate into a candle's flame without extinguishing it, by drawing a line on a chalkboard as long as the tone continues, or by recording the child's sound and having him continually attempt to better his previous performance.

Following these procedures, consonants can be introduced with the therapist demonstrating and the child imitating her verbal behavior. Sometimes a mirror is used as an aid to the child for imitation of the therapist and for correction of his own oral movements through the visual feedback it provides.

It is important to be aware of the fact that prior to sound production the child is trained in recognition of the sounds which are to be produced. He needs experience in perceiving and discriminating sounds within larger units, such as a sentence. This training can be given in the form of story telling, during which the child is asked to listen for specific sounds, or in guessing games, wherein pictures are shown to the child who must guess their sounds. Speech sounds can later be linked to sounds in the child's environment, such as "bong" for a bell, or "meow" for a cat.

Once sounds can be produced in isolation they are incorporated into phrases and sentences. These are typically brief and concerned with activities which are meaningul for the child, as in "I want to eat," and "Bye-bye." Each expression is encouraged and praised by the therapist, although not every one may be intelligible to the listener. Sounds produced by the child which interfere with intelligibility are selected for more intensive work by the therapist.

Voice

Control of variations in voice is often a serious difficulty for children with cerebral palsy, especially those of the spastic type. Greater variation may be obtained if the child is made aware of his inflections of pitch and is able to discriminate gross deviations.

The child is taught to produce sounds softly at first, then loudly, so as to both hear and feel the difference. He can be taught "scales" by having him go up and down "stairs" with his voice, first in stepwise fashion and then with increasing smoothness. While normal voice quality may never be achieved because of the child's neuromuscular involvement, improvements are possible. The child must often learn to accept efficiency of function as a substitute for perfection.

Language

Although the language development of the child with cerebral palsy is usually delayed or interrupted so that it lags behind that of a normal child, it still follows the same general course in its progression from undifferentiated vocalizations to the use of sentences.

The techniques which are employed with other language-handicapped children can be used with the cerebral palsied, emphasizing deficient areas and with modification of materials and procedures so that these are adaptable to the special motoric problems of this special group. The factor of chronological age must largely be ignored, since such a scale is meaningless as a criterion of language development for the cerebral palsied. Rather, the child's needs become the key guide in progression from one developmental level to the next.

Once the child has reasonably efficient sucking, chewing and swallowing patterns, breathing patterns which permit speech, sustained phonation, and babbling, language training is initiated. The early stages of treatment focus upon the increase of babbling through sensory recognition of objects, imitation of environmental sounds and voice recognition. The child then progresses to the symbolic use of meaningful words, vocabulary growth and sentence development. Training begins with nouns, followed by verbs, adjectives and prepositions. In the final phase of language training emphasis is placed upon muscular control and clear articulation.

A final point to be stressed with regard to the speech and language training of cerebral palsied children: the clinician who works in this specialty must be a very unique kind of person. She needs infinite patience, great empathy, considerable ingenuity and special skill. The road is long and hard and progress is slow. Yet the rewards are great. The satisfaction which is gained from the habilitation of a child, from helping a child to become an individual through language, from enabling a child to join a speaking society, is perhaps the greatest of any area of communication therapy.

GROUP THERAPY FOR COMMUNICATION DISORDERS

In some cases a speech clinician may feel that an individual whom she is working with might benefit from group participation and will introduce him into a group of patients with similar impairments who are at similar levels of training.

Group therapy is generally employed as an adjunct to individual treatment, and is seldom the only form of therapy given to a patient.

Group training has several values. It provides the patient with social experience. He gains motivation from peers. He learns through observation of others. He gains several, often highly critical, listeners. He learns to adjust to others while seeing how they adjust to him.

Group therapy provides an opportunity to be a teacher for those who are more severely impaired. It can be a reinforcing situation as the patient progresses. With children, where group training is often a play situation, frustrations which result from lack of adequate language can be expressed. Constructive toys requiring cooperation among children can be an aid in increasing communication.

There are certain shortcomings of group therapy. Some patients may be withdrawn and hesitant to speak in the presence of persons other than the therapist. The group's rate of progress may be too rapid for an individual. It is possible for a group to become dominated by one or two members while the other members remain passive unless the clinician is skilled in group leadership. Some individuals dislike having their peers hear their errors.

It is up to the speech clinician to decide which of her patients are suitable candidates for group participation and which are not, and to determine the appropriate time for introducing an individual into a group as well as ascertaining when a patient should be withdrawn from the group because of lack of progress or other factors.

Chapter 14

AUDITORY DISABILITIES

ONE OF THE IMPORTANT FUNCTIONS of the speech clinician in rehabilitation is the assessment and therapeutic remediation of hearing problems and the referral of such problems for medical treatment and prescription. Hearing evaluations are performed routinely as part of the screening procedure and more thoroughly during the initial evaluation.

Prior to discussing auditory disorders it is worthwhile to review what "hearing" actually is and how the human ear hears.

SOUND

A sound may be defined as a propagated change in the pressure and density of an elastic medium. Sound is created when a force sets an object into vibration so that molecular movements occur in the medium within which the sound is located and a sound wave is produced. When the characteristics of the wave fall within the limits of detection of the ear and the nervous system, the sound is heard.

While sounds can be produced by reeds or strings, as in the case of some musical instruments, by natural forces like the wind, and by mechanical devices, the speech clinician is concerned primarily with human sounds, specifically the sounds of communication. Such sound is produced through a series of muscular acts. The source of the human voice is the vibrating vocal folds in the larynx. These folds are brought together by muscular action and thus impede the passage of air through the larynx. Voice power is provided by air pressure which is built up below the vocal folds through the actions of the muscles of exhalation. When air pressure below the larynx becomes greater than the muscular tension of the vocal folds, the folds become temporarily separated. When the air pressure and muscular tension are almost balanced, the vocal folds are set in vibration. These vibrations are transmitted to columns of air in the throat, mouth and nose which act as resonators, reinforcing and amplifying them.

From the vibrating source the sound must travel through a medium to a receptor if hearing is to occur. The medium can be a gas, a liquid or a solid. Most of the sound which concerns us is conducted through air. By means of movement of molecules of air the sound is transmitted from its source to a receptor.

A sound wave is the motion of the air molecules, or particles. Following the production of a sound the molecules nearest the sound source are the first to be set into motion. These, in turn, set the molecules adjacent to them in movement, and so on until the sound reaches the receptor. A wave of particle movement emanates in all directions from a sound source, proceeding outward in concentric spheres at a set velocity which is determined by the temperature and density of the medium through which it is being transmitted. In an air medium of standard density and temperature the sound wave, or particle displacement, travels at a rate of approximately one thousand feet per second. Each vibrating molecule of air moves only a very short distance and then returns to its original position.

Sound has several attributes which are measurable and which are of importance to the clinician.

Frequency is measured in terms of cycles per second, or cps. Sound waves are comprised of repetitions of compressions and rarefactions which occur periodically at the same rate over a period of time. One successive compression and rarefaction constitutes one cycle of a sound wave. It is these cycles which are referred to in the measurement of frequency. In the compression cycle the particles of air move against each other while in the rarefaction phase they separate, or move away from each other.

Wavelength is inversely related to frequency. The wavelength of one cycle of a sound wave equals the frequency of the wave divided by one thousand feet. Thus, for a sound which has a frequency of one thousand cps, the wavelength is one foot. As the frequency of a sound increases, the wavelength decreases.

The normal human ear perceives frequencies of from approximately twenty to twenty thousand cycles per second. This is referred to as the audible range of frequencies. However, the ear is not equally sensitive to all frequencies within this range. It is most sensitive to frequencies between one thousand and four thousand cps. Sounds which fall outside of this range must be made more intense to be perceived, and the farther away they are in frequency towards either end of the scale the greater must the intensity be if hearing is to take place. Sounds which occur at frequencies which are above human limits of hearing are called ultrasonic, while those which occur below these limits are termed infrasonic.

Intensity refers to the rate of sound-energy transmission through a medium, or to the strength of molecular vibration in the medium. Intensity is dependent upon the force which a sound source sets into motion. It is measured either in terms of power, or flow of energy, and is then expressed in watts per square centimeter, or in terms of pressure expended, in microbars, or in dynes per square centimeter.

Pitch is a psychological dimension of sound. As the frequency of a sound becomes greater, the pitch becomes higher. As frequency is doubled, pitch is raised one octave. Conversely, as frequency is halved, pitch is lowered one octave. Pitch is the quality which enables us to arrange sounds on a scale from low bass to high treble and hence permits us to play a tune.

Pure tones are described in terms of frequency and intensity. These are, however, relatively rare and most of the sounds we hear consist of complex tones, which are a number of frequencies of various intensities occurring simultaneously. Complex tones can be analyzed into their component parts by a technique known as a Fourier analysis. When this is done the result is a tonal spectrum. The spectrum of a sound is related to the psychological sensation of quality. We are able to recognize voices because of the differences in the spectra of their sounds from those of others. Noise is characterized by irregular frequencies and intensities of sound. So-called "white noise," which is often employed as a masking noise in audiometry, contains a wide band of frequencies at intervals of one cps or less at approximately the same intensity.

Phase refers to the time relationship between two or more pure tones occurring together. If two tones of the same frequency and intensity are produced so that their periods of compression and rarefaction occur simultaneously, they combine into a tone with twice the amplitude of either one taken singly. These tones are "in phase." If, on the other hand, the tones are separated by half a cycle so that one is in compression while the other is in rarefaction, they will cancel each other out and the resulting amplitude will be zero. They are, therefore, "out of phase."

Differences in phase account for the acoustic phenomenon known as beats. If the ear receives two tones of slightly different frequencies simultaneously, a sensation of pulsing, or beats, is heard. The ear hears as many beats per second as there are cycles of difference between the two tones in frequency. If the tones are more than a few cycles apart in frequency the beats occur so rapidly that the ear does not detect them, but instead receives a sensation of two separate tones. If the tones are far enough apart, a difference tone will be perceived which is equal in frequency to the difference between the two tones in cps.

Loudness is a psychological attribute which is closely related to intensity. As the intensity of a tone increases, so does the loudness we hear. While just noticeable steps in loudness, as measured through psychophysical methods, are roughly constant in terms of decibels, a given physical intensity may sound much louder if the tone lies near the middle frequencies of audibility than if its frequency is very high or very low. (Note: A decibel is one-tenth of a bel, which is a dimensionless unit for expressing the ratio of two values of power, the number of bels being the logarithm to the base 10 of the power ratio. It is named, of course, for Alexander Graham Bell.)

THE ANATOMY OF THE EAR

For purposes of discussion, the human ear can roughly be divided into three main parts, the outer ear, the middle ear and the inner ear.

The Outer Ear

The outer ear is comprised of the pinna, or auricle, and the external acoustic meatus, or canal. The *pinna* is the external ear which we can see as a prominence on the sides of the head. It directs sound waves into the external meatus in a more concentrated way than they would be if the pinna were absent. While in animals the pinna can be moved by muscles so that sounds are more precisely located, this ability either never existed in man or has dropped out through evolutionary changes.

The *external acoustic meatus* is a roughly cylindrical or oval-shaped canal, approximately one inch in length, ending at the *tympanic membrane,* or eardrum. It serves the purpose of protecting the eardrum from dirt, dust and insects through the secretion of *cerumen,* or wax, and blockage by small hairs. The tympanic membrane is the external boundary of the middle ear and it completely closes the canal.

The Middle Ear

The middle ear, or tympanum, is a cavity of about one to two centimeters which lies between the tympanic membrane and the inner ear. It is actually an extension of the nasopharynx by way of the Eustachian tube and is lined with a mucous membrane which is continuous with the lining of the nasal cavities.

There are three small bones, collectively called the *ossicular chain,* which connect the eardrum and an opening in the bony capsule of the inner ear. These bones are the malleus, the incus and the stapes.

The *malleus* transmits the vibrations of the eardrum to the inner ear and also keeps the membrane tightly stretched and cone-shaped through the influence of the *tensor tympani,* a small muscle which is attached to it.

The *incus* has a socket into which fits the head of the malleus, and these two bones move together as a single unit. As the eardrum vibrates, these ossicles execute a rocking motion, rotating on a horizontal axis just behind the upper edge of the eardrum and perpendicular to the external canal. This axis is formed by projections from the malleus and the incus and they are attached by ligaments to the walls of the middle ear cavity. The incus ends in a long, slender tip near the center of the tympanum and contacts the head of the stapes.

The *stapes* is sealed by the *annular ligament* into the *oval window* which faces the inner ear. As the eardrum vibrates, the stapes rocks. The tendon of the *stapedius muscle,* which attaches to the neck of the stapes, pulls the stapes outward and backward, counteracting the pull of the tensor tympani. These two muscles keep the ossicular chain in a taut state.

The *round window,* just below the oval window, is another opening between the middle ear and the inner ear. It is closed by a thin, elastic membrane and serves as a termination of the acoustic pathway to the inner ear.

The middle ear and its structures increase the sensitivity of hearing for sounds in an air medium. The tympanic membrane receives energy which is delivered through the ossicles from a relatively large malleus to a relatively small stapes. This reduction of area makes for efficient transfer of energy to the dense fluid of the inner ear. The tympanic membrane and ossicles thereby considerably increase the sensitivity of the ear. If the eardrum and ossicles are lost there is a resultant slight hearing loss. If the ossicular chain is interrupted, sensitivity is decreased by about twenty-five decibels, or db. A hole in the eardrum may result in a hearing loss of from five to ten db. The middle ear also probably serves as a cushion to deaden loud sounds and hence, protects the inner ear from possible acoustic damage.

The Inner Ear

The inner ear serves both as an end organ for hearing and as the sensory organ for balance. It is composed of a series of chambers and passages in the temporal bone known as the *labyrinth,* because of its complicated shape. The outer hard shell of the inner ear is known as the *bony labyrinth,* and the inner membranous portion is called the *membranous labyrinth.* The latter is protected by a fluid, *perilymph,* which is, in fact, spinal fluid from the ventricles of the brain. Within the membranous labyrinth is another fluid, *endolymph.*

The central portion of the labyrinth, or *vestibule,* consists of the *utricle,* which is sensitive to gravitational forces and to acceleration, the *saccule,* which shares the functions of the utricle in humans, and the three *semicircular canals,* the *anterior* and *posterior vertical canals,* and the *horizontal,* or *lateral, canal.* These canals aid the body in maintaining balance and position sense in space.

That part of the inner ear which is concerned with hearing is the *cochlea.* This is a flat spiral, coiled like a snail's shell for two and one-half turns. The basal end of the cochlea lies nearest the middle ear, while the apical end is furthest from it. The canal within the cochlea is slightly over one inch long, ending at the apex. It is partially divided by a spiral shelf of bone into the *vestibular* (upper) and *tympanic* (lower) *scalae* (galleries). The division of the cochlear canal is completed by the *basilar membrane,* a fibrous, flexible membrane. On the vestibular surface of the membrane lies a membranous tube known as the *organ of Corti* which contains the sensory cells and their supporting structures. The basilar membrane is widest at the apex and narrowest at the base of the cochlea, being just over one inch in length. When fluid in the vestibule is pushed by the stapes into the vestibular gallery, the basilar membrane bulges into the tympanic gallery and, in turn, the membrane of the round window bulges into the air-filled middle ear.

Along the basilar membrane lie four parallel rows of *hair cells.* There is an inner row of about 3500 of these sensory cells, and three outer rows of approximately twenty thousand smaller cells. These cells make contact with the *tectorial membrane* above them which lies in contact with the upper surface of the organ of Corti. They are connected with nerve fibers which run into the central core of the cochlea and there they unite to form the acoustical nerve branch of the eighth cranial nerve. The acoustic branch joins with the vestibular branch coming from the utricle, saccule and semicircular canals, and the eighth cranial nerve proceeds to the brain.

THE PHYSIOLOGY OF HEARING
Air Conduction

Since the majority of sounds to which we attend are airborne, and because our system of air conduction is more sensitive than that of bone conduction, it is through the mechanism of air conduction that we normally hear.

Sound is produced by some source. The resulting sound waves travel through the air medium to the pinna which directs them into the external acoustic meatus. The sound waves then impinge upon the tympanic membrane, setting it into vibration. The eardrum then initiates action of the ossicular chain, since the handle of the malleus is imbedded in it. The ossicles vibrate as one unit, with a rocking motion of the stapes being produced in the oval window. A resultant wave of pressure is formed in the perilymph of the vestibule. The ossicular chain transforms the energy collected by the tympanic membrane into greater force and less excursion, matching the impedance of sound waves in air to that in fluid. If the sound which impinges on the eardrum is very intense, the stapedius muscle restricts the vibrations of the ossicles as protection for the inner ear.

The membrane of the round window responds to the rocking motions of the footplate of the stapes in the oval window, thus relieving the pressure in the inner ear caused by the action of the stapes. When the stapes pushes inward into the vestibule, the membrane of the round window is bulged outward towards the middle ear. If such reciprocal action did not take place, the incompressibility of the perilymph would resist the movements of the ossicular chain and prevent the eardrum from vibrating.

The motion of the fluid from the oval window to the round window is relayed through the cochlear duct. As the stapes is pushed into the perilymph of the scala vestibuli, the *vestibular membrane,* or membrane of Reissner, is bulged into the cochlear duct. This results in movement of the endolymph within and also movement of the basilar membrane. The hair cells on the basilar membrane detect this endolymphatic motion. The movement of the hair cells initiates nervous impulses which are carried by nerve fibers to the acoustic portion of the eighth cranial nerve and from there to the brain.

Bone Conduction

Hearing can also occur without vibrations proceeding from the eardrum and the ossicular chain. That is, sound can be transmitted by bone conduction. This is a far less efficient method since vibrations must be strong enough to set the bones of the skull into movement before they can be heard by means of bone conduction. In addition, sounds are not accurately transmitted through skin, tissue and bone since sounds of longer wavelength are more greatly impeded by these structures than are sounds of shorter wavelength. Thus, with bone conduction, our hearing is somewhat distorted as we hear certain sounds more clearly, or accurately, than we do others.

Generally, we are not aware of sounds heard via bone conduction since most of the sounds we perceive are airborne and because air conduction is a far superior mechanism. When we place our heads on objects, such as a desk, we receive vibrations and these are heard through bone conduction. We are aware of our own voices partly through bone conduction since vibrations of the laryngeal folds are transmitted to the air cavities in the head and neck, and thus to the bones of the skull, which directly sets the fluid in the inner ear into motion. When air conduction is impaired bone conduction can be utilized as an alternative method of hearing through the use of a hearing aid which amplifies sound.

DISORDERS OF HEARING

The concept of normal hearing is generally based upon the hearing ability of a young adult who has no known pathology. For such a person, the range between -10 and +10-15 db is considered to be normal. The condition known as "hard of hearing" begins at about 16 db, and what is usually termed "deaf" begins at 82 db. These figures mean that with 0 db representing average, normal hearing, a person with a 25 db level, or 25 db hearing loss, requires 25 db more sound pressure in order to hear than does a person with normal hearing.

While there are numerous types of hearing disorders the present chapter will be restricted to those auditory disabilities which are most commonly encountered in rehabilitation.

Conductive Hearing Loss

Any impairment of the outer or middle ear when the inner ear is normal is referred to as a conductive hearing loss. In such a case the problem lies in the failure of sound to be conducted to the inner ear because of interference of some sort in the external auditory canal, the eardrum, the ossicular chain, the middle ear cavity, the oval window, the round window, or the Eustachian tube.

Causes

A *congenital malformation,* such as *atresia,* or closure of the external canal is one possible etiological factor in conductive hearing loss. With atresia there is also frequent malformation of the eardrum and ossicles.

Impacted cerumen which blocks the auditory canal and prevents sound waves from reaching the eardrum can also result in a conductive loss. This can be a consequence of failure to clean the ear for a long period of time, although some individuals naturally produce greater amounts of wax than they need for ordinary protection and this tends to build up a plug which shuts out sound waves.

External otitis can cause a conductive impairment. It is produced by skin infections or fungus growth often as a result of the skin being scratched with a sharp object. Skin swelling or trapped secretions from an infection can close off the canal and keep out sound waves.

Otitis media, inflammation of the middle ear, is perhaps the most common cause of conductive hearing loss. The familiar earache of children is usually produced by otitis media.

The inflammation is typically associated with an upper respiratory infection in which nasal secretions travel along the Eustachian tube to the middle ear. When the lining of the Eustachian tube becomes inflamed the tube cannot be opened by swallowing and air pressure in the middle ear is no longer equalized. Oxygen in the air of the middle ear is absorbed by the blood and a partial vacuum is produced. The eardrum is forced inward, producing fixation of the ossicles and flow of clear tissue fluid from the mucous lining. When there are no bacteria in the fluid causing it to be pus, the condition is known as *nonsuppurative otitis media.* If there is pus present, it is termed *suppurative otitis media.*

While otitis media is most often caused by upper respiratory problems such as a cold, or an allergy, or mumps, or measles, it can also result from puncture of the eardrum with a dirty object.

When suppurative, or purulent otitis media persists for several months, or has an unpleasant odor, it is referred to as *chronic otitis media.* In such a case, infection can spread to the mastoid region resulting in *mastoiditis.* This represents a threat to life because infection here, in the temporal bone where the mastoid process is located, can spread to the meninges of the brain producing meningitis.

Cholesteatoma refers to a cyst which is lined with skin. It grows from the upper part of the eardrum as a pouch, or as a tumor-like growth within the inner ear. It may result from a marginal perforation of the eardrum which causes inflammation, or from chronic wetting of the deeper parts of the external auditory canal. Since the lining of the cholesteatoma is skin, when it desquamates it does so into the pouch, enlarging it. This eventually can erode the ossicles or other bony structures.

Otosclerosis is a disease affecting the bony capsule surrounding the inner ear. It turns the normally hard bone into soft, spongy bone.

It is most commonly found near the oval window and fixes the footplate of the stapes in the window. Thus, as the stapes becomes fixed, vibrations carried to it from the other ossicles are not properly transmitted to the fluid of the inner ear. The result is a hearing loss.

Symptoms of Conductive Hearing Loss

One sign of a conductive loss is softer speech on the part of the affected person. He hears himself with adequate loudness due to normal inner ear and bone conduction, but because of his air conduction loss is not aware of other noises which make it difficult for others to hear him.

The speech discrimination of the person with a conductive impairment is relatively unaffected. If speech is made loud enough for him to hear, he will understand it. He can also hear better in the presence of noise than can the individual with normal hearing. Since during conditions of noise speech must be produced at a greater volume, the person with a conductive loss hears the louder speech but not the background noise. This phenomenon is termed *paracusis willisiana*.

Furthermore, such an individual is able to tolerate sounds which, because of their loudness, are uncomfortable or unpleasant to the normal ear. His impairment serves as a screen, or ear plug, within the usual range of intensities of sound. That is, if the person with a conductive hearing loss has a twenty-five db level and the sound he hears is of fifty db, he will only hear what a person with normal hearing would for a sound of twenty-five db. However, at sound-pressure levels of 130 db or higher he responds as would a person with normal hearing.

The person with a conductive impairment tends to have about the same loss of sensitivity for sounds of all frequencies.

Frequently, the affected individual complains of head noises which may be localized in only one ear, may be bilateral, or may be unlocalized in the head. These noises are typically a "hissing" or "roaring" sound and are collectively called *tinnitus*.

The patient with a conductive hearing loss has a more favorable prognosis than does the person with a sensory-neural impairment since modern surgical techniques can cure or improve the great majority of cases. In addition, he can benefit from a hearing aid since his main need is for amplification of sound which such a device provides.

Sensory-Neural Hearing Loss

Sensory-neural hearing impairments have been called "perceptive impairments", "nerve deafness" and "retrocochlear hearing loss". This type of disorder occurs when there is damage either in the inner ear or to the auditory nerve. The prognosis for restoration of hearing is not nearly as favorable as it is for a conductive type of loss". With therapy there are improvements and spontaneous remissions do occur.

Causes

With the exception of congenital atresia, most children who are born with a hearing loss have a sensory-neural impairment. Congenital causes of hearing disabilities include hereditary factors, diseases of the mother during pregnancy, such as rubella, influenza and mumps, and Rh incompatibility.

Sensory-neural hearing disorders can be acquired at any time of life. By far, the most common cause of such loss is increasing age. After the age of thirty, acuity becomes progressively poorer with each succeeding decade. After the age of forty, some atrophy of the organ of Corti and the auditory nerve occurs. This progressive loss of hearing due to advancing age is known as *presbycusis* (or presbyacusia). While not all elderly persons exhibit a hearing loss, the vast majority do as a result of degeneration of the cells in the organ of Corti toward the base of the cochlea, and of their connecting nerve fibers.

Sensory-neural hearing impairments may be the result of disease, such as measles, mumps, scarlet fever, influenza, diphtheria, pertussis, and other viral infections. They produce a toxic effect on the nerve endings in the cochlea. Meningitis and encephalitis also can cause a sensory-neural hearing loss from cochlear damage.

Ménière's disease, or endolymphatic hydrops, is a disorder that can be included within this group as it is confined to the inner ear. Its symptoms are vertigo, tinnitus and hearing loss, caused by increased fluid pressure within the membranous labyrinth. This is probably a result of vascular changes in the inner ear which, in turn, are caused by an allergy. The disability resulting from Ménière's syndrome can be quite severe, forcing the patient to be incapacitated for weeks at a time with recurrent periods of vertigo accompanied by nausea, tinnitus and deafness. It usually occurs primarily in one ear.

Drugs, such as quinine and aspirin, have been known to produce sensory-neural hearing disability and there is a possibility that tobacco and caffeine also affect audition. Certain antibiotics are ototoxic, as are carbon monoxide, arsenic and lead, which in rare cases produces hearing loss. Tinnitus or hearing loss can be the result of hypersensitivity of the tissues of the inner ear to certain proteins in the air or blood stream. "Bacterial allergy", or sensitivity to bacteria, is common and occurs when certain foods are consumed.

Trauma accounts for a certain number of sensory-neural hearing problems. Mechanical injury, as in an automobile accident where the temporal bone is fractured and the inner ear damaged, is one type of traumatic accident which can result in hearing loss. Noise is another. When an individual is constantly exposed to loud sounds for a length of time he becomes temporarily hard of hearing. This condition may last for a few days with recovery being complete. It may be considered as fatigue rather than actual injury and is termed *temporary threshold shift*. There can, however, be permanent loss of hearing due to noise, such as from an explosion, or a gun blast, which ruptures the eardrum membrane or causes permanent sensory-neural hearing loss. This type of injury can also occur if a noise of sufficient intensity is prolonged. Ear injury produced by a single, brief exposure to a loud noise is known as *acoustic trauma*. It typically reduces auditory acuity of the high frequencies first, at about four thousand to six thousand cps, since the region of the basilar membrane which corresponds to these frequencies is most susceptible to injury.

Symptoms of Sensory-Neural Hearing Loss

The individual who suffers from a sensory-neural hearing impairment tends to speak more loudly than is required for ordinary conversation. Since his problem is in the inner ear he does not hear himself speak nor does he hear the voices of others. Hence, he speaks loudly to achieve what appears to him to be adequate volume for communication.

Sometimes a sensory-neural loss will cause problems in speech discrimination. While the words the patient is listening to may be spoken at well above threshold loudness, certain high frequency consonants might not be perceived because of his hearing loss, and consequently, speech is misunderstood.

The person with a sensory-neural disorder may speak loudly but react adversely when others speak loudly to him. This is because once his threshold of hearing has been crossed there is a rapid increase of the sensation of loudness. Thus, a patient with a db level of fifty may just be able to detect a sound of an intensity of fifty db above normal threshold, but hears a sound of fifty-five db intensity as of greater loudness than a normally hearing person hears a sound of five db. This sudden increase in loudness once the hearing threshold has been crossed, is known as *recruitment*.

Another symptom observed in the patient with a sensory-neural loss is tinnitus, but of a different kind than that which is experienced by the person who has a conductive impairment. He experiences a "ringing", or "buzzing", noise which may be localized in either ear or unlocalized in the head.

Other Hearing Impairments

A *mixed hearing impairment* is one is which a conductive loss is accompanied by a sensory-neural impairment in the same ear.

A *central hearing loss* is produced by damage to the pathways by which the auditory nerve fibers enter the cortex, and by damage to the cortex itself. It may result from a tumor, an abscess, vascular changes in the brain, brain trauma, and by kernicterus in erythroblastosis fetalis, a congenital hemolytic disease. The patient with a central hearing loss presents a similar symptom picture to the patient with auditory agnosia in that he has difficulty recognizing and interpreting what he hears.

In a *functional hearing disorder* the disturbance is of psychogenic origin or has psychological factors superimposed on a mild organic hearing loss which increase the extent of the disability.

THE EVALUATION OF A HEARING DISORDER

There are four crude tests of hearing which are administered to a patient when rapid testing is necessary and/or when there is no proper instrumentation available. They are better than no test at all, and therein lies their only advantage.

In the *watch-tick test* the clinician holds a watch next to the patient's ear and slowly moves it farther and farther away. The patient is asked to inform her when he no longer hears the ticking sound. Hearing loss is expressed as a fraction, with the distance at which the normal ear hears the watch as the denominator and the distance at which the patient hears it as the numerator.

The *coin-click test* involves the clinician dropping a large coin on a hard surface or striking two coins together. If the patient hears the sound as a "ringing" noise, his high frequency hearing ability is considered to be normal. If he hears a dull thud he is judged to have a high frequency hearing loss.

In the administration of the *conversational voice test,* the patient is placed at a prescribed distance from the examiner, usually from between fifteen to twenty feet away, in a manner so that first one ear and then the other is facing the examiner. The patient plugs the ear not being tested with his finger and he is then instructed to repeat the examiner's words. In a normal voice the examiner speaks some simple words, phrases and numbers. The patient who cannot correctly repeat what he hears is gradually moved closer to the examiner until he can. Hearing loss is expressed as a fraction, with the distance at which the normal ear hears being the denominator, and the distance at which the patient hears serving as the numerator.

The *whisper test* is quite similar, with whispering being substituted for conversational loudness. This test has an advantage over the conversational voice test in that it is relatively easy to standardize the loudness of a whisper by speaking only at the end of an expiration. It also represents a fairly even intensity at the frequency range needed for clear understanding of speech.

The problems with all such quick and rough measures lie with the necessity of providing a quiet test room and the lack of standardization of test stimuli. With modern audiology and other techniques these tests are becoming increasingly infrequent in their usage.

A step upward in auditory testing is *pure tone testing* with a tuning fork. While exact measurement is not possible much useful information can be gained through this method.

Tuning forks of various standard frequencies are used. They are octaves of "C" on a scale from sixty-four cps to 8192 cps. If a patient can no longer hear a tone, the clinician may place the fork to her own ear as a check. If she cannot hear it, or if it is very faint, the patient will be diagnosed as having normal hearing. If, on the other hand, the patient cannot hear the fork at its loudest, he has a hearing loss for that particular frequency.

A tuning fork can be employed to measure air conduction by holding the vibrating fork near, but not touching the patient's external auditory canal. Bone conduction is evaluated by holding the base, or handle, of the vibrating tuning fork directly on the skull, either on the forehead, or upper incisors, or mastoid bone, or closed mandible.

There are three commonly utilized tuning fork tests. The *Rinné test* is used to differentiate between a conductive and a sensory-neural hearing loss. The fork is set into vibration and held close to the patient's external ear. When he reports that he no longer hears the sound, the fork is placed quickly against the patient's mastoid process and he is asked if he now hears it. If he reports that he does it is indicative of a conductive loss, and this is called a Rinné negative. If the patient hears the fork longer by air conduction than by bone conduction it implies a sensory-neural impairment and is termed a Rinné positive. In a normal ear, results will be Rinné positive since we are ordinarily more sensitive to sounds which are air-conducted.

The *Schwabach test* is a quantitative test of bone conduction. The clinician places the handle of a vibrating tuning fork against the patient's mastoid process and the patient notifies her when he no longer hears the tone. She then places the handle of the fork against her own mastoid and counts the number of seconds during which she continues to hear the fork vibrate. Presuming normal hearing on the part of the clinician, the number of seconds longer than the patient during which she hears the tone is considered to be the amount of hearing loss which the patient has.

The *Weber test* is used in cases of unilateral hearing loss, or when hearing in one ear is superior to hearing in the other. It is a test which compares the hearing, by bone conduction, of the patient's two ears. The hilt of the vibrating tuning fork is placed in the center of the patient's forehead and he is asked where he hears the tone. If both ears are normal the sound will be heard as coming from the center of his head. If there is a conductive loss the tone will be heard better on the impaired side via bone conduction.

There are primarily two kinds of audiometric tests which can be performed by a speech clinician. The first to be discussed is *pure-tone audiometry*.

A pure tone audiometer has an electronic oscillator circuit which provides an alternating current of the desired frequency. Nearly all modern audiometers have a series of fixed frequencies based upon even thousands of cycles. The intensity of the tones is controlled by an attenuator dial which is usually graded in steps of five db according to the American Standards for Audiometers. Zero db represents average, normal hearing and thus, hearing loss is represented in terms of the number of db in excess of this point which the patient requires to hear.

In as sound-proofed a room as possible test tones are delivered

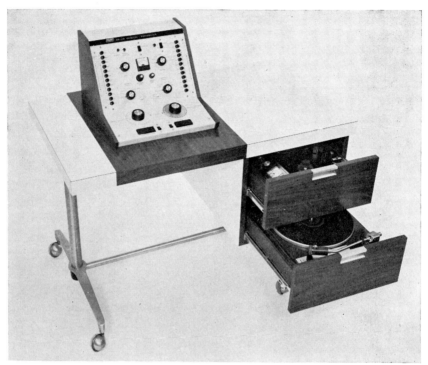

FIGURE 88. A two-channel clinical audiometer. (*Courtesy of Tracor, Inc.*)

to the patient's ear through earphones, or receivers, for air conduction tests and through a bone conduction receiver for tests of inner ear functioning. Receivers are padded for comfort and are placed against the patient's head. The test tone is turned on and off by the clinician. The clinician also controls an interrupter switch or special switching circuit which allows the current to fade in and out so as to avoid any audible clicks which might occur from a sudden start or stop. When the patient hears a tone which has been presented to him he raises a finger as an indication. There is also a masking noise which can be delivered to the ear not being tested at the moment. Masking may be required if the ear being tested is hard of hearing while the other ear hears well by bone conduction.

Modern audiometers are calibrated for frequencies of 250, 500, 1000, 1500, 2000, 3000, 4000, 6000 and 8000 cycles. This covers the range of speech which humans normally must hear for adequate communication. Usually, the 1000 cycle tone is tested first since it is the easiest one for which to establish a definitive threshold.

The frequency dial is set at 1000 cps and the intensity is set at about twenty db above estimated threshold. The interrupter switch is gently depressed for less than one second in duration. If the patient responds the intensity is reduced to zero or minus five db and the tone is presented again. Two responses out of three presentations at this level are generally considered far enough down the scale to record the patient's threshold at that level, although, of course, the examiner can continue if she wishes. If the tone was not heard at twenty db the intensity is increased to about forty db. If it is now heard the clinician will present the tone at intensities between twenty and thirty db to determine the threshold at that level. Then the frequency selector on the audiometer is moved to 2000 cycles and the thresholds are measured in the same way, and so on for all tones.

The *audiogram* is the written record of the audiometric performance. It illustrates the patient's hearing level as measured with the pure tones. The most familiar form of audiogram is a graph on which the frequencies are marked off on the horizontal axis and the tone intensities appear on the vertical axis. The patient's hearing loss, or threshold, at each frequency tested is plotted on the graph separately, by both bone and air conduction. The threshold represents the lowest sensation level at which the patient can detect the test tone fifty per cent of the time.

The audiogram is useful in that it provides information on the comparative sensitivity of the patient's air and bone conduction, and

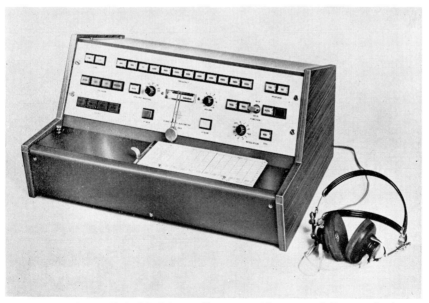

FIGURE 89. A clinical Békésy audiometer. (*Courtesy of Tracor, Inc.*)

it points up the need for rehabilitative measures such as auditory training. In addition, by examining the slope of the audiogram curve for air conduction the extent to which a patient can benefit from a hearing aid may be determined. The patient with a hearing loss which is approximately the same for all frequencies would be considered a good candidate for such a device.

The second type of audiometry to be considered is *speech audiometry*. Contrary to pure-tone audiometry, speech audiometry is performed in two rooms, the patient being in a sound-isolated room and the clinician in an adjoining room. Material is presented to the patient and his responses are recorded via a communication system. Another major difference between speech audiometry and pure tone techniques is in the materials employed. Whereas in the latter tones are used to test hearing, in the former it is speech which is employed as the test stimuli. Words or sentences are spoken into a microphone or played on a pre-recorded tape. The patient either wears earphones or listens to a speaker. The strength of the speech signal is varied by a calibrated attenuator and the listener determines when he can identify the words he hears. This is accomplished either by having him repeat them, or write them down, or check them on a printed form or multiple choice list. Another technique involves having the patient merely listen to the material and set the volume control himself.

If the testing is aimed simply at determining the hearing level of the patient for speech, the actual materials used and the voice inflections of the speaker do not have to be standardized. If actual identification of the material is required then this must be standardized and there are several standard tests which are commercially available. Speech audiometry is employed to measure the patient's threshold for speech reception, his tolerance for loud speech, and his articulation or word discrimination ability.

THERAPY FOR THE HEARING-IMPAIRED PATIENT

While certain kinds of hearing loss, particularly of the conductive type, are amenable to medical and surgical treatment, this section will focus upon the techniques which are employed by the speech clinician in the training and rehabilitation of patients with auditory disorders.

Speechreading

Speechreading, or lip reading as it is still occasionally called, is usually a beneficial technique regardless of the age of the patient or the extent of the hearing loss. Even persons with normal hearing

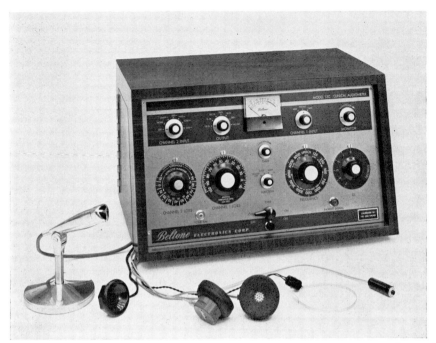

FIGURE 90. A two-channel pure tone and speech audiometer. (*Courtesy of Beltone Electronics Corp.*)

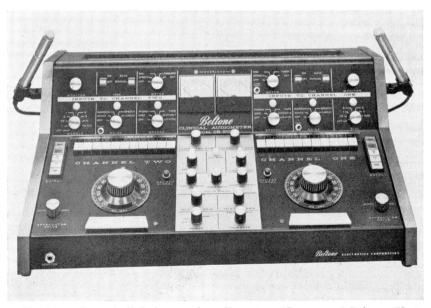

FIGURE 91. A two-channel clinical research audiometer. (*Courtesy of Beltone Electronics Corp.*)

rely, to an extent, on visual cues to improve communication, albeit without awareness.

The principle underlying speechreading is a simple one, namely that when one avenue of communication, the auditory sense, is impaired the loss can at least be partially compensated for by using another pathway, the visual sense. In fact, one indication that an individual may be hard of hearing is an intense concentration on his part on the speaker's oral movements. Speechreading is the method which develops a person's skill at observing the speaker and thereby increasing his understanding of spoken language.

Spoken language consists of approximately forty phonemes, divided into vowels and consonants. Some of these phonemes are visible when they are pronounced and others are not. The phonemes are produced by changing the positions of the peripheral speech mechanisms, the articulators, and it is these changes which the speechreader must note. Since about two-thirds of all sounds we produce are not clearly visible, the speechreader must learn to fill in the gaps. This is done partly by utilizing clues provided through kinesthetic feedback as he imitates the speaker, partly by knowing the context in which the gaps occur, partly by observation of rhythm, stress and accent on the part of the speaker, and partly by analyzing gestures, facial expressions and other non-verbal facial movement.

The task is, as it appears to be, a difficult one. The speechreader must learn to recognize and interpret oral movements instantly since possibilities for review are nonexistent. Poor lighting can be a hindrance, and the more severe the aural handicap, the more difficult the job. As the extent of hearing loss increases, so does the need to use visual cues. Thus, the mildly impaired individual does not need to concentrate on observing the speaker as intently as does the more severely disabled person. Many of the problems of speechreading are greatly helped through the use of a hearing aid. Of course, the technique of speechreading presumes a knowledge of language on the patient's part. If he does not have familiarity and facility with the language, he will not become a speechreader regardless of the effort expended.

Speechreading is not a perfect substitute for hearing, and in teaching speechreading the clinician attempts to have the patient utilize his remaining auditory powers as well as his visual modality. Some voice is employed by her during the lessons, but not at a loudness which would enable the patient to understand by hearing alone since this would interfere with his development of speechreading skill. The clinician speaks in a way which is barely audible to the patient, making listening difficult. She thereby simulates what he probably experiences in his daily contact with others and, at the same time, forces him to rely on his abilities of observation.

In training adults it may be useful to begin with numbers since they play a significant role in our life and daily routines. The clinician may say a number such as "8:30", and have the patient set the hands of a clock to correspond to it. This can be done for various times and the patient given practice in speechreading numbers from one to sixty. Dates are practiced, first in sequence, such as using the days of the week or months of the year, then in random order, and finally in combination with numbers, as in "Ten o'clock, Wednesday, November 13, 1968." Lessons are planned around money, as when the clinician names a coin or a bill's denomination and the patient chooses it from an array on the desk or points to a picture of it. The patient is taught to repeat the numbers as well, since a variety of different numbers can appear alike when spoken. In real life situations, where accuracy is often highly important, repetition of a number by the reader allows the speaker to correct him if necessary.

Situations such as interviews, shopping dialogues and the like are used for instruction since they are both utilitarian and of interest to the patient. Short anecdotes provide good material since whether or not the patient "gets" the "punch line" is an indication of his comprehension of what was said. Patients are always told to relax and to keep their minds clear and flexible. To be effective, they must not have a preconceived idea of what the speaker is saying, or should say. This tends to put words into the speaker's mouth which may be incorrect and interfere with understanding.

With children it is often believed important that they begin training by learning to match. This is initiated by having them match exact objects, then similar objects, then objects to pictures and finally, words as spoken by the clinician, or written on cards to objects and pictures.

The child is thus taught, through a series of progressive abstractions, the names of things, and that these names can be spoken or written, both of which can be understood by him. Lessons are planned using materials which are appropriate to the child's age and using games as an integral part of learning. Initially, lessons are restricted to words which are familiar to the child, with new words being added gradually as his speechreading skill increases.

The illumination of the therapy room is designed so that light falls on the therapist's face. She speaks naturally, without over-exaggeration of articulation. Longer words and phrases are preferred to short ones since this gives the child more time to observe and comprehend. Thus, "It is now time to go to bed" is preferred to "bedtime". Words are repeated as often as is necessary for the child to understand them. Speechreading is integrated with auditory training. A great deal of rewarding praise is given for each successful performance by the child.

Group Speechreading

Group speechreading is often a useful experience if the group is relatively homogeneous in speechreading abilities and the interests of its members. Group work enables the individual patient to realize that others are "in the same boat" as he is. It can provide a motivating force for improvement due to a spirit of competition which such groups often tend to generate. Group members can help each other attain higher levels of speechreading competence.

In a group, which is usually small in number of its members, each individual can take a turn speaking so that the other members have the opportunity of speechreading several different speakers. Dialogues are set up as the group progresses, forcing members to constantly shift attention from one speaker to another as well as having to observe speakers from different visual angles.

Group lessons are an interesting and practical supplement to individual instruction but they are not a substitute, particularly in beginning therapy or for the very slow or very superior patient.

Auditory Training

Auditory training is the term used to denote the techniques of therapy which enable individuals to improve their ability to correctly discriminate sounds.

There are primarily three kinds of auditory discriminations which we make. Gross discriminations are those made between very dissimilar sounds, such as an automobile's horn and a baby's cry. Simple speech discrimination refers to the recognition of sounds of speech under favorable listening conditions. Difficult speech discrimination is the recognition of speech sounds under adverse conditions, such as the presence of background noise or in situations where every phonetic element must be precisely heard. Obviously, auditory discrimination is impaired by a hearing loss.

The adult with a hearing loss does not require as extensive auditory training as does the child because he has already had experience with hearing. Gross discriminations generally do not require training unless the patient has suffered almost total loss of hearing. It is most often found that the adult has difficulty with consonant sounds, most particularly the high frequency voiceless consonants. The adult with a hearing aid which compensates him for a loss may need little or no auditory training. The test of whether or not auditory training is required is the patient's ability to understand speech, with or without the amplification provided by an aid. If he does wear a hearing aid the therapy program is designed around the instrument. Maximum use of residual hearing is always encouraged.

Training often begins with listening exercises. The therapist speaks certain sounds which are moderately difficult to distinguish between, such as *mo-lo, al-at* and *in-an,* and the patient repeats what he hears. Each time he errs the pair is repeated for him by the clinician. Such lessons progress from simple to more difficult distinctions. When the patient can distinguish contrasting pairs, single words and phrases can be provided which are printed in a list. The clinician reads the list several times, in a different order each time. The patient numbers the words in the order which he thinks the clinician has said to them. His paper is corrected at the conclusion of the task and the list is repeated so that he can review the words which he confused. From single words the patient progresses to sentences and then to paragraphs. The therapist reads sentences aloud which contain key words. If heard correctly, these words will make the sentence correct. The patient is asked to repeat the sentence or write it down. A similar procedure can be employed using numbers, beginning with one digit and two digit numbers and advancing to higher numbers as the patient progresses.

Since it is important for patients to be able to make rapid, as well as precise recognitions of sounds, drilling is conducted which presents an item, such as a word, a sentence or an anecdote, only once. Although the patient is given the opportunity to check on the accuracy of his hearing, the emphasis in this procedure is on a variety of auditory experiences.

While most adults do not require training in gross discriminations, some can benefit from such work. Furthermore, not all important sounds are speech sounds. With the aid of a phonograph and sound-effects records a personalized training program can be devised for the individual patient who needs such treatment.

In the case of some patients who have a sensory-neural hearing loss there may be a very narrow range between the threshold of speech recognition and that of discomfort so that a hearing aid is contraindicated. Auditory training can be employed to increase the patient's level of tolerance and thus enable him to wear an aid. Using an auditory training unit, recorded speech materials are played at a volume which corresponds to the patient's ability to tolerate intense speech. The patient increases the volume himself until it becomes unbearable to him. Gradually, as he becomes more accustomed to amplified speech, he becomes more and more able to tolerate higher levels of intensity and, in time, becomes able to tolerate and adjust to the amplification furnished by a hearing aid.

Since everyday life situations often require hearing to take place under adverse conditions, part of the auditory training program consists of practicing listening under different acoustic circumstances. One form of exercise involves listening under conditions in which background noise masks out some of the auditory cues provided for discrimination. Drills, such as those described above, are given to the patient in the presence of the noise, which is controlled by the therapist. A second type of task involves discriminating sounds which are presented via records, tapes, radio, television or loudspeakers, since such reproducers lack perfect fidelity and require slightly greater discrimination than do voices which are actually present. A third technique requires listening over a telephone and training for the patient with a hearing aid in the use of the telephone for maximum benefit from both instruments. Such formal instruction may be supplemented by practice in the home and, in fact, should be so supplemented if the pateint's discrimination ability is to be fully restored.

Auditory training with children differs from that given adults to the extent that the child has not had the years of hearing experience which the older patient brings to therapy. When the impairment is present at birth, or occurs shortly thereafter, the child does not progress through the normal developmental stages in learning discrimination. Some of these children acquire the habit of behaving as if they were totally deaf. Thus, the sounds which they are able to hear are ignored and they become less conscious of them and less able to discriminate. Teaching awareness of sounds and sound discrimination can overcome this handicap, particularly if it is done in conjunction with the use of a hearing aid.

A child may have good hearing for low tones and be deaf for tones of high frequency. Since he can hear the low frequency components of sounds he is usually aware of them. He can learn to discriminate sounds, but his hearing loss produces confusion because of the components he misses. Auditory training can be of much value for such a child.

There are other children who have a partial, but relatively uniform, hearing impairment. If sounds are loud enough they are perceived. However, many sounds are not of significant enough intensity to stimulate the child aurally, and, as a consequence, his auditory discriminations develop more slowly than normally. Such a child may come to rely upon other senses to help him perceive sounds. Auditory training encourages him to make as much use of his hearing as possible. A hearing aid is often valuable for this type of problem.

The person who sustained a hearing loss in late childhood has had the effect of a disturbance of once adequate auditory discrimination ability. He can no longer use all of the auditory cues which he once did in his perception of sounds. If the loss persists for a long time the confusions resulting from impaired hearing can lead to progressive deterioration of his ability to discriminate.

Auditory training with children is begun by developing an awareness of sound in the child. The child is taught to know when a sound is present and to direct his attention to that sound. In addition, he is taught the meanings of the sounds he hears. The clinician, therefore, employs sounds which are of sufficient loudness to overcome the child's hearing loss and which have some meaning for him in his life. Play situations, using musical instruments, are useful because they are enjoyable for the child as well as therapeutic. Loud sounds, and even unpleasant ones can be used to overcome the child's resistance to hearing. Responses to particular sounds are indications for repetition of those sounds as an introduction to other sounds which elicit less, or no responding.

Children are next taught that sounds differ from one another. The clinician uses a set of selected noisemakers, such as horns, bells, cymbals, whistles, rattles, and the like. The child watches as she lifts each object and makes its characteristic sound with it. Then it is the child's turn to repeat her act. A game may be played wherein the child turns his back as the therapist produces a sound and then has to choose the object she used. If he is correct, he can then make the noise himself. If he chooses incorrectly he watches while the therapist makes the sound again. Once gross discriminations of this kind are made, finer ones are introduced, such as using a set of horns, each of which produces a slightly different sound in terms of pitch and quality. The object of all such training is to provide the child

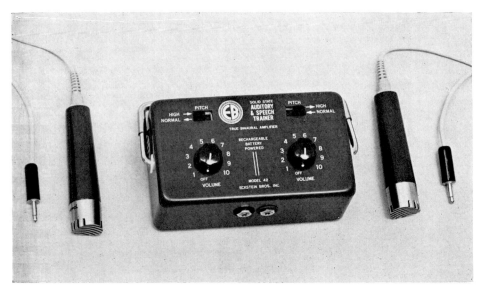

FIGURE 92. Binaural speech and auditory trainer. (*Courtesy of Eckstein Brothers, Inc.*)

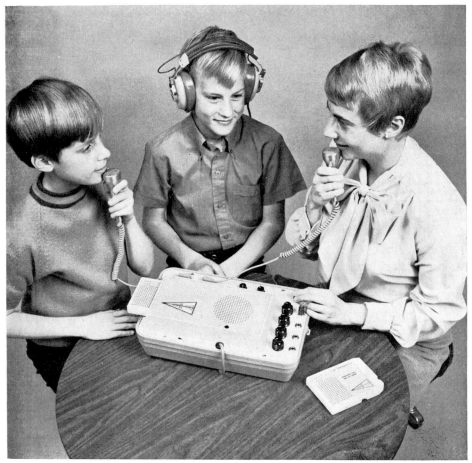

FIGURE 93. Phonic Mirror®. (*Courtesy of HC Electronics, Inc.*)

with a solid, broad foundation upon which finer discrimination abilities can be built.

Following his learning of differences of sound, the child is introduced to speech. Usually, differences in vowels are taught first, by stressing them within a word, such as h*o*t and m*e*, and then consonants are introduced into the lessons. Familiar phrases such as "Hello, Mommy" and "I want to eat" can be used to aid the child in recognizing the meaning of an entire group of connected words without analyzing it into its parts. This has the advantage of relating to the child's everyday life, and also of reproducing the normal manner of learning.

The last stage of auditory training is directed at teaching increas-

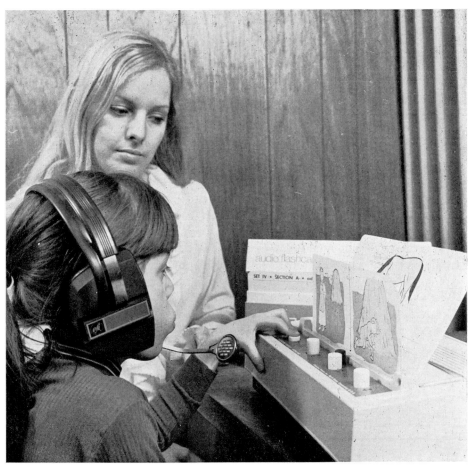

FIGURE 94. Audio Flashcard Reader® being used by a child who has difficulty in auditory discrimination. (*Courtesy of Electronic Futures, Inc.*)

ingly finer discriminations of speech sounds. The child is given repeated drill work which requires him to recognize the more subtle phonetic differences, such as between *s* and *sh*, and *f* and *th*. He is taught to know and to recognize a large vocabulary which contains a variety of spoken words and phrases. He is given training in following connected speech, integrating his vocabulary so that sentences which are rapidly spoken are understood. Stories, phonograph records and conversation are useful tools in building these skills. The child is thus guided, not only in the actual wording, but also in the use of normal intonation, reflection and rhythm, which are so difficult for the hard of hearing person.

Some children, for whom audiometric testing has found a hearing loss severe enough to require the use of a hearing aid, and who are of the type which would benefit from such an instrument, need some auditory training prior to receiving the instrument. This is typical of the child with a severe loss, for whom the sounds of everyday life are not heard and thus not attended to. He is first taught that sound vibrations can have a meaning for him. This is accomplished through training in the gross discrimination of sounds as previously described. Once he learns that sounds can provide information about his world, a hearing aid can be considered.

Some audiologists believe that as soon as it has been established that a child has a profound hearing loss, an aid should be provided, even prior to any auditory training. Others feel that without any experience with amplified sound, or without knowledge of what he is hearing, the child may reject the aid. It is perhaps the latter view which is gaining greater acceptance today.

If a child is given a hearing aid he is trained in its operation so that he can make a satisfactory adjustment to it. He is taught the most comfortable way of wearing it, how to operate its controls, and how to change the battery when necessary. Some trial and error experimentation may be warranted in the setting of the volume control. The child with a sensory-neural loss may suffer further inner ear damage from acoustic trauma if amplification is too great, even though he may feel no discomfort. The audiologist demonstrates the proper volume setting to the child.

It should be borne in mind that not all children with a hearing problem require a hearing aid. Those children who suffer hearing losses less than the minimum for which an aid is indicated, and children with sensory-neural losses who have good hearing through five hundred cps, or possibly one thousand cps, but with a severe drop in hearing sensitivity at higher frequencies, will not have a hearing aid prescribed for them. However, these children are still able to benefit from auditory training.

Since it is primarily language which sets Man apart from phylogenetically lower organisms, the importance of a speech pathology service in rehabilitation cannot be overemphasized. The patient with impaired speech, or language, or hearing, who has not significantly improved or regained his lost abilities, leaves the rehabilitation hospital as an unhappy person, while the individual who has recovered his communication skills returns to the community as a functioning, self-satisfied person able to meet the demands of life. Only with proper therapy can the patient be truly rehabilitated.

———————————

Section IV

References

1. Achilles, R. F.: Communicative anomalies of individuals with cerebral palsy. Part 1. *Cerebral Palsy Review, 16*: 15, 1955.
2. Achilles, R. F.: Communicative anomalies of individuals with cerebral palsy. Part 2. *Cerebral Palsy Review, 17*: 19, 1956.
3. Agranowitz, Aleen and McKeown, M. R.: *Aphasia Handbook for Adults and Children.* Springfield, Thomas, 1964.
4. Berry, Mildred and Eisenson, J.: *Speech Disorders. Principles and Practices of Therapy.* New York, Appleton–Century–Crofts, 1956.
5. Cruickshank, W. M. (Ed) : *Cerebral Palsy: Its Individual and Community Problems,* 2nd ed. Syracuse, Syracuse University Press, 1966.
6. Davis, H. and Silverman, S. R.: *Hearing and Deafness.* New York, Holt, Rinehart, Winston, 1966.
7. de Reuck, A. V. S. and O'Connor, Maeve: *CIBA Foundation Symposium. Disorders of Language.* Boston, Little, Brown, 1963.
8. Gray, G. W. and Wise, C. M.: *The Bases of Speech,* 3rd ed. New York, Harper, 1959.
9. Hirsh, I. J.: *The Measurement of Hearing.* New York, McGraw–Hill, 1952.
10. Johnson, W., Darley, F. L. and Spriestersbach, D. C.: *Diagnostic Methods in Speech Pathology.* New York, Harper & Row, 1963.
11. Krusen, F. H., Kottke, F. J. and Ellwood, P. M.: *Handbook of Physical Medicine and Rehabilitation.* Philadelphia, Saunders, 1966.
12. Luchsinger, L. and Arnold, G. E.: *Voice–Speech–Language. Clinical Communicology: Its Physiology and Pathology.* Belmont, Wadsworth, 1967.
13. McDonald, E. T.: *Articulation Testing and Treatment: A Sensory–Motor Approach.* Pittsburgh, Stanwyx, 1964.
14. Mecham, M. J., Berko, M. J. and Berko, F. G.: *Speech Therapy in Cerebral Palsy.* Springfield, Thomas, 1960.
15. Newby, H. A.: *Audiology: Principles and Practice.* New York, Appleton–Century–Crofts, 1958.
16. Osgood, C. E. and Miron, M. S.: *Approaches to the Study of Aphasia.* Urbana, University of Illinois Press, 1963.
17. Penfield, W. and Roberts, L.: *Speech and Brain Mechanisms.* Princeton, Princeton University Press, 1959.
18. Rusk, H. A.: *Rehabilitation Medicine: A Textbook of Physical Medicine and Rehabilitation.* St. Louis, Mosby, 1964.
19. Sataloff, J.: *Hearing Loss.* Philadelphia, Lippincott, 1966.
20. Schuell, Hildred, Jenkins, J. J. and Jimenez-Pabón, E.: *Aphasia in Adults.* New York, Hoeber, Harper, 1965.
21. Taylor, Martha L.: *Understanding Aphasia: A Guide for Family and Friends.* New York, Institute of Rehabilitation Medicine, 1958.
22. Travis, E. L. (Ed) : *Handbook of Speech Pathology.* New York, Appleton–Century–Crofts, 1957.
23. Van Riper, C.: *Speech Correction: Principles and Methods.* Englewood Cliffs, Prentice-Hall, 1963.

24. Van Riper, C. and Irwin, J. V.: *Voice and Articulation*. Englewood Cliffs, Prentice-Hall, 1958.
25. Wepman, J. M.: *Recovery from Aphasia*. New York, Ronald, 1951.
26. West, R. (Ed): *Childhood Aphasia*. Berkeley, California Society for Crippled Children and Adults, 1962.
27. Westlake, H.: Muscle training for cerebral palsied speech cases. *Journal of Speech and Hearing Disorders, 16:* 103, 1951.

THE PSYCHOLOGY SERVICE

Chapter 15

ASSESSMENT PROCEDURES

A LTHOUGH PSYCHOLOGY IS a relative newcomer to the field of rehabilitation medicine, there is hardly a rehabilitation institution
today which does not provide psychological services for its patients.

A BRIEF INTRODUCTION TO REHABILITATION PSYCHOLOGY

Psychologists are unique among rehabilitation personnel in that
they typically come from fields of study which have not prepared
them directly for work with the physically disabled. Thus, while
other disciplines, such as, for example, physical therapy, train their
students for rehabilitation work, there are comparatively few university graduate programs in rehabilitation psychology. Psychologists, therefore, come from backgrounds of clinical psychology, child
psychology, developmental psychology, physiological psychology, experimental psychology, social psychology, counseling psychology,
educational psychology, psychopharmacology and human engineering. The rehabilitation psychologist is usually one who applies his
knowledge of his particular field of specialization to the problems of
the disabled.

The psychologist is also unique from other rehabilitation professionals in that a fairly large proportion of the patients' problems
which he deals with existed prior to the onset of a disability or a disease. It is true that there are many difficulties which a patient can
experience as a direct consequence of a physical disorder, but it is
often the case that the patient had a previous psychological disturbance which has only been exacerbated by his disability. There
are also cases where the psychological disorder has been unaffected
by the physical handicap and these two variables must be dealt with
separately.

Psychology in a rehabilitation setting is primarily an *applied*
clinical service. While many rehabilitation psychologists function as
researchers, the very nature of rehabilitation is such that the greatest

demands are in the areas of patient care and service. This section, therefore, will not discuss psychological research in rehabilitation, despite its importance, but will be concerned with the main role of the rehabilitation psychologist, that of a clinician.

The majority of rehabilitation psychologists perform such duties as interviewing, testing, counseling, diagnosing, consulting, and conducting psychotherapy. It follows from this that the greatest number of psychologists in the rehabilitation field have a history of clinical training and experience, as the term is broadly used to denote diagnostic and therapeutic work with humans.

It is not quite correct, as in sometimes assumed, that a psychologist without specific training in rehabilitation can enter the field and immediately apply his knowledge successfully to the broad range of new problems he faces. There are a multiplicity of difficulties and situations which are unique to the disabled population, making special training and/or experience necessary. An internship in rehabilitation psychology is an important prerequisite and, in addition, only years of actual work in such a setting can provide the knowledge and experience required for satisfactory functioning.

Often, the role of psychology in rehabilitation is unclear to the other team members, and the psychologist is frequently called upon to perform services which are not a part of his professional responsibility. This section is intended to orient the reader to the role and duties of the rehabilitation psychologist.

THE INITIAL PSYCHOLOGICAL EVALUATION

As is true for all professional staff members in the rehabilitation services, the psychologist evaluates each new admission to the hospital. The purpose of the psychological evaluation is threefold. It serves to determine which patients are not able, because of serious psychologic dysfunction, to participate fully on an active rehabilitation program, thus obtaining maximum benefit from their hospitalization, and also which patients will, as a result of their psychologic impairments, disturb others or prevent other patients from being rehabilitated. The information gained during the initial evaluation is also used by the psychologist to inform other members of the rehabilitation team of the patient's status and of any special procedures or methods which should be employed in working with him. Finally, the evaluation session provides data for the psychologist concerning the need for further diagnosis and/or treatment once the patient has been admitted to the rehabilitation institution.

In the initial evaluation the psychologist is concerned with several variables. These include the patient's general state of consciousness, general orientation, confusion, memory, attentiveness, concentration ability, ability to comprehend and follow directions, intelligence, learning ability, cooperativeness, independence, social adjustment, perceptual-motor abilities, attitudes toward his disability and hospitalization, motivation for rehabilitation, emotional reactions, behavioral reactions and signs of psychopathology.

It must be remembered that the most important aspect of the initial psychological examination is the assessment of the candidate's qualifications for rehabilitation. The two basic questions which the psychologist is attempting to answer are these: Should the individual be admitted as a patient to the rehabilitation program? And what type of patient will he be during his hospital stay and in rehabilitation activities? All initial evaluation procedures are directed at obtaining information which will answer these key questions.

Areas of Assessment
State of Consciousness
Since, by definition, patients being considered for physical rehabilitation must be in a conscious state, very few, if any, comatose or semi-comatose patients are evaluated by the psychologist. Although a patient may receive passive range of motion exercises from a physical therapist while the former is still comatose from a cerebrovascular accident or other brain injury, from the psychologist's point of view there must be at least some minimal state of wakefulness if he will consider the patient to be a rehabilitation candidate. The more alert the patient appears, the better rehabilitation prospect he is felt to be, although, of course, this is but one criterion for acceptance.

A judgement of consciousness may be made on the basis of several points. Observation of the patient is of primary importance. The way in which he sits in his wheelchair is noted. Does he sit upright or slumped over? The former is a favorable prognostic sign while the latter is not. Is his head held upright or does it lean forward onto his chest? The upright position is naturally the more desirable one, although the psychologist must be aware of certain disabilities which predispose a patient to various head and body positions. Only if the patient's disorder is such that it does not preclude maintenance of an erect head position, does a failure to do so indicate a deficit in alertness. The patient's eyes should be open and focussed primarily on the interviewer. A patient with a post-CVA hemiplegia may be unable to open his eye on the affected side, but his uninvolved eye should be as fully opened as possible.

Latency in responding is another variable which the psychologist observes in assessing a patient's level of consciousness. A markedly long latency between the examiner's inquiry and the patient's response may indicate that the latter is less than fully alert, although lack of attention on the patient's part might also account for this latency. In certain disorders, such as advanced multiple sclerosis, or in specific types of brain damage, a longer response latency may be expected but the experienced psychologist is aware of how much of this can be attributed to the disorder. If the latency is considerably beyond these limits, inferences can be made regarding consciousness.

This is also true of unusually slow speech. The right hemiplegic who has sustained a CVA may speak more slowly than the normal person but, even in such a case, there are limits to the reduced rate which are a direct consequence of the physical condition.

The evaluation of a patient's state of consciousness is important because unless he is alert he will experience difficulty in functioning on an active rehabilitation program.

Orientation

There are three "spheres of orientation" which are typically evaluated by the psychologist.

ORIENTATION FOR PERSON. Of concern in this sphere are the patient's knowledge of his own name, of the names and relationships of family members, of the physician and/or nurse on his ward or floor, of his age, sex, occupation, physical characteristics, required medication, and of other variables which pertain to and describe him as an individual. Should the patient fail to correctly answer the majority of questions asked of him regarding this aspect of his orientation it becomes questionable as to whether he will be able to participate fully in rehabilitation. This is mainly because severe deficits in personal orientation are often indications of either serious brain damage or psychopathology, either of which can hamper rehabilitation efforts.

ORIENTATION FOR PLACE. The psychologist wants to know whether or not the patient knows where he is, whether he is aware that he is in a hospital, and which one, and whether he knows the ward or floor which his bed or room is on. He should also be cognizant of the fact that during the evaluation sessions he is not on his own floor, but is on another floor or in another part of the hospital, if such is the case. He should also have been aware that he was being taken from his floor or ward and conveyed elsewhere while he was so transported. In addition, it is determined if the patient recalls his home address and the name and location of the hospital from where he was transferred to the rehabilitation institution.

Questions directed at the patient to gain this type of information are necessary if the patient is to be presumed to be a rehabilitation candidate. The patient who is unaware that he is in a hospital, or does not know where his bed is located, for example, cannot be expected to report regularly for his therapy classes and return to his bed area unassisted. Deficits in this area of functioning do not necessarily preclude a patient from rehabilitation, but rather inform the psychologist that he needs to alert other staff members, particularly the nursing staff, that the patient requires supervision in travelling from place to place within the hospital.

ORIENTATION FOR TIME. The well-oriented individual will know the date at the time of his evaluation, including the year, season of the year, month and day of the week. Initially, the psychologist may just ask him to give the date, but should he be unable to respond correctly, further detailed questioning is employed, including providing the patient with multiple choices from which he can select the one he thinks is correct. Such a technique is often used with the expressively aphasic patient who cannot speak, but is able to nod or gesture upon hearing the right choice.

Perfection of responding is not necessarily to be expected of the patient. If the patient has been hospitalized for a prolonged period or has been out of contact with the public media he may not know the exact date and should not be negatively regarded because of this. But even in such a case, a gross orientation, such as knowing the current year or the season of the year may be expected of him.

Failure to know whether it is morning, afternoon or evening, or whether it is Wednesday or Sunday may result in later difficulty for the patient in keeping to his schedule of therapy classes, or in taking medication.

Memory

Since a relatively good memory is so important in most, if not all activities of daily life, this becomes an area of focus for the psychologist. There are many concepts of memory and a number of theories as to what elements and functions compose memory. The following is a description of three main components of general memory which this author has observed as very frequently assessed in determining a patient's candidacy for rehabilitation.

REMOTE MEMORY. Included in this area are items and events which have been well learned and are familiar to the patient, and also those materials which have passed out of daily meaningfulness for him but are of significance in his life or were at one time important to him.

Such memory items include his place and date of birth, his place of schooling and number of years of education, his employment history, past hospitalizations and illnesses, and past friendships and family relationships. Even in cases of brain injury or disease where memory losses are common, the events and materials which the patient has learned and lived with for many years tend to be the ones best remembered. Deficits in the recall of these kinds of items may generally be considered a poor diagnostic sign.

RECENT MEMORY. As the term implies, recent memory items are those which are relevant to the patient's current and near-current pre-morbid life. It is difficult to always determine precisely where remote memory ends and recent memory begins. One rule of thumb which may be used is to define recent memory as recall of events which occurred within six months prior to the onset of the disability, or to the patient's admission to the hospital.

In this category then, the patient should remember his last home address and telephone number, the last hospital he was in, the events surrounding the onset of his disability and admission to the hospital, the names of the members of his immediate family, the name of his house of worship, his place of employment, the type of work he does and his employer's name, as well as what he ate that day, where he had been, whom he had seen, and his activities prior to being interviewed by the psychologist.

Losses of recent memory items may be considered a serious sign because they can interfere with attendance at therapy classes, with learning and with continuing various therapeutic exercises outside of class.

IMMEDIATE MEMORY. The main question to be answered in assessing a patient's immediate memory is: Can he recall material from minute to minute, or even from one second to the next?

The patient may be required to repeat a series of digits immediately upon hearing it, or to repeat sentences following a single reading, or to answer questions based upon his reading of a paragraph on a test or in a book or magazine. In addition to recording responses on these tasks, the psychologist observes whether, in the absence of a hearing loss, the patient requests questions and directions to be repeated because he did not remember them long enough to respond, or, if he is interrupted during a narrative, whether he is able to resume at the point where the interruption occurred.

When a patient demonstrates marked impairment of immediate memory ability this has implications for the rehabilitation therapists. In such a case, they must remain with the patient during his exercises and activities rather than assume that he can be given a series of instructions to carry out on his own while the therapist devotes attention to another patient.

Confusion

The word "confusion" has a variety of meanings for psychologists. In rehabilitation it is best to relate the term to the patient's awareness and understanding of the nature of his disability and the consequent need for rehabilitative hospitalization.

In determining a patient's knowledge of his condition the psychologist must be aware that many persons do not know the etiology of their disorder, nor are they always aware of the implications or prognosis of a disease process. A complete, technical understanding of the disability, therefore, is not required. However, the patient is expected to be informed enough to realize that he is hemiplegic, or, on a more general level, unable to move an affected upper extremity, or unable to ambulate.

The great majority of rehabilitation patients are able to state with fair accuracy the nature of their disability. When they cannot even grossly describe their condition this must be viewed as one variable which may contraindicate acceptance to the rehabilitation program.

There are two reasons for this. First, if a patient does not have any awareness of what is wrong with him he probably has brain damage to the extent which would make learning on a rehabilitation program very difficult. Second, unless an individual has some understanding of his physical losses it is unlikely that he will view the rehabilitation therapies as necessary and important for him. For example, the hemiplegic may be unwilling to undergo fatiguing, perhaps even painful, muscle strengthening exercises unless he realizes that his extremities are weak and require such exercise if strength and function are to be regained.

The issue of the patient's knowing why he is hospitalized in a rehabilitation institution is thus related to participation on the therapy program. It cannot be expected that the patient who is not aware of his condition, nor understands the reasons for his rehabilitation program will be as active a participant as one who possesses such knowledge.

(Note: By this point the reader will have noticed some overlap in the information obtained by questioning the patient with regard to his orientation, memory and confusion. That is, the patient's knowledge of his disability relates to his personal orientation, his orientation for place coincides with his recent memory ability, and so on. This is a natural consequence of the nature of the interview and is not necessarily to be construed as unnecessary duplication of data. Rather, it may be interpreted as a "check" which provides verification of findings between the various phases of the evaluation and as a means of gaining additional supportive material for the psychologist's conclusions about the patient.

Since much of the above segments of the initial evaluation is geared toward obtaining factual information, the question arises as to the validity of the material supplied by the patient. There are some patients who deliberately omit or distort certain aspects of their responses for a variety of reasons, as well as patients who, because of brain dysfunction or other medical reason, cannot recall events at all or cannot recall them accurately. Because of such possibilities it is incumbent upon the psychologist to carefully review the patient's medical chart and records prior to the evaluation session. By reading all pertinent data and becoming familiar with the patient and his history via the chart, the psychologist can judge whether or not the patient is presenting a true picture of himself. Omissions and distortions can then be focussed on in detail during the initial assessment so as to gain an understanding of the individual in question.)

Intelligence and Learning Ability

While it may be true that participation on a rehabilitation program and performance of therapeutic exercise do not require a high level of intelligence, it is also true that determining the intellectual capacity of a patient serves several important purposes.

To begin with, the possibility of intellectual retardation must be considered. If, upon testing the patient, it is learned that he is retarded, this does not necessarily mean that he will not be accepted to the rehabilitation service. If the individual is profoundly, severely or moderately retarded he probably will be unable to learn what is taught in therapy classes, and in such a case rejection is likely. On the other hand, the mildly retarded or borderline patient can be accepted to the program if the staff is made aware of his limitations and works with him accordingly. The psychologist must explain the nature of the patient's difficulties to the staff and advise on the approach which should be used with him if he is to profit from his experiences.

There are also certain tasks required during the rehabilitation process, particularly some which are part of speech and language training, which demand a higher intelligence than other activities. Based upon intelligence test findings the psychologist will be able to advise others regarding the feasibility of employing these tasks or, if such are deemed necessary by the patient's therapists, the most fruitful way of proceeding with the particular individual.

The nursing staff should be given a report on the intellectual capabilities of the patient. They need to know whether or not the patient can be relied upon to care for his morning and evening ADL, to perform certain activities on the ward, and to take medication as directed, and whether or not supervision is required in all or any of these activities. The physical therapists and occupational therapists who work with the patient must know if the patient can learn to put on and take off prostheses or orthotic devices unassisted or if this must be done for him. Again, high intelligence is not required, but the patient should be functioning within the normal range or only slightly below in order to perform certain tasks.

If the patient is of school age and placement in the hospital school is being considered for him while he is in residence at the institution, a measure of his intellectual ability is important. Such a measure can serve both as a guide to grade level placement and as data for the instructors concerning the most appropriate teaching methods to employ.

Additionally, many patients seek vocational placement following discharge from the hospital. The majority of these cannot, due to their disability, return to their former type of employment. Therefore, the rehabilitation counselor must work with them in finding new jobs. By knowing the patient's intellectual strengths and weaknesses the counselor can plan with him and find placement for him in a job which is both equal to his abilities and personally satisfying.

It is not always possible for the psychologist to obtain a complete profile of a patient's intelligence during the initial evaluation. This is primarily due to lack of time. A complete intelligence test requires approximately one to one and one-half hours to administer and the psychologist typically has this time or slightly longer (or perhaps slightly less) for the entire evaluation, during which he must obtain a great deal of information in addition to the patient's intelligence level. Therefore, at first, he must estimate the patient's intelligence. This can be done in several ways, and all of these ways are used in combination.

From the number of academic years completed and the patient's report of his achievements in school a rough idea may be formed of his ability. The inherent fault in this is that many patients reach only a relatively low level of formal academic training, not because of lack of intellectual capacity, but because other circumstances forced them to leave school. By questioning the patient, the psychologist may learn the reasons for an incomplete education and modify his judgements accordingly.

In addition, the psychologist notes the patient's comprehension of his vocabulary and questions, and the patient's own vocabulary as a further indication of intelligence. He may also question the patient as to what he has read, or usually reads, his activities, his hobbies and his interests.

The best method of rapidly estimating intellectual ability is administration of a standardized test or subtest, such as the Vocabulary subtest of the Wechsler Adult Intelligence Scale or the Wechsler Intelligence Scale for Children, both of which will be discussed in detail later in this section. The Vocabulary subtest has the highest positive correlation of any of the subtests of these intelligence scales with the total IQ score and thus can provide a fairly reliable measure. Following the acceptance of the patient to the rehabilitation program the psychologist can administer a complete intelligence test, since time will not be as limited as it is upon the patient's initial hospital admission.

From the patient's intellectual performance, the psychologist can infer his capacity to learn new information. Obviously, the patient with a low intelligence rating will not learn as quickly, nor perhaps as well, as the patient with a greater intellectual reservoir. Furthermore, there are differences between patients based upon age, educational experience and type of disorder. Thus, for example, the older patient may not learn as swiftly as his younger associate but, given more time for learning or completion of a task, he can usually do equally well. The patient with little formal education may have more difficulty initially grasping new concepts than will the more educated individual but, eventually, if he is of comparable intelligence, he will equal the performance of the latter. Also, some types of brain injury will predispose a patient to limited learning potential. Concrete thinking, for example, as opposed to the ability to reason abstractly, is a prognostic indicator of learning difficulty and this is a fairly common finding among certain forms of brain damage.

When the psychologist concludes that the patient will have difficulty learning new tasks or materials, he conveys this to the therapists who will be working with him. He may generally describe the problem to them or may, because of certain specific information which he has obtained, suggest definite approaches and training methods.

The Ability to Follow Instructions

It is not as vital for the psychologist to determine the new patient's ability to comprehend and carry out instructions as it once was believed to be. There are two reasons for this. First, the majority of tasks which the psychologist asks the patient to perform in his office are different, and often only indirectly related to those which he will actually be engaged in on a therapy program. Second, during the initial evaluation period the psychologist is not the only rehabilitation team member who assesses the patient. The patient is also evaluated by the physician, the physical therapist, the occupational therapist, the speech clinician, etc., all of whom give numerous instructions to the patient and all of whom require a variety of responses. Thus, were the psychologist not to evaluate the patient's ability to understand and follow directions, the other team members would be able to report on how the patient responded to their commands, and on tasks which are directly concerned with the actual therapy he will be receiving.

There are still valid reasons for the psychologist to test this ability in the patient. When other therapists evaluate a patient for admission to the rehabilitation program, they are not primarily interested in his ability to follow commands. Rather, the physical therapist is concerned with range of motion, and muscle strength in the lower extremities and with ambulation, and the occupational therapist focusses on ADL, and muscle strength, range of motion and sensation in the upper extremities, to name a few examples. Evaluation of comprehension of instructions is not paid a great deal of attention but, instead, is a secondary finding which becomes noticed only when there are marked deficits. Therefore, the psychologist, who considers this to be a prime area of focus, may be able to provide the most complete information.

Furthermore, although the tasks which are presented by the psychologist for the patient to carry out are not those in which he will engage during his rehabilitation, the psychologist is able to judge from the patient's performance how well the patient will succeed in other areas. That is, the patient's general capacity is tested and from this inferences can be made to other tasks which, although dissimilar in nature, have the similarity of basic comprehension ability.

The psychologist can evaluate the patient's ability to follow instructions in a number of ways. He gains an initial impression of the patient through speaking with him. If the patient understands all of the questions put to him and responds relevantly the impression gained is more favorable than if the opposite were true. Next, the psychologist gives the patient simple commands involving the use of body parts, such as asking him to raise and lower each arm, clench and unclench each hand, close and open his eyes, nod his head, open his mouth, protrude his tongue, and the like. He then proceeds to more complex body-part commands, as in requesting the patient to clap his hands, to touch his left ear with his right hand, to touch his right knee with his left hand, and to raise one upper extremity and the contralateral lower extremity simultaneously.

Following this series of instructions the patient is directed to perform first simple, and then complex functional tasks. These can be initiated by asking him to hand over objects which the psychologist names, or to take objects and move them from one place to another on the desk. Then multiple-step commands are given, such as requiring the patient to pick up a pencil, place it in a box, go to the office door, open and close the door, return to the desk, remove the pencil from the box and give it to the psychologist. The performance of these tasks depends, of course, upon the physical abilities of the patient.

From observation of the patient's capacity to carry out these and similar instructions the psychologist is able to inform the other members of the rehabilitation team of the extent to which the patient is able to comprehend and follow directions.

Cooperation, Attention Span and Concentration

Cooperation, attention span and concentration ability are three behaviors which are not necessarily assessed directly by the psychologist. That is, they are observed in the patient throughout the evaluation session as he engages in various tasks and are not typically measured with specific psychological instruments.

In determining the cooperativeness of the patient the psychologist initially notes whether or not the patient was willing to attend the evaluation session. There may be several reasons for a patient's refusal or unwillingness to see the psychologist, including fatigue, pain, fear, anxiety, etc., but the psychologist must determine the validity of these reasons and make a judgement based upon this determination. If the patient has been evaluated by other services just prior to the psychological screening he may be weary or tired of being examined by so many new and unfamiliar people. If the patient is in pain, either because of the nature of his disability, as might be the case with an arthritic, or because of some procedure to which he has recently been subjected, he may want relief from the pain before he feels able to spend some length of time in an evaluation session. Some patients, due to lack of adequate knowledge, may fear the psychologist or be anxious about meeting him because of some "powers," or "superior intelligence," or "magical" ability which they believe that he possesses.

All of these reasons are, from a patient's point of view, valid and are accepted as such by the psychologist. On the other hand, the patient who refuses to attend the initial evaluation session because he is "too busy," or "can't be bothered," or feels it is unnecessary, or because he "doesn't like to be tested" is considered differently. For such a patient, future difficulties may be anticipated during his hospital stay.

A patient's willingness to cooperate is also assessed during the evaluation interview. The patient who does all that is required of him, who answers questions directly and who generally cooperates with the psychologist may be judged to present the same characteristics with others. The patient who refuses to answer many queries or answers reluctantly, who complains about having to perform tasks or is unwilling to take tests may be considered to be one who will present problems to the staff working with him in therapy activities.

One difficulty in estimating a patient's cooperativeness in such a way is that the tasks given him by the psychologist are typically not as fatiguing nor as painful as some of the activities and exercises which he will engage in once he is on a rehabilitation program. Thus, a patient may be quite pleasant and agreeable in the psychologist's office but prove to be the opposite in other, more taxing situations. Nonetheless, it is incumbent upon the psychologist to assess this factor and to report his conclusions to others, since his findings are, in general, reliable.

Furthermore, the psychologist must follow up his report by speaking with the patient's therapists after the latter has been on a training program for a while to confirm the accuracy of his conclusions and, if necessary, modify his evaluation procedure.

Attention and concentration are interrelated functions. One must be able to attend to a task before he can concentrate on it, and concentration is impaired when attention is distractible.

Attention span and concentration ability vary considerably between individuals of the same age and between persons of different ages. They are, to an extent, a matter of training, and therefore a person with such training, as one with many years of academic experience might be, will perform better on tasks requiring these abilities than will one who has not had such experience. A very young child will have a shorter attention span than will a young adult. Certain forms of disability which involve brain damage—e.g. hemiplegia resulting from a CVA, or brain damage consequential to trauma, or advanced multiple sclerosis—reduce attention span. The elderly individual with arteriosclerotic brain disease is less able to attend and concentrate than is the patient not so affected.

The psychologist assesses a patient's ability to attend and to concentrate in two main ways. One is through observation. He notes whether or not the patient attends to questions and directions as evidenced by the latency between question or instruction and response, and by the relevancy or appropriateness of the response. In addition, the psychologist can have the patient perform on a subtest of a general test, such as the Wechsler scales, which requires prolonged concentration, and note the patient's ability to remain at the task until completion without discontinuing at some point of being distracted by extraneous stimuli.

The information gained during this segment of the evaluation may be crucial for the rehabilitation therapists to know once the patient is on program. A patient with a short span of attention may need to have directions repeated to him several times before he can follow them, simply because he could not attend well enough or long enough when they were first given to him. The individual who lacks the ability to concentrate for long periods on a given activity will require the therapist to remain with him in constant supervision if he is to benefit from completed therapy sessions.

Social Adjustment

Determining whether or not a patient is well adjusted socially is not an easy matter during the initial evaluation session. The psychologist must both accept the patient's statements regarding the number and intensity of his interpersonal relationships, and also look beyond these verbalizations to interpret the meanings of what the patient relates as well as "read between the lines."

When a patient says that the only real friend he has is the "dollar bill," or that people are only friends as long as one has money, it may be assumed that this individual is not highly sociable nor does he value friendships to a great extent. By making such statements he is revealing something important about his value system. A patient who reports that he had many friends until he became ill or disabled and dependent, whereupon his friends deserted him is also indicating a lack of a high level of sociability. The questions which the psychologist must answer in such a case are: Did this person actually have many friends? Were they really friends or only acquaintances? Did he, upon becoming sick or disabled, become so demanding, so in need of support, so complaining, or so withdrawn that he did, in fact, turn others away from him? Was he the kind of individual who turned from others when they were in need and therefore, is now receiving similar treatment from them in retaliation? The patient who lived alone and "needed no one" may also be viewed as asocial.

On the other hand, there are those patients who claim to have many friends, who provide evidence of their social relationships by stating that they belonged to a variety of community and religious groups, and who cite a long list of their friends, acquaintances and social activities. These persons can, in all likelihood, be accepted at their word as generally having had no difficulties in interpersonal relationships, simply because of the evidence which they provide and firmness with which they give their statements.

In the above examples, the pictures presented by the patients are rather clearcut. There are many cases, however, in which a patient's report is ambiguous or vague in nature and requires further clarification. When an individual says merely that he "has friends," or has "lots of friends" without further elaboration, or avoids a direct answer to this type of questioning, the psychologist must do additional probing. This can be accomplished through further, more detailed questioning concerning how the patient spends his time and with whom, the types of activities which he enjoys, both alone and with others, the number of people he expects will visit him while he is hospitalized, his conception of a "friend," and so on. It can also be achieved through more formal psychological testing. Often, by observing the individual's responses to the stimuli of certain tests such os the Rorschach Test, or Thematic Apperception Test, or Rotter Incomplete Sentences Blank, or Minnesota Multiphasic Personality Inventory, all of which are described later in this section, or other test or subtest, the psychologist can draw meaningful conclusions about his sociability.

The psychologist is able to at least partly verify his conclusions by observing the patient's interactions with other patients and staff members and by noting the number of visitors and the frequency of visits made to the patient by persons whom he knows.

One reason for determining a patient's sociability is for possible future reference should he be considered a candidate for some group activity, such as those which are organized by recreation workers, or group psychotherapy. The individual with a history of asocial, with-drawn behavior would probably best be dealt with in an individual situation. In addition, the person with pronounced antisocial tendencies may present problems on his floor or ward which the nursing staff should be alerted to.

Perceptual-Motor Ability

Perception may be defined as a hypothetical construct residing within the organism which is controlled primarily by the sense receptors but is also influenced by other factors which have their origins in the life history of the organism, such as his past reinforcement history. On a practical level, it is the translation which the brain makes of information received by the sensory organs.

The term *perceptual-motor* refers to the performance of an overt motor response, which is not primarily verbal, when a concrete, non-verbal stimulus situation is presented. It is, therefore, the integration of the perception and the motor response to what is perceived.

The psychologist is not the only rehabilitation team member who is concerned with perceptual-motor skills. The physical therapist and occupational therapist particularly are also interested in this behavior. However, the psychologist makes this an area of concentration and tests it somewhat differently from other paramedical personnel.

There are certain disabilities, particularly hemiplegia, which tend to demonstrate losses in the perceptual-motor sphere. Patients so affected, notably those with hemianopsia, are prone to ignoring stimuli which are presented on their involved side, and this results in incorrect responding. Patients with peripheral neuropathy may have sensory losses which interfere with their perceptual-motor functioning. Individuals with ataxia of the upper extremities tend to do poorly on perceptual-motor tasks because of impairments in motor coordination. Children who have spina bifida have difficulty in perceiving stimuli correctly and in perceptual-motor learning.

The psychologist should, upon completion of the initial evaluation, be able to inform other staff members as to the deficits which an individual possesses in this area and be able to offer suggestions as to the most effective ways of presenting materials to such a patient.

Testing of perceptual-motor ability is best done through the use of standardized instruments such as the Bender-Gestalt Test, the Trial-Making Test, the Tweezer Dexterity Test, or certain subtests of the Wechsler scales. These are described in the section dealing with psychological testing.

Motivation and Related Factors

Motivation is perhaps one of the most important patient variables in rehabilitation. Despite a good medical and physical prognosis, if an individual is not motivated towards improved functioning the chances of such are greatly reduced.

Motivation is frequently defined as the nonstimulus variables which control behavior. It is the general term employed for the fact that an organism's acts are partly determined in intensity and direction by its own internal state. The external features of motivation are those reinforcers and punishers which exist in the environment and exercise behavioral control.

Motivation is typically considered to have two "anchor points," need and goal. The term *need* refers to a lack in the organism, usually a lack of what would generally be considered a positive variable. *Goal* refers to an end result, a state or condition which, when achieved, concludes a directed course of behavior or action. In physical rehabilitation the question is one of whether or not the patient wishes to improve his condition and how badly he wants this, or what effort he is willing to expend toward this goal.

Motivation for rehabilitation is a very difficult variable to assess in an initial evaluation session. The psychologist uses two main approaches. One is direct questioning. That is, he simply asks the patient if he wants to improve. The great majority of patients will reply in the affirmative, although some will state that they can "manage" as they are and would prefer to return home without going through the rehabilitation process. Once the psychologist receives a positive reply to his question, he can then describe some of the rehabilitation therapies to the patient, emphasizing such aspects or byproducts of therapy as pain, fatigue, arduousness, and slowness of recovery. He then inquires of the patient as to whether or not he is willing to sustain these discomforts in order to achieve the desired goal. Should the patient answer affirmatively, as the majority do, the psychologist may point out to him that he seems to be doing well in a wheelchair, or on crutches with braces, and could probably continue in that way, thus giving him the option of difficult rehabilitation or remaining wheelchair-bound, or crutch-bound without having to work hard. Positive responses on the part of the patient to this type of inquiry point to a good level of motivation.

The other approach used to determine a patient's motivation is through inference from related variables. These include the patient's degree of independence, his attitudes toward disability, his current adjustment to his disability, his expectations of rehabilitation, and his own potential and future life plans.

A person who has led a relatively independent life, maintaining steady employment, heading a family and being relatively self-reliant will have a better chance for success in rehabilitation than one who has been comparatively dependent upon others for support, both economic and psychological. Similarly, the patient whose attitude towards his disability and his adjustment to and acceptance of his condition, is one of tolerance but not of satisfaction, nor of complete resolution and acceptance, will be judged to demonstrate greater motivation than one who readily accepts his status as a natural conse-quence of life, or "God's will," or fate which must be borne because "that's the way life is," as some patients do, indeed, believe. The patient who refuses to accept or adjust to his condition at all or who uses denial of reality as a defense mechanism presents another type of problem, particularly if he will be permanently disabled, but such an individual may be expected to be motivated toward self-improve-ment.

The belief that rehabilitation will be either a very rapid process or one which leads to complete return of function, or another such unrealistic expectation, can lead to certain motivational difficulties when these expectations are not met. The psychologist can provide a patient who has these ideas with correct information and can regularly meet with the patient to discuss discrepancies between his views and the reality situation, easing the transition from expectation to fact.

One indicator of what may be expected of a patient with regard to motivation is his future plans. If a patient is planning on returning to school or work following his discharge from the hospital, whether or not the school or employment is the same as that which he formerly engaged in, this is a sign that he will want to improve his condition to the point where these plans can be fulfilled. This is particularly true if the patient has a definite career to pursue or a family to support. Patients who do not have such plans are not necessarily to be viewed negatively, especially young children whose lives would not include these goals, but where they do occur in a patient's thinking they can be considered positive.

There are some difficulties in assessing motivation in the ways just described. A patient's verbal report, when he is not actually being put to the test, may not correlate highly with his performance when demands are being made upon him. It is quite a different matter for a person who has not experienced the pain of having a contracted joint stretched, or the fatigue of repetitive weight-lifting with a weakened upper extremity, to say that he will do anything to improve, from actually undergoing such therapy activities. Thus, at times, patients express high motivation only to later fail to report for therapy classes once the full implications of the rehabilitation program are realized and experienced.

A problem with judging a patient's motivation from his previous life style is that many patients have not faced the crises and severe hardships that are concurrent with a marked physical disability. Thus, a man might be the head of a family and an independent, industrious worker, and be able to manage his life successfully in the absence of great challenge. However, the kinds of difficulties which must be faced with the onset of serious disease or disability may be such that the individual is unable to cope with them and loses his sense of independence and motivation.

The psychologist must regularly follow up the patients he has evaluated to determine the accuracy of his predictions.

Behavioral Reactions

Evaluating the behavioral reactions of a patient and inferring the bases for them constitute a fundamental role of the psychologist. When the psychologist concludes that a patient is not a candidate for rehabilitation and should not be accepted to the program, it is very often on the basis of his findings in this area that a judgement of this nature is made.

Some of the more frequently observed behavioral reactions of rehabilitation patients are described below.

Denial, or the mechanism by which a patient denies, falsifies or distorts the reality of his condition, usually because acceptance of the truth would be psychologically traumatic. Some conditions in which this is most commonly seen are multiple sclerosis, in the early stages, Hansen's disease, or leprosy, in the early stages, paraplegia and quadriplegia. The patient either refuses to admit to himself and/or others that he, in fact, has the disease or condition, or that the prognosis is unfavorable.

Grandiosity, in which the patient describes magnificent, unrealistic plans or unrealistic notions of his own importance or abilities. This is observed in some psychotic disorders, such as paranoid schizophrenia, and in certain brain disorders, such as general paresis associated with syphilitic infection.

Impulsivity, or acting out without delay or reflection, or obvious differential control by the stimulus situation. The behavior may be elicited by a stimulus but the determining condition for the act is the individual's own state or condition. The impulsive person appears unable to suppress his actions. An individual may be impulsive because of a neurosis, psychosis, personality disorder, or brain dysfunction.

Isolation and Withdrawal are terms which are employed to describe the individual who tends to avoid social contacts and who demonstrates an exaggerated indifference to his environment. Isolation is often believed to be common in obsessive-compulsive neurosis. The withdrawn, seclusive individual may remove himself from frustrating or conflict-arousing situations and obtain satisfaction through daydreaming, drowsiness, alcoholism, narcotic addiction or even strenuous work. Marked withdrawal is generally considered one characteristic sign of the schizoid personality which can develop into schizophrenia. In physical rehabilitation, isolation and withdrawal are observed in patients with traumatically produced disabilites who have not yet accepted nor adjusted to their condition or to the hospital.

Low Frustration Tolerance is not necessarily associated with a psychopathological disorder but can occur in certain types of individuals who do not deal with stress, frustration, pressure or conflict in an effective way. These persons are easily frustrated and can react either by abandoning a task, physically leaving a situation, acting out in anger, weeping, becoming humorous, fearful or compulsive, or psychologically withdrawing and then obtaining gratification in the ways which are characteristic of the withdrawn individual.

The psychologist can assess a patient's level of tolerance for frustration through his responses and behavioral reactions to questions, and through observation of his behavior on tests which require concentrated effort and which challenge his abilities.

Opposition refers to resistance of an idea of another person or group without the accompaniment of anger or hostility. Thus, in physical rehabilitation, the oppositional patient may refuse certain medications or forms of therapy. The refusal is made from fear, ignorance, or the belief that he, the patient, is the best judge of which treatment modalities he requires. Oppositional behavior is usually a life-long characteristic of the individual and as such presents some difficulty in management. Understanding the nature of the patient's contrariness and the reasons for it, plus psychological assistance and a tactful approach by the rehabilitation team can, in most cases, overcome the problem.

Rigidity of thought or behavior is characterized by a relative inability to change actions or attitudes even when objective conditions require it. This type of individual clings to ways of feeling or behaving even when they are no longer appropriate. He tends to perceive himself and situations in a stereotyped way despite reality changes which have occurred. The rigid person may use denial as a mechanism which permits him to maintain his views and may behave in an oppositional or compulsive manner.

Not infrequently, rigidity is encountered in the teen-aged patient who has sustained a spinal cord injury and who persists in viewing himself as he was premorbidly. He refuses to accept his prognosis, refuses to recognize the extent of his disability and refuses to reorganize his future plans and goals. This problem is typically observed during the first several months following injury, and psychotherapy is of great value in helping such a patient to eventually adjust to the new realities of his life.

Self-depreciation, where the patient expresses feelings of lack of self-worth, usefulness, loss of manhood, and the like is also met with in the young, traumatically-injured patient. Once again, the psychologist must work with the patient during this period of thought.

Similar views are seen among patients with chronic disabilities— e.g. multiple sclerosis, rheumatoid arthritis, Parkinson's disease, post-poliomyelitic paralysis, and occasionally, hemiplegia and amputations. Often, the patient expresses these ideas because he is seeking reassurance that he is, in fact, incorrect and is still a useful, worthwhile person with much to contribute to himself and his loved ones. There are, however, patients who fully believe their self-depreciating verbalizations and in these cases the possibility of suicide attempts must be seriously considered.

There are a number of behavioral observations which the psychologist makes from which a patient's emotional condition can be determined. Perhaps the two most common affective, or emotional states of new rehabilitation patients are anxiety and depression.

Anxiety is best defined as an unpleasant emotional state characterized by a feeling of fear, threat without knowledge of the exact nature of the threatening event, autonomic nervous system activity, such as palmar sweating, increased heartrate, blood pressure and respiration rate, pupil dilation, stomach contractions and headaches, and a suppression of responses typical to a situation with substitution of other responses, such as avoidance behaviors, which appear appropriate to the individual but are usually inappropriate to the situation. Anxiety can be manifested in a variety of ways, including agitation, rapid speech, irregular breathing, perspiration, wringing of the hands, compulsive behaviors, changes in vocal tone and quality, habits, tics, weeping and facial expressions, loss of appetite, insomnia, and more.

Patients who are new to a rehabilitation hospital exhibit anxiety for several reasons. In the usual case, they have recently been severely injured or recently diagnosed as having a serious disease. They are therefore anxious about their condition and their future. Many do not fully understand the nature of their disability or the meaning of the disease and its associated complications. Thus, being in a state of relative lack of knowledge, they are nervous and fearful. This fear can be detected in the questions which they ask. Will I die? Will I be permanently crippled? What will happen to me? What will happen to my family?

Most patients do not understand what rehabilitation means—what is involved in the rehabilitation process, what it will do for them, what they will have to do, and what they can expect. For these patients, anxiety is a natural consequence of sudden crippling disease or disability and should not be looked upon as pathological. Only when the anxiety persists beyond the point where it is expected to be a natural reaction to the onset of physical dysfunction is it considered to be a problem in need of psychological amelioration.

Depression is a psychological state of lowered initiative, decreased accessibility to stimulation, and dejection which is observed fairly frequently in the physical rehabilitation population.

The loss of a limb, or of bodily function, or the onset of a disability, or the consequences of chronic disease are depressing concepts and patients who are affected reveal their depression in numerous ways. These include reduced rate of speech, latency of responding, insensitivity to environmental stimuli, slow motoric reactions, drowsiness, gloomy ideation of thought, sad facial expressions, weeping, easy fatigability, and an apathetic and pessimistic outlook towards both the present and the future.

A depression can be situational, in which it is related to specific environmental and personal events and/or situations, or it can be chronic, in which it characterizes a patient's life style and is of several years' duration. In the rehabilitation patient population, both forms are encountered although the former is observed far more frequently than the latter. The situational depression is generally anchored to the disability, the hospitalization, and their associated variables. It usually is amenable to psychotherapy and tends to have a brief course except in extreme cases. Chronic depression, however, is more serious, is not as clearly defined with regard to its eliciting stimuli, and is more difficult to deal with therapeutically.

Two other types of depression which may occasionally be seen upon the initial admission of a patient are *agitated depression,* marked by restless overactivity, despair, apprehension and self-condemnatory delusions, and *psychotic depressive reaction,* which is characterized by severe depression and gross distortion of reality, including delusions and hallucinations. In either of these types the patient would not be accepted to a rehabilitation institution because the nature of his depression is such that participation in therapy activities to any meaningful extent would be highly unlikely.

At opposing poles of the affective scale are the apathetic patient who exhibits listlessness, indifference, and a lack of interest or feeling in situations which usually arouse strong reactions, and the excitable patient who overreacts to stimuli and is aroused by a great variety of stimuli, many of which would not usually be arousing.

With the exception of psychotic extremes of such emotions and behaviors, and the disability-related stimuli which can evoke them, these affective states are usually long-standing habit patterns of the individuals in whom they are observed. They can present certain difficulties for the nursing staff and for the therapists working with such patients, but essentially can be dealt with effectively in a therapeutic milieu.

PSYCHOPATHOLOGY

As in the evaluation of behavioral and emotional reactions, the psychologist is the key figure and, in fact, is the only staff member who can assess a pathological condition in a patient. Since this rubric encompasses abnormal behavior based upon brain disorder and physiologic dysfunction as well as functional psychopathologies, it is primarily in this area that a psychologist's conclusions regarding acceptance of a patient to a rehabilitation program are made.

There are a great many psychological disorders and, theoretically, a patient who enters a rehabilitation institution can exhibit symptoms of any one or more conditions. However, from a practical and experiential standpoint, not all are actually seen in rehabilitation settings. This is primarily because some disorders are so psychologically disabling that the affected individual would not even be considered as a possible candidate for a rehabilitation therapy program, or because many seriously incapacitated persons are hospitalized in psychiatric institutions or in acute medical hospitals.

This section will discuss in most detail those psychopathological disorders which are more frequently encountered upon the initial evaluation of a patient for rehabilitation, and will briefly describe other conditions which are only occasionally observed in this type of patient admission.

Brain Disorders
Chronic Brain Syndrome, Alcohol Intoxication

Alcoholism and the disorders which are associated with it may lead to both acute and chronic brain syndromes. In a rehabilitation setting, where the treatments are not directed towards curing the alcohol addiction problem, it is the chronic brain syndrome which comes to the attention of the psychologist. The patient who enters the rehabilitation hospital because of the consequences of long-term alcohol ingestion is usually treated for the weakness and incoordination of peripheral neuropathy produced by chronic drinking.

Korsakoff's syndrome occurs in both acute and chronic alcoholic patients. It is characterized by amnesia, particularly for recent events which the patient tries to conceal by falsification, and by disorientation for time and place. Often what seem to be hallucinations or delusions are attempts to fill in the gaps of an impaired memory. There is an inability to form new associations and thus, new events are not retained and related to past data. This disorder is most typically observed in older, chronic alcoholics and it is most probably a result of a vitamin B deficiency.

Alcoholic deterioration refers to the general personality disintegration of the person who has consumed excessive amounts of alcohol over a prolonged period. Symptoms include disturbances of memory and judgement, reduction of concentration ability, impulsivity of behavior, loss of sense of responsibility, neglect of personal appearance and of family, feelings of hostility, resentment and guilt, attempts at deception, loss of affection, defensiveness, irritability, and intellectual and moral deterioration.

The brain damage which is produced by chronic alcoholism is most likely a result of avitaminosis. In severe cases there is a progressive, chronic parenchymatous nervous disintegration, sometimes affecting much of the neuraxis, and a progressive atrophy of the frontal cortex.

Alcoholism is treatable in a variety of ways. The patient who is admitted to the rehabilitation hospital may not, at that time, be using alcohol but therapeutic intervention is important during his stay as a preventive measure against future indulgence following his discharge. In the more severe chronic cases of alcoholism the psychological deterioration may be of such magnitude that the patient cannot be accepted to the rehabilitation service because his condition precludes fruitful participation on the program.

Chronic Brain Syndrome Associated with Trauma

The psychopathology which follows brain injury is often regarded not only as a manifestation of the changes produced in the person by the lesion but also as an expression of the efforts of the individual to adapt to his deficits and to the demands which can no longer be met, or met only with difficulty, because of the neurological damage. The so-called "catastrophic reaction" is an example of this. When a brain-injured person is confronted by a problem which is insoluble for him he may become anxious, agitated and appear dazed. Irritability and aggression or anger may result. One consequence of this may be withdrawal and restriction of the environment so that the patient avoids tasks which are challenging, while at the same time he becomes meticulous with regard to activities which he can perform.

The symptoms of *post-concussion syndrome* include headaches, vertigo, fatigability, oversensitivity to strong sensory stimuli, insomnia, memory losses, reduction of concentration span, narrowing of interests, lessening of spontaneity, exacerbation of symptoms resulting from temperature extremes, exertion or excitement, reduced tolerance for alcohol and anxiety, which is the primary symptom.

The diagnostic problem is one of differentiating organic causes for the symptoms from psychogenic origins. If the patient's headaches are throbbing, paroxysmal and aggravated by alterations in body posture and of physical effort, and if his intellectual functioning is slow, his emotional status is not one of depression, apprehension or irritability, and if the symptoms persist and are unamenable to psychotherapy and the patient indicates high motivation for rehabilitation, the conclusion may be drawn that the difficulties are not psychogenic. Recovery may take place over a one to two year period.

Post-traumatic personality disorder of adults is characterized by irritability, quarreling, impulsivity, outbursts of rage and aggression, loss of interest in family and other obligations, loss of ambition, resentfulness, selfishness, withdrawal from social contacts and, occasionally, depression and paranoid reactions.

Post-traumatic personality disorder of children is evidenced as disobedience, behavior problems, impulsiveness, antisocial acts, shortened attention span, loss of interest in school work, hyperactivity, aggression and deficits in the perceptual and perceptual-motor spheres. The younger the child is at the time of injury the more favorable is the prognosis. Proper training can do a great deal to overcome the difficulties.

Chronic Mental Disorder Secondary to Head Trauma: Psychoneurosis

Neurotic reactions can develop following a subjectively disturbing post-concussion syndrome or other post-traumatic symptoms can facilitate neurotic attitudes. Anxiety is the most common reaction. A patient's pre-morbid life is a key factor in determining whether or not neurotic problems will follow brain injury.

Headaches, vertigo, memory deficits, ready fatigability, irritability, fear, apprehension and hypochondriacal behavior may result. Presenting symptoms are generally vague, numerous and inconsistent. Rehabilitation, including psychotherapy, is of much help.

Brain Syndromes Associated with Chronic Arteriosclerosis

Arteriosclerotic brain syndrome usually has its onset between the ages of fifty and sixty-five. In over half the cases a sudden attack of confusion is the first psychological sign. Frequent symptoms include episodes of confusion or excitement, or a combination of the two, during which consciousness is clouded and the patient is incoherent and restless. In other cases the onset is more gradual and is manifested as ready intellectual fatigability, reduction of initiative, impairment of memory, loss of affective control, and a tendency toward depression. Some patients become meddlesome, obstinate, irritable, quarrelsome, jealous and paranoid. Memory becomes increasingly impaired. Some patients tend towards garrulousness. Nocturnal bewilderment, anxiety and delirium are sometimes observed. As the disease progresses the patient becomes more forgetful, careless of his personal appearance and cleanliness, and expresses delusions of hypochondriasis and grandeur.

SENILE PSYCHOSIS. This geriatric disorder results from several factors, including cerebral atrophy, primarily of the frontal lobes of the cortex, a reduction in the number of brain cells, and the presence of tissue degeneration scattered throughout the cortex, mainly in the frontal lobes and Ammon's horn.

The disease progresses insidiously. It may begin with periods of depression following a specific event and be exacerbated by illness or emotional disturbance. The individual evidences a declining interest in his environment, loss of recent memory, limitations in new learning and abstract reasoning, complaints, hostility, resentment of change, reduction in ambition and activity, selfishness, irritability, self-isolation, carelessness of habits and dress, hoarding, delusions, loosening of morals, defective judgement and losses in orientation.

There are several types of senile psychosis, including simple deterioration, delirious and confused, depressed and agitated, paranoid and presenile, but these categories overlap to such an extent that they are largely academic and assignment of a patient to any one is an arbitrary matter.

Chronic Brain Syndromes Associated with Diseases of Unknown or Uncertain Causes

MULTIPLE SCLEROSIS. The general nature of the symptoms, while having exceptions, appears to be dependent upon the premorbid behavior of the patient. Thus, one can observe complacency, cheerfulness and euphoria in some patients, and denial, depression and paranoid behavior in others. There is a general emotional instability with loss of full control over crying and laughing. As the disease continues, memory defects and intellectual losses become manifest.

PARKINSON'S DISEASE. While most patients do not present psychological symptoms until the disease has progressed for several years and memory, reasoning, learning ability and intellectual functioning become impaired, some individuals react negatively to their disability. These reactions are typically those of anger, irritability, dissatisfaction, depression, fear and anxiety. Obsessive-compulsive neurotic features are among the most frequently observed behavioropathic signs in Parkinson patients.

HUNTINGTON'S CHOREA. The initial psychopathologic symptoms of this disease may be irritability, obstinacy, moodiness, lack of initiative or euphoria. Esthetic and ethical senses later become blunted, and many patients become faultfinding, irascible, spiteful and even destructive and assaultive. There is a decrease of spontaneous activity. Suspiciousness, jealousy, and even delusions of persecution may appear. Attention span, concentration ability, memory and judgement become increasingly impaired as the disease progresses. In later stages the patient may function as a psychotic or intellectually retarded person.

LUPUS ERYTHEMATOSIS. Patients affected by this disease can present either neurotic or psychotic symptoms. Phobias may develop. Depression is a common finding. Schizophrenic patterns may be seen. Psychiatric disorders are believed by many to be related to the use of steroid therapy during the course of illness, but steroid therapy *per se* is probably not directly related to the disturbances since exacerbation of the disease itself seems to increase the psychopathological symptoms.

Psychogenic Disorders
Psychotic Disorders

The psychoses represent the most serious functional psychologic disturbances. They are characterized by varying degrees of intellectual and behavioral disorganization. Generally, they mean a break with, or a dissociation from, reality and a failure to test and evaluate reality correctly. Individuals with psychotic disorders fail to relate themselves appropriately and effectively to other people and to their environment. As a result, their ability to meaningfully function in the real world is temporarily or permanently impaired.

There are three symptoms which are generally associated with psychosis although they are not necessarily observed in all the psychoses, nor in combination in any one patient.

An *hallucination* is a false perception, a perception without object, which has the compulsive sense of reality of objects although relevant and adequate stimuli for such perceptions are lacking. That is, the person perceives, through one or more sensory modalities, stimulus objects and situations which are not actually present. Examples of psychotic hallucinations include hearing accusatory voices, seeing crawling insects, smelling gaseous substances, and the like.

A *delusion* is basically a false belief. It is a belief which is maintained despite contradictory evidence. Some frequently encountered psychotic delusions include believing that voices transmitted through the radio are directed at, and contain messages for the patient, believing that everyone in the environment is a foreign spy, and believing that one's brain or other organs are rotting away.

An *illusion* is a mistaken perception. There is always an object present but it is incorrectly perceived by the patient. Some examples of psychotic illusions are perceiving the rustling of leaves as approaching, menacing footsteps, interpreting the slamming of a door as the sound of an executioner's axe, and perceiving the sensation of a breeze as the touch of a human hand.

There are other symptoms of psychosis and these will be described within the context of the disorders in which they most frequently occur.

Disorders Due to Disturbances of Metabolism, Growth, Nutrition or Endocrine Function

INVOLUTIONAL PSYCHOTIC REACTIONS. The involutional psychoses tend to be of two types, one characterized by depression and the other by paranoid ideation. Since the latter form of the disorder is rarely, if ever, observed in admission of a patient to a rehabilitation institution, discussion will center about the depressive form.

Involutional depressive reaction occurs most frequently in women in their late forties and in men in their late fifties. It is two to three times more prevalent in women than in men. The term "involutional" in the description of this disorder comes from the fact that it occurs during the period of the beginnings of decreased endocrine and reproductive gland function, the age generally known as the involutional period of life.

The problems which are caused by changes in metabolic and vegetative body activities, cessation of ovarian activity and increased irritability of the sympathetic nervous system are only a part of the etiology of the psychotic disturbance. More important, perhaps, are the psychological implications of these physiological and chemical changes, such as the feelings which are engendered in the individual as a consequence of loss of biological function.

The major component of this psychotic reaction is depression manifested in motor behavior and speech. Other symptoms include hypochondriasis, pessimism, insomnia, loss of appetite, inability to concentrate, doubt and indecision, lack of initiative, narrowing of interests and withdrawal from the environment. The most conspicuous symptoms in a "typical" case are profound depression, anxiety, agitation, hypochondriasis, guilt-laden delusions of sin, feelings of unworthiness, delusions of having a disease, and a sense of, or belief in, impending death. Premorbid life has much to do with the type and severity of symptoms during the illness.

About forty to fifty per cent of patients with involutional depression recover. The patient who does not evidence much psychotic behavior, such as delusions, or who does not exhibit extreme depression or hyperagitation, may be accepted to a rehabilitation program for her physical disability, but obviously, the more seriously disturbed individuals cannot be considered.

Disorders of Psychogenic Origin or Without Clearly Defined Tangible Cause or Structural Change

AFFECTIVE REACTIONS. This group of psychoses include those disturbances in behavior which are characterized primarily by increased or decreased activity and by thoughts of either elation or depression.

Manic-Depressive Psychosis. This group of psychoses are typically thought of as presenting alternating mood and behavior swings between profound depression and euphoria. This is actually incorrect.

There is the *cyclic type* which does present this symptom picture, but there is also the *manic type,* in which only the elation is seen, and the *depressive type,* which exhibits only the depression.

Because of his verbal and motor behavior, the manic individual, or the cyclic patient with a manic component, is not seen in rehabilitation since his extreme hyperactivity precludes taking part in therapy and presents difficult problems of management outside of therapy classes. Similarly, the severely depressed type would also be unable to participate on an active program. The depressive phase of manic-depressive psychosis, in which there is a mild depression, permits physical rehabilitation activity and thus possibly the patient in such a phase may be considered as a candidate.

Mild depressive phases tend to be characterized either by a period of fatigue and inertia, or by one in which the patient has physical complaints for which no organic basis can be found. In the first group, the primary symptoms are feelings of fatigue and inadequacy, need for isolation, doubts, fears, anxiety, slowness of intellectual function, latency of responding and, occasionally, hostility and anger. The most typical symptom of the latter group is hypochondriasis. There are also losses of weight and appetite, disturbed sleep, feelings of weakness, worry over small details, insomnia, headaches and undue attention paid to bodily sensations. The main features which would serve to make either type questionable for rehabilitation are lack of initiative, lack of motivation and easy fatigability.

Psychotic Depressive Reaction. While the depressions of manic-depressive psychosis usually develop in the absence of an experience which would logically elicit them, those of the psychotic depressive reaction arise as a result of the individual having been confronted with an extremely stressful situation.

There is a definite pathological depression, often associated with gross misinterpretations of reality in the form of delusions, suicidal ideation or attempts, feelings of guilt, and sluggishness of thinking and psychomotor activity.

An example of this disorder recently seen during an evaluation for rehabilitation admission is the case of a young woman who, in addition to being rendered quadriplegic from an automobile accident, lost her husband and two children in the same disaster. This patient exhibited nearly all of the symptoms just described and was not accepted to the rehabilitation program. She eventually recovered from her psychotic condition, was re-evaluated and accepted to the institution for therapy.

SCHIZOPHRENIC REACTIONS. Schizophrenia is among the most common of the serious psychologic disorders yet its etiology is still largely unknown. Theories have been propounded regarding direct genetic inheritance, genetic predisposition, biochemical and neurophysiological dysfunction, family upbringing and home environment, and inappropriate or faulty learning, but no explanation has proven satisfactory. There is still no conclusion, in fact, as to whether schizophrenia is a single disease entity or a group of related disorders.

Schizophrenia usually has its onset between late childhood and late middle age although it can occur in children as young as two years old and it is not excluded from the geriatric population.

The group of disorders within the general category called schizophrenia are manifested by characteristic disturbances of thought, behavior and affect. Thinking disturbances are marked by alterations of concept formation leading to misinterpretations and distortions of reality, including hallucinations, delusions and illusions. Mood changes include inappropriate emotional responses, loss of empathy with others, ambivalence and constricted affect. Behavior may be withdrawn, regressive, expansive and bizarre.

The withdrawal, affect disturbances, depersonalization, hypochondriasis, lack of logical thought and association of ideas, delusions, hallucinations, impulsivity and lack of behavioral control, avoidance of spontaneous activity, negativism, stereotyped mannerisms and general detachment from reality which characterize schizophrenia make patients with this disorder unlikely to be accepted to physical rehabilitation. This section will describe only those types of schizophrenia which would be considered as possible candidates for admission to a rehabilitation institution.

The *simple type* has a slow, insidious development marked by disturbances of mood, emotion, interest and activity. Apathy and indifference lead to impoverishment of interpersonal relations, intellectual deterioration and adjustment at a reduced level of functioning. Hallucinations are rare and brief, and delusions do not play an important role.

The *paranoid type* is characterized by numerous illogical delusions, generally either of a persecutory or a grandiose nature, hallucinations, negativism, disturbances of association, ideas of reference and emotional changes. Behavior is often aggressive and consistent with the delusions. Mannerisms, apathy, incoherence and neologistic speech, or the coining of new, unique words, are often observed.

The *schizoaffective type* evidences combinations of schizophrenia and affective psychosis. For example, behavior and thought may be so divorced from reality that the patient appears schizophrenic, while the elated or depressed affect indicates a manic-depressive psychosis.

The *pseudoneurotic type* is one in which the schizophrenic disorder is concealed by a façade of neurotic manifestations. Such a patient usually exhibits anxiety, phobia, obsessive-compulsive neurosis, depression and hypochondriasis in various combinations and to varying degrees. Brief psychotic episodes may occur and about one-third of these patients develop into a true schizophrenia. This type is sometimes referred to as latent schizophrenia.

Schizophrenia, chronic undifferentiated type is the diagnosis for persons who show mixed schizophrenic symptoms and who present definite schizophrenic thought, affect and behavior patterns but who are not classifiable within a distinct category.

Schizophrenia, childhood type presents a wide variety of symptoms. Affected children exhibit regression, intellectual retardation, mutism, withdrawal or overactivity, precocious language development and excessively abstract thinking. The older the child, the more the clinical picture resembles adult schizophrenia. Thus, in the older child, there is not only withdrawal but also hallucinations and delusions, loss of affective contact with people, regression, obsessive rumination, posturing, aggression and flights of ideas.

The term *early infantile autism* refers to the child who has an inability to form emotional ties with his parents and other persons, lacks reponsivity to stimuli in the environment, prefers objects to people, has stereotyped mannerisms or postures, usually lacks language, demands sameness of the environment, and has unpredictable, unwarranted temper tantrums.

This disorder usually can be detected between the ages of two and three, and sometimes, even earlier. It is frequently confused with mental retardation, but the trained psychologist can make a differential diagnosis.

Although it was stated at the beginning of this section on schizophrenia that only those types which might be considered as possible rehabilitation patients would be described, it must be added here that out of the types which have been discussed, only the less severe cases would be admitted to a rehabilitation hospital. The seriously disturbed, acting-out paranoid schizophrenic, or the schizoaffective type whose emotional states are extreme, or the chronic undifferentiated individual whose symptom picture is one of bizarre, irrational behavior, or the autistic child whose behavior problems are such that he cannot be dealt with in therapy or in his bed area, would not be accepted to the rehabilitation program and, likely, would not even be considered as a candidate.

Psychophysiologic Autonomic and Visceral Disorders

The reactions which are included within this group are those which are frequently referred to as "psychosomatic." Anxiety leads to disturbances which are primarily expressed through physiological processes.

There are three main groups of patients within this general classification. In the first are those patients who suffer from various physical symptoms but who do not have a bodily disease which serves as a cause of these symptoms. In the second group are individuals who have a physical disease, but the origins and causes were primarily of an emotional nature. In the third class the patients do have organic disease but certain symptoms or exacerbations of the disease arise not from the disease itself but from psychological variables. Disorders which can be found within one of these groups include those of the cardiovascular system, the alimentary system, the respiratory system, the endocrine system, the genitourinary system, the nervous system, the musculoskeletal system and the skin.

Certain disabilities which require physical rehabilitation may have psychological components and it is these which the psychologist sees in his initial evaluation.

RHEUMATOID ARTHRITIS. It has been frequently observed that the onset of, or exacerbations of, the symptoms of rheumatoid arthritis are related to periods of emotional stress. The patient with this disease has often been described as a person who is emotionally composed, seldom expressing his feelings overtly, and who derives gratification from being of service to others. He masks his dependence on others and usually is active and competitive, both physically and intellectually. Death of, or separation from, a loved one, miscarriage of pregnancy, rejection by important figures, and severe personal disappointments are among the events which can precipitate the arthritic condition.

MULTIPLE SCLEROSIS. It is a common finding among patients with multiple sclerosis that emotional upset or psychological stress will result in exacerbations of the disease.

HUNTINGTON'S CHOREA. There is a condition which is known as "pseudochorea" in which the patient does not have the actual disease, Huntington's chorea, but behaves as if he did. This is primarily due to the hypersuggestibility of the individual. Such cases occur among the offspring of parents who have the disease, since it is inherited as a monohybrid dominant with the result that one half of the children of an affected parent develop the disease. Thus, when an individual's parent has Huntington's chorea the person may begin to suspect that he has inherited it and each minor body dysfunction which occurs becomes interpreted as an indication of the presence of the disease. (Note: While it is not exceptionally uncommon for a person to "think himself into symptoms," it is interesting to note that in true chorea the symptoms are exacerbated by anxiety.)

PARKINSON'S DISEASE. The symptoms of Parkinsonism, such as tremor and shuffling gait, are often heightened by emotional stress or periods of anxiety.

PARAPLEGIA. Occasionally, a patient will be evaluated for admission to a physical rehabilitation institution who evidences all of the symptoms of true paraplegia resulting from spinal cord injury but who, upon medical examination, is found to have no spinal cord lesion. The issue then becomes one of psychosomatics, and it is frequently learned that the individual is, albeit without purposeful awareness, "using" the disability as a means of avoiding an unpleasant or feared task or situation.

A similar observation is often made in the case of chronic low back pain where the patient complains of disabling pain in the lower lumbar, lumbosacral and sacral areas in the absence of medical causation. The psychologist usually can determine what secondary gain the patient is receiving from his symptoms and disability.

Psychoneurotic Disorders

The psychoneuroses are disorders of psychogenic origin, or without clearly defined tangible cause or structural change.

Anxiety is generally believed to be the chief characteristic of the neuroses. This anxiety may be expressed directly or it may be controlled without awareness and automatically by various psychological symptoms, or reactions. The neuroses are relatively benign disturbances which arise from efforts to deal with specific, private, internal and stressful situations that the patient is unable to master without tension or disturbing psychological devices caused by the anxiety aroused. The mechanisms which are employed by the neurotic person generally produce symptoms which are experienced as subjective distress from which the individual desires relief.

The psychoneuroses do not manifest the gross distortions and misinterpretations of reality, nor the gross behavioral and intellectual deteriorations which typify the psychoses although they can be severe enough to seriously impair or limit an individual's functioning. Studies have revealed that approximately two-thirds of all severe neuroses show complete remission, or nearly complete remission, within two years following onset of the symptoms without the benefit of therapeutic intervention.

There are six primary psychoneurotic reactions, or disorders, and any one of them might be encountered by the psychologist during his evaluation of a patient.

ANXIETY REACTION. In this disorder the characteristic symptom is one of a pervading, chronic anxiety. It is often described by the patient as a constant, unpleasant sensation, an "uneasiness of mind," a state of heightened tension accompanied by inexpressible dread, a feeling of apprehensive expectation. The patient often cannot describe exactly what is wrong but reports that he "just feels nervous all the time."

The anxiety is not restricted to specific objects or situations. Autonomic nervous system signs of anxiety include tachycardia, palmar sweating, stomach contractions, headaches and rapid, shallow respiration. In addition to the chronic condition, acute anxiety attacks occur during which there is an exacerbation of the symptoms. Insomnia is also a frequent symptom.

PHOBIC REACTION. The phobias are characterized by an intense fear of an object or situation which the individual usually is not cognizant of as a real threat or danger to him. Phobic reactions to such stimuli include feelings of faintness, fatigue, nausea and palpitations, perspiration, tremor, escape and avoidance behaviors, and, at times, panic.

Some common phobias among adults are fear of height, fear of confinement, fear of open spaces, fear of travel, fear of snakes, fear of blood, fear of germ contamination and fear of cancer. In children, other phobias are more frequently encountered, such as fear of the dark, fear of school, fear of dogs, fear of strangers and fear of separation from parents.

While phobias formerly required years of psychotherapy and were considered difficult to entirely remove, since the advent of the newer behavior therapies they are easily and rapidly eliminated.

DISSOCIATIVE REACTION. Dissociative reactions are often classified as some form of hysteria. Anxiety is so overwhelming in the patient with this disorder that certain aspects of his personality become dissociated from each other. There are four dissociative reactions.

Amnesia is a partial or total inability to remember past experiences. In dissociative amnesia there is a blotting out of awareness of particular unpleasant events. While the individual may remember basic habits, such as how to talk, walk, write, read, calculate, ride a bicycle, or play the piano, he often cannot recall his name, age, place of residence, friends and family. Periods of great stress, terror, shame and guilt tend to be forgotten.

The *fugue reaction,* or *fugue state* is one in which the patient takes flight as a defense. He wanders away from home and then days, weeks, or even years later he suddenly "awakens" to find himself in an unfamiliar place with amnesia for how he got there and for the total fugue period. He often forgets his identity during the fugue state and assumes a new one, remarrying and living a new life.

In a patient with *somnambulism,* or sleepwalking, certain thoughts able to be blocked from memory during wakefulness are strong enough to determine behavior during sleep. Somnambulistic episodes may occur only infrequently or with regularity.

During sleep, the person may arise, go into another room or even out of the house and perform certain acts. His eyes are usually at least partially open, he avoids obstacles, hears when spoken to and obeys commands, including those requesting that he return to bed. Upon being awakened during the period of sleepwalking he will be surprised and bewildered as to his situation. If he returns to bed on his own volition he will not recall the events of the previous night upon awakening. Sleepwalking episodes are usually of from fifteen to thirty minutes in duration.

Multiple personality is rare. It is a dissociative reaction to stress in which the patient manifests two or more complete personalities, each with its own habits, morals, beliefs, emotions and behaviors. The personalities are usually markedly different from each other. The popular book, *The Three Faces of Eve,* is a dramatic example of this disorder.

CONVERSION REACTION. In a conversion reaction, or conversion hysteria, as it is occasionally called, the anxiety of neurosis becomes "converted" into functional symptoms in organs or body parts. A physical illness appears in which there is no underlying organic pathology. There may be sensory symptoms, such as loss or impairment of sensitivity, hypersensitivity, loss of pain or temperature sense, and exceptional sensations such as tingling or burning. There are losses of sense organ function, as in partial or complete blindness or deafness, or disturbances of these functions. There are also motor hysterias, such as paralysis and loss of speech.

The conversion reaction is one in which the individual obtains some type of secondary gain from his "illness," such as not having to meet certain people, or work in an unpleasant job situation, or perform undesirable tasks. By assuming an illness role he can avoid these experiences without suffering the reprimands and accusations of others and without feeling guilty. As a "sick" person he is not expected to function normally.

The psychologist has several criteria for distinguishing between organic illness and neurotic conversion disorders.

1. The hysteric typically exhibits a lack of concern over his illness. Some worry may be expressed but complaints are presented in a matter-of-fact way with little of the anxiety that is expected from one who has become blind or paralyzed.

2. The conversion dysfunction usually does not follow a feasible anatomic pattern of actual nerve distribution. That is, a hand might be paralyzed without involvement of the rest of the arm, which is not neurologically possible. In addition, except in cases of many years' duration, paralyzed extremities do not show atrophy.

3. The disorder is usually selective in its dysfunction. The hysterically blind person does not collide with objects, the hysterically deaf patient hears the warnings of automobile horns, and hysterical joint contractures disappear during sleep.

4. Under hypnosis or narcosis the symptoms can be removed, induced or shifted from one body location to another.

5. Patients with this disorder are highly suggestible. Thus, if told that within a week their paralysis will begin to dissipate, or that pain will begin to occur ten days following onset of the primary symptoms, such are likely to occur. In addition, if the patient is suddenly awakened from a sleep, he may be tricked into using the paralyzed arm.

OBSESSIVE-COMPULSIVE REACTION. The patient with an obsessive-compulsive reaction is aware of the irrationality of his behavior but he is unable to control it. He is compelled to think about something which he does not wish to think of or to carry out actions which he does not want to perform.

There are three clinical forms of this neurosis.

1. The persistent recurrence of an unwanted and often unpleasant or distressing thought.

2. A morbid and usually irresistible urge to perform a certain repetitive, stereotyped act.

3. An obsessively recurring thought accompanied by a compulsion to perform a repetitive act.

DEPRESSIVE REACTION. The general appearance of the neurotically depressed individual is one of dejection, sorrow and discouragement. There is self-depreciation, diminished activity, anxiety, lowered self-confidence, loss of initiative and restricted interests. Sometimes, somatic complaints and even feelings of vague hostility are exhibited. In many cases the depression has its onset following the loss of, or separation from a loved one, or a defeat in the personal or economic sphere.

As stated earlier, the rehabilitation psychologist may observe any one of the psychoneurotic reactions during his initial interview session. However, some are seen more frequently than others. These include depressive reaction and anxiety reaction. Less often encountered are phobic reactions, conversion reactions, and mild forms of obsessive-compulsive reaction. Dissociative reaction is rarely encountered.

A patient with a psychoneurosis generally will not be denied admission to a rehabilitation medicine institution, but some severe forms of obsessive-compulsive reaction, dissociative reaction and, occasionally, phobic reaction, depressive reaction and anxiety reaction will preclude acceptance because the psychological disability will interfere markedly with participation in rehabilitation therapies.

Once a neurotic individual is admitted to the hospital, it becomes encumbent upon the psychologist to treat his disorder and to advise other staff members with regard to management and approach.

Personality (Character) Disorders

The group of character disorders also have no clear, tangible cause or structural change apparent and are considered to be of psychogenic origin.

This class of disturbances is characterized by deeply ingrained maladaptive behavior patterns which are qualitatively different from either the psychoses or the neuroses. These patterns usually are of life-long, or many years' duration and are frequently identifiable by the time of adolescence, or even sooner. Persons who are affected by a personality disorder are generally not in need of hospitalization for their problem and are able to function in the various spheres of their lives without coming to the attention of a psychologist. Often, however, their disturbance is of a magnitude which produces problems for them in one or more areas of living, for which they seek, or are referred for, professional help.

PARANOID PERSONALITY. The behavior pattern presented by this disorder is one of hypersensitivity, rigidity of thought, unwarranted suspicion, jealousy, envy, excessive feelings of self-importance, and a tendency to blame others and ascribe ulterior motives to others. Such characteristics obviously can tend to impair the individual's social and interpersonal relationships.

CYCLOTHYMIC PERSONALITY. This character disturbance is marked by recurring, alternating periods of depression and elation, with the associated thoughts and behaviors of each phase being manifested as the affective pendulum swings towards one mood or the other.

SCHIZOID PERSONALITY. The schizoid individual exhibits shyness, hypersensitivity, seclusiveness, avoidance of close relationships, and at times, eccentricity, Daydreaming, autistic thinking, and the inability to express ordinary aggressive feelings are common. Disturbing experiences and conflicts are generally met with detachment.

EXPLOSIVE PERSONALITY. An individual diagnosed as being in this category demonstrates gross outbursts of rage or of verbal or physical aggression. He is generally excitable and over-responsive to environmental pressures.

OBSESSIVE-COMPULSIVE PERSONALITY. This behavior pattern is characterized by excessive concern with conformity and adherence to standards of conscience. Thus, the person may be rigid in his thinking, over-inhibited, over-conscientious, concerned with details, perfectionistic and unable to relax easily.

HYSTERICAL PERSONALITY. An hysterical person is excitable, emotionally unstable, over-reactive and dramatic. He seeks attention, is self-centered and vain, and usually dependent upon others. Somatic complaints are frequently offered.

ASTHENIC PERSONALITY. The behavior of the asthenic individual is typified by easy fatigability, a low level of energy, lack of initiative and enthusiasm, incapacity for enjoyment, and hypersensitivity to physical and emotional stress.

ANTISOCIAL PERSONALITY. Formerly termed a psychopath, now more commonly referred to as a *sociopath,* such an individual is one who is basically unsocialized and whose behaviors repeatedly bring him into conflict with society. He is incapable of loyalty to individuals or groups or social values. He is grossly selfish, callous, irresponsible, impulsive and unable to feel guilt or remorse or to learn from experience and punishment. He functions without a conscience and lives by his own value system. Frustration tolerance is low. He tends to blame others or offer rational explanations for his behavior. Chronic lying and frequent difficulty with the law are common characteristics of the sociopath.

PASSIVE-AGGRESSIVE PERSONALITY. This type of personality is characterized both by aggression and passivity. The aggression is passively expressed, as in obstructionism, procrastination, intentional inefficiency and stubbornness. Thus, hostility is expressed by the person who dares not express it more openly.

INADEQUATE PERSONALITY. The behavior pattern here is one of ineffectual responses to emotional, social, intellectual and physical demands. While the patient is of normal physique and intelligence he exhibits inadaptability, ineptness, poor judgement, social instability, lack of physical and emotional stamina, and generally fails at whatever he attempts, or succeeds only in a minimal way.

SEXUAL DEVIATIONS. Within this category are placed individuals whose sexual interests and efforts are directed primarily towards objects other than persons of the opposite sex, towards sexual acts not usually associated with coitus, or towards coitus performed under bizarre circumstances.

Disorders of this group include the following: *homosexuality,* where the predominant mode of sexual expression is with a person of the same sex; *pedophilia,* the pathological sexual interest in children; *fetishism,* in which sexual interest becomes attached to a material object or a part of a person rather than to the whole individual; *transvestism,* or the impulse to dress in the clothing of the opposite sex; *exhibitionism,* or the exposure of one's genitals to others; *voyeurism,* wherein sexual gratification is sought through observing others in undress or engaged in sexual acts; *sadism,* in which sexual satisfaction is obtained through the inflicting of pain; *masochism,* wherein the receiving of pain is sexually gratifying, and others.

ALCOHOLISM. This category is for persons whose alcohol intake is of sufficient quantity to damage either physical health, or personal or social functioning, or where it has become a prerequisite for normal functioning. The alcoholic individual may become intoxicated four times per year, twelve times per year, or may be entirely dependent upon alcohol, or dependent to a degree where he cannot function on a daily basis without it and must therefore be considered addicted.

DRUG DEPENDENCE. The term *drug dependence* refers to patients who are addicted to, or dependent upon drugs other than alcohol, tobacco and ordinary caffein-containing beverage. Dependence upon medically prescribed drugs is also excluded if the individual restricts his intake to the prescribed dosages and frequencies of administration. Habitual usage or a clear sense of need of the drug is required for a diagnosis of addiction. Withdrawal symptoms are not a sufficient diagnostic clue because they are absent in the case of some drugs, such as cocaine and marijuana, although always present when opium derivatives are withdrawn.

Transient Situational Disturbances

This classification is reserved for the more or less transient disorders of any severity which occur in individuals without apparent psychological disorders, and which represent an acute reaction to great environmental stress. It includes the adjustment reactions of infancy, childhood, adolescence, adult life and later life. Those which are observed in a rehabilitation setting are usually reactions to the sudden onset of a disability and/or separation from loved ones because of the need for prolonged hospitalization.

Behavior Disorders of Childhood and Adolescence

Included within this category are disorders which occur during the childhood and adolescent years which are more stable, more internalized, and more resistant to treatment than transient disburbances.

Characteristic manifestations include *hyperkinesis,* or hyperactivity, withdrawal, shyness, feelings of rejection, over-aggressiveness, delinquency and habit disturbances such as tics, nail-biting, thumbsucking, and *enuresis,* or involuntary passage of urine, particularly the nocturnal type.

The psychologist may find any of these disorders in a rehabilitation candidate. It is unlikely that a patient would not be accepted to a therapy program because of such diagnoses. There are, however, certain disorders which would tend to make the individual a relatively unsuitable rehabilitation patient. These are the paranoid, cyclothymic, explosive, asthenic, antisocial and passive-aggressive personalities. The schizoid patient is of questionable regard as a rehabilitation candidate. Alcoholic and drug dependent patients would not be seen in a physical rehabilitation hospital while still addicted, although the difficulties which led to their addiction would be treated psychotherapeutically during their stay in the institution. Patients with the other personality disorders would, in all likelihood, be accepted to the rehabilitation program and the psychologist would follow up his diagnosis by speaking with the patients, with the goal of providing therapeutic help if they so desired.

ACCEPTANCE AND REJECTION OF A REHABILITATION CANDIDATE

When, on the basis of his findings during the initial evaluation session, does the psychologist decide to recommend rejection of a potential patient for the rehabilitation program? What constitutes the criteria for acceptance of a patient to the rehabilitation services? The answers to both of these questions are relatively simple, although the determination of such answers is relatively complex. As mentioned earlier in this chapter, the rehabilitation psychologist should be concerned with one main factor during his evaluation of a patient, namely, the ability of that patient to function meaningfully on an active rehabilitation program. Therefore, with this in mind, a patient is judged as acceptable to the program if his memory, orientation, perceptual-motor ability, learning ability, ability to comprehend instructions, motivation and lack of serious psychopathology enable him to participate in and benefit from the various rehabilitation services. If these variables are of a nature which prevent him, or prevent others, from profiting maximally from therapies, he is not considered a suitable candidate and rejection will be recommended.

Such criteria do not include a diagnosis *per se* of psychopathology. Patients with neuroses, personality disorders, psychopathology resulting from organic causes, and even psychoses may be admitted to the rehabilitation program, if only on a tentative "trial" basis. The primary criterion, again, is the ability of the individual to adequately function in rehabilitation and gain from therapy. Thus, a psychotic person may be accepted, providing that he is not judged to be harmful to himself or to others, is not considered likely to create a disturbance in therapy classes or on his ward or floor, is not felt to be a nursing management problem, and is not so divorced from reality in his thinking that he will be unable to comprehend new information or learn new skills. The neurotic patient whose disorder is not of a magnitude which will seriously impair his functioning is also accepted, as is the patient with a chronic or transient personality disturbance. Once an individual is accepted to the rehabilitation program, the psychologist carefully observes him, particularly if he has been diagnosed as having a psychopathologic disorder, and attempts to initiate psycho-therapy if there is a need for such treatment.

On a more specific level, criteria for rejection of a rehabilitation candidate include the following: serious memory impairment, so that instructions which are given to the patient by a therapist on one day will be forgotten by the next day or sooner; marked disorien-tation, whereby the patient cannot find his way to and from his bed, therapy areas or other hospital sections, cannot keep appointments and has lost his sense of time; intellectual retardation, or low level of intellectual functioning, so that the patient cannot comprehend any but the most simple directions and cannot learn new tasks and skills; confusion, which is severe enough for the patient to be un-aware of his disability and reasons for rehabilitation; lack of moti-vation, to the extent that the patient is apathetic about improvement or actually prefers his dependent condition; attention and concentra-tion spans which are so short as to preclude learning; lack of desire to cooperate with the rehabilitation staff; aggressive or hostile attitudes towards staff, other patients, or rehabilitation in general; and serious psychopathology, such as marked psychotic reactions.

With the exception of a serious psychosis, the demonstration of only one of the above signs by a patient does not necessarily contra-indicate acceptance to the rehabilitation hospital. Rather, com-binations of several of these symptoms must be observed before the psychologist will recommend rejection. If at all possible, a patient will be recommended for acceptance. No one should be denied the opportunity for rehabilitation. However, when a multiplicity of contraindicating behaviors are observed, the psychologist must decide for rejection of the candidate. Not only is the patient in question considered, but other patients on the ward or floor must also be thought of. If their rehabilitation will be interferred with by the admission of a new patient, then that new patient cannot be accepted.

Sometimes a patient who fails to meet the criteria for acceptance will exhibit such high motivation that he will be recommended for a trial period of rehabilitation of from four to six weeks duration. In general, however, a patient must be relatively psychologically intact to be considered a good rehabilitation candidate.

THE PSYCHOLOGICAL RE-EVALUATION

The psychologist is in a unique position from the other rehabil-itation disciplines when it comes to the re-evaluation of patients.

While physical therapists or occupational therapists, for example, see all of the active rehabilitation patients on a daily, or near daily basis, the psychologist usually sees only a small percentage of the total rehabilitation population on a regular schedule. All patients enter the hospital for physical, not for psychological treatment. It is the decision of the psychologist which patients are in need of, and can benefit from, his services. Thus, his regular caseload of ongoing therapy patients can range from one patient who is seen once a week to ten or more patients who are seen two or three or more times per week. Since the psychologist is not in daily intimate contact with all of the rehabilitation patients as are many of the other services, he must truly re-evaluate each patient in his charge prior to the periodic re-evaluation conferences.

It must be pointed out that, while the psychologist may not be engaged in psychotherapy with all of the patients in his assigned area, this does not mean that he is unfamiliar with them. In addition to the evaluation which he conducted upon their initial admission to the institution, he has become familiar with each patient during their hospital stay through numerous ways. Daily ward, or bedside rounds, observations of patients in their living areas and therapy classes, informal discussions with them, discussions with other rehabilitation team members, consultations upon request from medical and other personnel, conferences with patients at their request, and daily interactions with patients have all provided the psychologist with the opportunity to know the patients and to observe their progress. However, when a patient is scheduled for presentation at a re-evaluation conference, the psychologist must still interview and/or test that patient and compare his findings with those obtained upon the patients admission and/or with the data gained during the previous re-evaluation.

During the initial evaluation session the psychologist determined what further work was required with the patient. If further psychological testing was indicated, it was carried out following the patient's admission and the findings are reported at the re-evaluation meeting. If psychotherapy was felt to be necessary and if the patient entered into a therapeutic relationship with the psychologist, this too is reported to the other team members although the psychologist is obligated to respect the confidentiality of the patient's verbalizations. He may report as to the general nature of the problem, the frequency of therapy sessions and the progress being made by the patient, but other information is generally kept confidential.

If the psychologist has not been seeing the patient on a regularly scheduled basis, he must re-assess the patient's function prior to the time when the latter is to be discussed in a team conference. Any deficits which were observed during the initial evaluation or at a previous re-evaluation are re-examined to determine if changes have occurred. Even if there were no dysfunctions previously noted, the psychologist generally evaluates the patient as a "check" that new problems have not arisen. His data are presented to the rehabilitation team, along with any new recommendations which he feels are necessary because of changes which have taken place in the patient.

When the question arises during a re-evaluation meeting concerning the possible discharge of a patient from the rehabilitation hospital, the psychologist is a key professional involved in making such a decision. If he feels that because of marked impairment in one or more areas of psychological functioning a patient cannot, or should not, be discharged to the community, other arrangements are usually made for the patient. The physician has the primary and legal responsibility for the welfare of the patient, but the psychologist's report is crucial to his final decision.

Chapter 16

PSYCHOLOGICAL TESTING
AND PSYCHOTHERAPY

T HERE ARE A GREAT NUMBER and variety of psychological tests available today, including tests of general intelligence, aptitude, interest, achievement and personality, which can be administered to individuals or on a group basis. Some are very frequently employed while others are rarely used. In considering the physically disabled, it is important to remember that not all tests, regardless of their general value, are applicable to the rehabilitation population. Often, both administration of a test and interpretation of its results must be modified so that the strict criteria stated in the test manuals cannot be followed. In many cases a test cannot be used at all because of the nature of the disability of the testee.

PSYCHOLOGICAL TESTING

In testing the physically handicapped individual with standard psychological instruments, certain assumptions must be made by the psychologist if he is to place any credence in the obtained results. The first is that the patient who is being tested does not differ from the standardization population except for his physical disability. Second, that impairment of function, as measured by the test, is not, with the exception of certain types of disability, a result of physical handicap. The exclusions include those patients with either a marked speech, language or hearing impairment who cannot comprehend or respond to orally presented material, and patients whose physical limitations prevent them from performing on motor tasks. Therefore, for example, an intellectual deficit in a patient with a hip fracture would not be attributed to his physical disability, while such a deficit in an aphasic patient might be so related. Third, that despite the fact that the test was not initially standardized on a rehabilitation population, a meaningful interpretation of the results can still be made for the patient being assessed.

Tests of General Intellectual Ability
The Wechsler Adult Intelligence Scale (WAIS)

The WAIS is designed to measure general intelligence in persons aged sixteen and older. It is based on a definition of intelligence as the global capacity to act rationally, think purposefully, and deal effectively with the environment. The WAIS is divided into two sections of six verbal and five performance subtests.

VERBAL SECTION. The *Information* test consists of twenty-nine items and contains questions similar to the following: *How many wings does a bird have? How many nickels make a dime? What is steam made of? Who wrote "Paradise Lost"?* And, *What is pepper?*

These questions have been formulated to tap the subject's range of information and this is believed to provide a good indication of intellectual capacity. This subtest has the second highest correlation of all of the subtests with the total WAIS score. The main criticism of such a test is that it is valid only if the testee has had the usual opportunities for experience and learning.

The *Comprehension* test contains thirteen items and asks questions which are similar to these: *What should you do if you see someone forget his book when he leaves his seat in a restaurant? What is the advantage of keeping money in a bank? Why is copper often used in electrical wires?*

It is a test of common sense. Success depends upon the possession of a certain amount of practical information and a general ability to evaluate past experience.

The *Arithmetic* test is made up of fourteen items resembling the following: *Sam had three pieces of candy and Joe gave him four more. How many pieces of candy did Sam have altogether?* Or this question: *Three men divided eighteen golf balls equally among themselves. How many golf balls did each man receive?* Or, *If two apples cost fifteen cents, what will be the cost of a dozen apples?*

The ability to solve arithmetic problems is a sign of mental alertness and a good measure of global intelligence. This test can also specifically be used as an indicator of attention span, concentration ability and abstract reasoning skill. Responses are timed.

The *Digit Span* subtest is subdivided into Digits Forward and Digits Backward, and measures both attention span and immediate rote memory span.

In the first part of the test the subject must repeat back to the examiner a series of digits which have been orally presented to him. It begins with a three-digit sequence and ends with a nine-digit sequence. In the second section, the testee must repeat, in reverse order, the digits which the examiner presented to him. It begins with a two-digit series and ends with a eight-digit series.

The test is considered good for lower levels of intelligence and for the detection of brain damage when considered with other factors.

The *Similarities* subtest is composed of thirteen items, each one consisting of two constructs or objects for which the subject must state the common concept which underlies both members of the pair. Some sample questions from this type of test are: *In what way are a lion and a tiger alike? In what way are a saw and a hammer alike? In what way are one hour and a week alike?* And, *In what way are a circle and a triangle alike?*

This test is a reliable indicator of intelligence and specifically measures intellectual maturity and abstract reasoning ability.

The *Vocabulary* test contains forty words which the subject is to define. The person is simply asked: *What is a*——————*?* or *What does*——————*mean?* The words cover a wide range of difficulty or familiarity.

This test measures general intelligence and reasoning ability and thought processes. It has the highest correlation with the total WAIS score of any of the subtests.

PERFORMANCE SECTION. In the *Digit Symbol* test the subject is required to associate certain symbols with their matching digits as indicated by a code key. He must write the symbol belonging with digit in the appropriate space within a specified period to time.

Concentration span, visual-motor coordination, perception and visual memory are tested.

The *Picture Completion* test has twenty-one pictures which are shown to the subject one at a time. Each one has a significant feature of the picture missing and the testee must identify the absent part.

This subtest measures perception and the ability to differentiate essential from nonessential details.

There are ten items in the *Block Design* subtest and performance is timed. The subject must create designs with nine colored blocks by following a picture in which the lines formed by the edges of the cubes have been omitted.

The test measures the ability to analyze and synthesize, abstracttion ability, visual-motor coordination, perception, concentration span, preseverance and impulsivity.

The *Picture Arrangement* test consists of eight series of pictures which, when arranged in the proper sequence, will tell a story. The subject must, within a given period of time, rearrange disordered pictures so that they are in logical sequence.

This subtest measures the ability to comprehend and evaluate a total situation, and "social" intelligence.

In the *Object Assembly* test there are four forms, or figures, each of which has been cut up into asymmetrical pieces. The testee must put these forms together, much like a jig-saw puzzle, so that they form a completed object. The test is timed.

Object Assembly measures perceptual-motor function, the ability to perceive and recognize a whole situation from its component parts, and the method of approaching a problem used by the subject.

The WAIS yields a Verbal IQ, a Performance IQ and a Full Scale IQ. It is, without doubt, the most frequently employed individual measure of adult intelligence.

The Wechsler Intelligence Scale for Children (WISC)

The WISC is a downward extension of the WAIS for use with children from five to fifteen years of age. It has the same basic subtests as the WAIS, although with simpler items, and these subtests measure the same abilities in children that the WAIS tests do in adults.

In the WISC, the Digit Span test is made optional rather than being included as a regular part of the scale because of its low correlation with the rest of the test. In addition, a *Maze test* has been added as an optional performance subtest. It requires that the child follow a drawn maze to a goal. The Digit Symbol test of the WAIS has been replaced by a *Coding* test which requires the association of variously positioned lines with geometric figures.

The Stanford-Binet Intelligence Scale

The latest revision of this test was made in 1960 and is known as Form L-M. It is designed for use with children from the age of two years through the age of fourteen, and also has four sections for adults. It is, however, primarily a test of children's intelligence.

Some examples of test items are as follows: *At the two-year level:* A formboard in which geometric shapes must be fitted into the proper holes; a paper doll for which body parts must be identified; a picture vocabulary where the child must name the pictures he is shown. *At the five-year level:* Folding a square of paper into a triangle; identifying similarities and differences between pictured items. *At the nine year level:* Determining the fallacy in absurd statements; re-peating orally-presented digits in sequence. *At the fourteen-year level:* A vocabulary test; logical reasoning; a directional orientation test.

The Stanford-Binet scale tests memory, perception, motor skills, verbal abilities, abstract reasoning, concentration, attention span, visual-motor coordination, calculation ability, logical thinking and general knowledge. It yields both a mental age (MA) and an intel-ligence quotient (IQ).

The Peabody Picture Vocabulary Test (PPVT)

The PPVT consists of a series of 150 cardboard plates, each con-taining four numbered pictures, one in each quadrant of the plate. The examiner presents a stimulus word orally with each plate and the subject must point to, or in some way indicate, the picture on the plate which best illustrates the meaning of the stimulus word.

The plates and stimulus words progress with increasing difficulty until the subject can no longer respond correctly, and the test is then terminated. Thus, one plate may contain pictures of a banana, a doll, an automobile and a pencil, and the examiner says "Put your finger on (or show me) the banana," while a more difficult plate would illu-strate a minister at the pulpit, a woman smiling while speaking on a telephone, a younger woman on horseback and a man pondering a move in a game of chess, and the tester says "Tell me the number of incertitude."

The age range for use of the Peabody is from two and one-half years to eighteen years. The PPVT tests perception, vocabulary, reasoning and general knowledge.

Raven's Progressive Matrices Test

This test consists of sixty matrices, or designs, printed on cards, from each of which a part has been removed. The testee selects the missing insert from five or six alternatives which are printed below the design. The items are grouped into five series of twelve matrices each, of increasing difficulty but of similar principle. There is no time limit and the test can be used with groups as well as with individuals, and with both children and adults. Eight years of age is generally considered the earliest starting point for this test.

The Ravens test assesses perception, logical reasoning, ability to concentrate and ability to perceive spatial relationships.

Intelligence Testing with the Physically Disabled

Since there are no tests which are specifically designed for the phys-ically disabled, the psychologist must decide which of the current measuring instruments are most appropriate for use with such a population and what modifications are necessary for their administration.

With the WAIS or the WISC, the entire Verbal portion may be given to all patients except those with a speech or language impairment which seriously interferes with, or prevents, either comprehension of questions or responding to them, and those whose hearing loss precludes them from an orally administered examination.

The Performance part of the Wechsler tests presents problems for any patient who has paralysis, paresis, marked tremor or motor incoordination involving the upper extremities. Nonetheless, with the exclusion of the quadriplegic or quadriparetic patient, the advanced Parkinson's patient, the patient with advanced multiple sclerosis, the child with muscular dystrophy or severe cerebral palsy, and patients with similar conditions, the performance tests of the WAIS and WISC can be attempted. With patients who have tremor, paresis, ataxia or other motor incoordination of the upper extremities, the Performance section items may be administered as a "power" test. That is, they are not timed and the purpose of administration is to determine whether or not the patient is able to do the task. Omitting the time factor on these tests ignores the criteria of their design, but there is no choice. On subtests such as Block Design, Object Assembly and Picture Arrangement, the examiner may even do the task at the direction of the patient. Testing in this manner is obviously much slower than when the tests are given in the standard, prescribed manner.

Geriatric patients can be tested with the WAIS since it has been standardized with that group. Brain damage or suspected brain damage is not a contraindication for giving the Wechsler scales because there are certain response patterns, or profiles, which such an individual will exhibit on these tests, and this is known and accounted for. Both tests are, in fact, fairly good diagnostic instruments for the assessment of brain damage.

The Stanford-Binet Scale is generally unsuited to a rehabilitation population. This is because almost all year-level tests contain at least one item which involves motor activity, particularly for the years prior to age eleven. Thus, anyone with a motor disability involving the upper extremities could not take this test. In addition, the Binet items are so designed that many cannot be performed by the psychologist at the direction of the patient and still retain any meaning. Whereas with the WAIS and the WISC many instructions can be nonverbally given to patients who are either deaf or lack oral comprehension, this is generally not true of the Stanford-Binet.

The Stanford-Binet has been revised for use particularly with cerebral palsied children. The examiner manipulates the materials while the subject responds by a head gesture.

Both the Peabody Picture Vocabulary Test and the Raven's Progressive Matrices test are better suited for use with the disabled since they are not timed and do not depend upon verbal ability for successful achievement. Therefore, the patient with motor incoordination or paresis can still respond appropriately, the quadriplegic patient can use finger gestures or give verbal responses, and the aphasic individual can merely point to indicate his response.

Personality Tests

Projective Techniques

The chief characteristic of projective techniques is that they present the subject with a relatively unstructured task. That is, instructions are minimal and the task permits an unlimited number and variety of possible responses. Test stimuli are generally ambiguous and allow free reign to the individual's fantasies.

The assumption underlying projective techniques is that the way in which the subject perceives the test material or provides structure to it reflects basic aspects of his own psychological functioning. In other words, the testee projects his own thoughts, feelings, anxieties, conflicts and self-concepts onto the stimulus materials.

Projective techniques are "disguised" tests in that the subject is usually unaware of the interpretations that will be made of his responses. They are also characterized by a global approach to personality rather than being employed to assess specific traits. Projectives are considered, by their proponents, to reveal unconscious, latent, or covert elements of personality.

THE RORSCHACH TECHNIQUE. The Rorschach is the most popular and most frequently used projective technique. It consists of ten cards, or plates, on each of which is printed a bilaterally symmetrical inkblot. Some of the inkblots are totally achromatic, some are completely chromatic, and some combine both chromatic and achromatic features.

The cards are presented individually to the subject who is asked to tell or describe what he sees, what the inkblot represents to him. The psychologist records his responses, latency of responding, positions in which the cards are held and general motor and verbal test behavior. Following presentation of all ten cards, the subject is questioned regarding the features of each stimulus which elicited the associations.

Interpretations of the patient's responses are made based upon the content of the percepts, general test behavior and an elaborate scoring system. The Rorschach is untimed and can be administered to any age group although its use is generally restricted to persons over the age of ten.

THE THEMATIC APPERCEPTION TEST (TAT). The TAT is another widely used projective technique. It differs from the Rorschach in that it presents more highly structured stimuli and requires more complex and more meaningfully organized and integrated responses.

The test consists of twenty cards, nineteen of which illustrate vague or ambiguous pictures of people and scenes, and one of which is blank. The cards are presented singly to the examinee who must make up a story to fit each picture. He must tell what is happening at the moment in the picture, what events preceded or led up to the current scene, and what the outcome will be. In the case of the blank card, the subject is asked to imagine a picture on it, describe it and then tell a story about it.

The test is usually given in either two sessions of ten cards each or in an abbreviated form during a single session. It is not timed and is used primarily with persons over the age of fourteen. Children are given a relatively comparable test, the Children's Apperception Test, or CAT, in which the figures on the cards are animals engaged in human-like activities.

THE ROTTER INCOMPLETE SENTENCES BLANK (ISB). All incomplete sentences tests use a sentence beginning, or stem, with the subject required to complete the sentence. Here are examples of this type of projective test: *I feel. . .; What bothers me most. . .; If I could. . .;* and *Women. . . .* The Rotter ISB is the most popular of this type of technique. It contains forty sentence stems, including: *When I make a mistake. . .;* and *My mother. . . .* The subject is asked to complete all of the sentences and to try to express his "real" feelings as honestly as he can. Each response is rated on a scale according to the degree of adjustment or maladjustment exhibited.

The ISB is designed for use with individuals in the ninth grade or above, although it was standardized on the college level only.

Personality Inventories

THE MINNESOTA MULTIPHASIC PERSONALITY INVENTORY (MMPI).

The MMPI is the most widely used general personality inventory. In consists of 550 affirmative statements to which the subject responds either "True," "False," or "Cannot say." Some of these statements are as follows: *I am worried about sex matters; I believe I am being plotted against; When I get bored I like to stir up some excitement;* and *I wish I could be as happy as others seem to be.*

The test was developed to determine the traits which are commonly associated with disabling psychopathology. It provides ten clinical scales on which to rate subjects—hypochondriasis, depression, hysteria, psychopathic deviate, masculinity-femininity, paranoia, psychasthenia, schizophrenia, hypomania and social introversion.

The MMPI is designed for administration to persons of about sixteen years of age and older.

THE EDWARDS PERSONAL PREFERENCE SCHEDULE (EPPS). This test is comprised of 210 paired statements, and the subject must select one statement of each pair as being more characteristic of himself. A sample item is:

A. *I like to talk about myself to others.*

B. *I like to work towards some goal that I have set for myself.*

The EPPS is a general personality test for use with adults. It yields fifteen scores on need for achievement, deference, order, exhibition, autonomy, affiliation, intraception, succorance, dominance, abasement, nurturance, change, endurance, heterosexuality and aggression.

Personality Testing with the Physically Disabled

With little exception, personality tests which have been designed for use with a nondisabled population can be employed with the physically handicapped. With the exception of special cases, such as spastic torticollis, orthopedic and neuromuscular disabilities should not interfere with the patient's ability to take these tests. There is nothing which the patient must do but look at the stimuli and give a verbal response. With tests such as the MMPI, the Rotter ISB, or the EPPS, the examiner can read the statements to the patient who may respond verbally or by gesture.

Patients who would not be able to perform satisfactorily on these tests include, in the case of projective techniques, those with impaired vision, as from cataracts or post-CVA hemianopsia, those with severe auditory loss who could not hear the basic instructions, those with marked perceptual deficits, and those with a speech or language disorder, such as expressive aphasia or apraxia, and in the case of the personality inventories, those with marked hearing loss, receptive aphasia, severe brain damage, and expressive speech and language dysfunctions.

The difficulty, then, with using standard personality measures with the disabled is not so much in their administration, but in the *interpretation* of results, and this is a matter of the psychologist's judgement. The physically disabled patient who scores highly on the hypochondriasis scale of the MMPI, or gives many anatomic responses to the Rorschach cards, or evidences somatic complaints on the ISB would not be judged in the same way as would the non-disabled individual who gives the same responses.

Other Psychological Tests

THE BENDER VISUAL-MOTOR GESTALT TEST. This test is sometimes classed as a test of perception or perceptual-motor ability, sometimes as a projective personality technique and sometimes as test for diagnosing brain damage. Theoretically, it is supposed to measure all three.

Nine simple geometric figures, each with a different pattern of organization, are presented individually, on cards, to the subject. He must copy each design exactly, or as perfectly as he can. Following presentation of all nine cards, they are withdrawn and the subject is asked to reproduce as many of the designs as he can from memory.

The Bender-Gestalt is not timed. It is meant to be administered to persons four years of age and older.

DRAWING TESTS. There are three main tests in use today which require that the subject draw something on paper.

The Goodenough-Harris Drawing Test requires that the examinee draw a man, then a woman, and then a picture of himself. Credit is given for the inclusion of body parts, clothing details, perspective and proportion. It is intended as a test of intelligence for children.

The Machover Draw-A-Person Test (D-A-P) is a projective personality test. The subject is asked to draw a person and then to draw a person of the opposite sex. The drawings are scored for absolute and relative size of the figures, their position on the page, the quality of the lines, the sequence of parts drawn, stance and position of limbs, clothing and other effects.

The House-Tree-Person Projective Technique (H-T-P) is also a projective personality measure. The testee is asked to draw, to the best of his ability, a house, which is supposed to arouse associations concerning his home and family, a tree, which is meant to evoke associations about his life role and ability to derive satisfaction from his environment, and a person, which should elicit associations concerned with interpersonal relations.

THE MARIANNE FROSTIG DEVELOPMENT TEST OF VISUAL PERCEPTION. This instrument is designed to assess the various kinds of abilities which together constitute visual perception.

There are five separate tests which make up the Frostig. They each seek to measure a different operationally-defined perceptual skill.

a. *The Test of Eye-Motor Coordination* involves the drawing of a continuous straight or curved or angled line between boundaries of various widths or between points without guide lines.

b. *The Figure-Ground Test* requires the subject to perceive figures against increasingly complex backgrounds. Intersecting and concealed geometric forms are used as stimuli.

c. *The Constancy of Shape Test* involves the recognition of certain geometric forms presented in a variety of sizes, positions in space and shadings, and the discrimination of these figures from other geometric shapes.

d. *Position in Space* is a test requiring the discrimination of reversals and rotations of figures, i.e. schematic drawings of objects presented in series.

e. *Spatial Relationships,* the fifth test, concerns the analysis of simple forms and patterns. The subject must copy lines of various lengths and contours using pre-printed dots as guide points.

The Developmental Test of Visual Perception is employed in testing children between the ages of four and eight and can be administered individually or as a group test. Results yield a perceptual age and a perceptual quotient (PQ).

INTEREST INVENTORIES. Interest inventories are usually employed for purposes of vocational and/or educational guidance and as such are typically administered by vocational rehabilitation counselors rather then by psychologists. However, some rehabilitation institutions, because of their relatively small size, may not have a rehabilitation counseling service and in such cases the burden of vocational assessment falls on the psychologist. There are two main interest inventories used today.

The Strong Vocational Interest Blank (SVIB) consists of 399 items grouped into eight parts. In the first five parts the subject records his preference by encircling the letter "L" "I" or "D," signifying "Like," "Indifferent" or "Dislike".

The categories involved in these five parts are occupations, school subjects, amusements, activities and types of people. The remaining three parts of the SVIB require the examinee to rank given activities in order of his preference, compare his interest in pairs of items, and rate his present abilities and other characteristics.

The test is scored with a different scale for each occupation. There are fifty-four occupational scales for the men's form and thirty-two scales for the women's form, with new scales being developed periodically. Interests are rated from a low of "C" to a high of "A."

The Kuder Preference Record is composed of forced-choice triad-type items. The individual taking the test must respond to each triad by marking the item he likes most and the one he likes least, leaving the third alternatives unmarked. Some examples of items to be selected from the Kuder Preference Record are: *Visit an art gallery – Browse in a library – Visit a museum; Collect autographs – Collect coins – Collect butterflies; Develop new varieties of flowers – Conduct advertising campaign for florists – Take telephone orders in a florist's shop.*

There are ten interest scales or clusters of occupational interests. They are Outdoor, Mechanical, Computational, Scientific, Persuasive, Artistic, Literary, Musical, Social Service and Clerical. From the subject's scores a profile of his interests is developed.

Testing the Disabled

Tests which involve drawing, such as the Bender-Gestalt, the Goodenough-Harris, the Machover or the H-T-P obviously cannot be administered to certain upper extremity amputees, quadriplegics, the severely involved cerebral palsied, or any patient whose upper extremity function is seriously impaired. While these tests presumably do not depend upon artistic ability for success, the performance of any of these types of patients would be such that scoring could not be satisfactory or might reveal abnormalities which would not be due to brain damage or personality factors, but rather would be a consequence of the physical dysfunction. However, patients who are not too severely handicapped and who are able to grasp and use a pencil can be given these tests if allowances are made for their physical limitations in scoring and interpretation.

Frostig claims that her test can be administered to children with cerebral palsy, but the nature of some of the tasks makes performance by severely impaired persons impossible. Thus, what might ordinarily be interpreted as a perceptual deficit might actually be a consequence of motoric disability, resulting in low and misleading scores.

The interest inventories can be given to all patients except those with severe hearing loss or receptive aphasia, since the test items can be read to the subject by the examiner. The former can indicate his answers verbally or by gesture.

THE PSYCHOLOGIST AS A CONSULTANT

In addition to his other diagnostic work the rehabilitation psychologist is often called upon by other professionals to act as a consultant. Those who seek the help or advice of the psychologist are not only the medical and paramedical personnel of the rehabilitation medicine services but may also include hospital staff members outside of the rehabilitation department, particularly in institutions which are primarily rehabilitation centers but which also provide additional patient services. In such cases it may be that all, or most psychologists are in the rehabilitation medicine service and therefore, other personnel turn to them when a psychologist is needed. Since referrals for psychological consultation from non-rehabilitation professionals occur with less frequency than those which come from members of the rehabilitation team, this section will be devoted to a discussion of the latter.

The kinds of problems which psychologists are called upon to help alleviate are of a great variety. The following examples were culled from the experiences of two rehabilitation psychologists during a six-month period: a patient refusing to take prescribed medication; a patient refusing to permit his temperature to be taken; a patient refusing to permit a blood sample to be taken; two patients having acute psychotic episodes; two patients expressing suicidal ideation; a patient refusing needed surgery; three patients appearing markedly depressed; a case of acute anxiety attacks; failure of four patients to regularly attend therapy classes; two patients disturbing others on their ward by lewd verbalizations; difficulty in communication between nursing staff and a patient; refusal of a patient to wheel his wheelchair; inability of a patient to accept his prognosis; fearfulness of two patients during ambulation training in physical therapy class; two patients requiring a diagnosis for suspected brain damage; apparent alcoholism on the part of two patients; a patient in need of psychological support while on methadone treatment for drug addiction; a patient requiring a diagnosis for suspected psychosis; a patient requiring a diagnosis for suspected neurotic conversion reaction; problems with three children who refuse to wear braces on their lower extremities; difficulty of a child in adjusting to separation from his parents; lack of progress in speech therapy of four patients with aphasia and one with apraxia; the need for new techniques in teaching patients in the use of a hearing aid; the need for the application of learning procedures in occupational training; assessment of six patients for possible vocational training; assessment of five patients regarding their ability to live alone following discharge; and management of chronic pain which is interfering with rehabilitation.

It often happens that a referral for a psychological consultation is inappropriately made. That is, the problem for which help is being sought does not fall within the province of the psychologist. The reason for this is primarily that some staff members do not really understand the role of the psychologist. Thus, the psychologist may receive a consultation request to investigate whether or not a patient is dealing in narcotics, or because a patient refuses medication. The psychologist is not a policeman nor an enforcer of hospital policy, and such requests are inappropriate to him.

In addition, many referrals are worded so that they have no meaning to the psychologist, or in a way that the problem, or reason for referral, is unclear. Requests worded like "Please see patient and evaluate behavior status," or "Diagnose current level of functioning," or "Assess need for therapy," do not provide enough useful information. The psychologist must then go personally to the individual who asked for the consultation and determine exactly what the problem is and what he expects from the psychologist.

Every consultation request requires first a diagnosis, and second, action by the psychologist or recommendations by the psychologist regarding actions that others should take.

Once the psychologist has received a request for a consultation and has investigated the purposes of the request, he must make the decision as to how to best deal with it. He may decide that the patient about whom there is a diagnostic question requires only a thorough interview, or he may believe the matter to be one which requires a complete battery of psychological tests. A behavior problem may be handled by speaking to the person (s) involved in the situation and then to the patient, and may be resolved by scheduling a series of therapy appointments with the patient. A request for initiating psychotherapy with a patient can be answered by interviewing the patient, determining his need for and desire for such therapy and arriving at a mutual decision with him.

Problems of other therapists, such as a patient's lack of progress in speech therapy, or fear during ambulation training in physical therapy, or lack of motivation in ADL of occupational therapy, may result in the psychologist discussing these problems with the respective therapists and observing the patients in their rehabilitation classes. He may then correct the problem in the actual therapy situation, or work it out with the patient outside of therapy class, or train the therapists in the techniques of behavioral engineering.

The point is that the psychologist must decide how to answer the consultation request, how to deal with the problem.

There are occasions when the psychologist feels that the referral is not within his capabilities because the issue involved is not a psychological one. In that case he will return the request to the sender with the recommendation that it be forwarded to the appropriate person.

PSYCHOTHERAPY

One of the crucial functions of the rehabilitation clinical psychologist, and the one to which he probably devotes the majority of his time, is psychotherapy. There are many definitions of psychotherapy. The one to which the term will refer whenever it is used in this text is as follows: Psychotherapy is the treatment of psychologic disorder, or maladaptive behavior, through the use of psychological techniques. The object of psychotherapy is the elimination, alleviation or retardation of the maladjustive behavior and the promotion of psychological growth and health.

Psychotherapy may involve a close interpersonal relationship between the therapist and his patient, or it may even be performed by a machine. It can be conducted on an individual or a group basis and therapy sessions can last from thirty minutes or less to several hours. The therapist can be very directive and didactic in his approach with a patient, or he may remain relatively passive and non-directive. Sessions may be held on a weekly basis or even more widely spread apart, or on a schedule of five or more times per week. Psychotherapy is employed to treat the severest disorders, such as the psychoses, and the mildest difficulties, such as thumb-sucking. It can be conducted in a hospital, clinic, private office or in the patient's home, or, in fact, anywhere it is needed and possible. In rehabilitation it is naturally most often conducted within the confines of the institution, usually in the psychologist's office or in the patient's living area.

The number and variety of psychotherapeutic techniques is quite large and there are probably over fifty different methods or approaches in use today. With few exceptions, the techniques of psychotherapy which are employed with adult patients can be, and have been utilized with children, sometimes with modifications appropriate to the population. Most, if not all, psychotherapies are based upon a theory or theories of behavior or personality. Naturally, it is beyond the scope of the present chapter to discuss all of the psychotherapies even if they were all relevant to rehabilitation, which they are not. Therefore, this section will describe those therapeutic approaches which are currently most frequently employed with the physically disabled.

Techniques of Psychotherapy

Behavior Therapy

The methods of behavior therapy stem, primarily, from psychological learning theory and experimental psychology.

The focus of behavior therapy is the current behavior of the individual and its relationship to the contingent consequences in the environment. The group of behavior therapies, for there is more than one behavioral technique, deal with overt, observable, measurable behavior. Contrary to a medical-model approach to behavior which postulates an underlying, usually unconscious, cause for the problematic symptoms, the behavioral approach regards the symptoms as being learned and furthermore, as not being "symptoms," but as being the problem itself. Once the symptoms have been eliminated, the disorder is eliminated. Intrapsychic and "dynamic" interpretations of psychopathology are avoided, and the question which the therapist asks is this: What are the contingencies of the maladaptive behavior which are causing and maintaining it and how can these contingencies be altered, or modified, so as to bring about behavior change?

There are many techniques which can be enumerated within the framework of behavior therapy, the majority of which stem from the learning theory approaches of Pavlov, Skinner and Hull. Those methods which have not been drawn directly from a systematic theory or set of assumptions have been adapted from the body of knowledge of experimental psychology. Procedures are based upon scientific data and demonstrated laboratory results.

The following is a description of some of the more frequently utilized behavioral procedures.

TECHNIQUES BASED UPON OPERANT CONDITIONING. A *positive reinforcer* is any stimulus contingent upon a response, the presentation of which produces an increase in the frequency of that response's occurrence. A response which has been positively reinforced tends to occur with increased frequency thereafter. Thus, if a particular behavior is to be increased in the frequency of its occurrence, it will be positively reinforced by the behavior therapist. Conversely, if it is learned that an undesired behavior is being maintained by positive reinforcement, the therapist will attempt to alter the contingencies so that this relationship between response and reinforcement is discontinued.

An example of the former case would be the child with a phobia of water who is given candy each time he more closely approaches a water or water-related situation. An example of the latter is the child for whom attention is reinforcing temper tantrums. The attention is withdrawn for such behavior and it is decreased.

Positive reinforcement is highly successful, not only with children but with adults as well, and is of great value with many rehabilitation behaviors such as improving speech and language, instating language in verbally impaired patients, increasing social interaction among patients, improving ambulation, training the hard of hearing, increasing motivation for therapy, improving ADL skills and many, many more.

A *negative reinforcer* is any stimulus contingent upon a response, the withdrawal of which produces an increase in the frequency of that response's occurrence. With this method—i.e. use of negative reinforcement—a patient can be placed in a noxious, or unpleasant stimulus situation which can be terminated by his responding in a desired way. If, for example, stuttering is the behavior to be eliminated, a loud, unpleasant tone or noise can be played, via earphones, into the patient's ear while he speaks or reads aloud. Every time he completes a phrase or a word fluently the tone will be shut off. Or, hot, flashing floodlights can be used surrounding a hallucinating patient and, whenever he ceases his hallucinations, the lights are turned off.

This approach is employed less often than positive reinforcement primarily because of difficulties in using apparatus in many settings and problems which arise as a consequence of using noxious stimuli with patients. When used, however, it is extremely effective.

The term *punishment* technically refers to the withdrawal of a positive reinforcer or the presentation of a negative reinforcer. In practice, it most often implies presentation of a noxious stimulus contingent upon a response which is to be eliminated. Electric shock, for example, made contingent upon a compulsive behavior or a habit disturbance such as a tic, will effectively eliminate or reduce the problematic behavior.

Time-out from all sources of reinforcement, such as placing an autistic child with temper tantrums or an adult psychotic who screams, in a small, perhaps darkened room for a brief period each time the undesirable behavior occurs, is another form of punishment.

Escape behavior is that which permits an individual to leave or to terminate a noxious situation. If an attempt is being made by a therapist to increase movement in an upper extremity of a hemiplegic patient, shock can continuously be delivered to the nonaffected upper extremity until the plegic arm is moved, thus terminating the shock.

In an *avoidance* situation the patient can perform the correct response prior to the onset of the noxious stimulus and thus postpone or avoid it. Thus, for the example of the hemiplegic patient just cited, a brief tone or light flash would precede the onset of the shock by a few seconds and, if the patient responds correctly between this signal and the scheduled onset of the shock, he can entirely avoid receiving the shock.

Punishment and escape and avoidance procedures can be successfully employed with almost any behaviors which are to be respectively decreased or increased and are most feasible in an institutional setting.

THE RELAXATION-BASED THERAPIES. The group of therapies within this category are, in the main, based upon the theory that anxiety is incompatible with relaxation. Thus, the therapist trains, or induces in the patient a state of deep muscle relaxation as an important step in therapeutic alleviation of a problem. Relaxation may be produced by progressive tension and relaxation of the muscles of the body, by suggestion, or "pseudohypnosis," by hypnosis, or even by drugs.

In the technique known as *systematic desensitization,* the therapist and patient construct a hierarchical list of feared or anxiety-provoking objects or situations, and then, while the patient is relaxed, the therapist verbally presents each situation to him, individually, beginning with the least feared and progressing to the most feared stimulus on the list. Each situation is presented until the patient can clearly visualize it without experiencing anxiety. Following such treatment, when the patient is actually confronted by these stimuli in his daily life, he will no longer be threatened by them.

With the employment of *in vivo desensitization* the actual feared object is presented to the patient while he is relaxed, or in the presence of the therapist who uses himself as a source of relaxing stimuli.

Emotive imagery requires that the patient envision stimuli and responses which are incompatible with anxiety, such as viewing a beautiful, calm natural scene or engaging in a favorite activity. The stimuli to which maladaptive responses are made, or which arouse fear or anxiety, are presented to the patient by the therapist as woven into the context of the pleasant activity.

Covert sensitization involves the therapist's verbally presenting to the patient the undesirable behaviors which the latter wants to eliminate from his repertoire. While doing this the therapist also presents punishing stimuli contingent upon these behaviors. For example, the obese patient will be asked to imagine himself eating a meal and, when he envisions eating the dessert, the therapist encourages him to think of himself becoming nauseous and vomiting, soiling his food and himself. The same procedure can be used for the treatment of homosexuality, alcoholism, cigarette smoking and the like.

During *covert reinforcement* therapy the patient imagines himself in a feared situation or engaged in a feared activity and, after successful completion of the task, is asked to visualize a stimulus which is reinforcing to him, such as eating a favorite food or listening to a favorite piece of music.

In the procedure known as *thought stoppage,* the patient is requested to think of the behavior or thought which is causing him difficulties. When he has clearly fixed this in mind the therapist shouts, "Stop." This is repeated often and the pateint is told to do the same.

With the exception of systematic and in vivo desensitization, relaxation may not always be a necessary condition to treatment although it is generally helpful and valuable.

The relaxation-based therapies have their greatest value in the elimination of anxiety and phobias with neurotic patients. But, as some of the above examples illustrate, they can be successfully employed with a large variety of problems, including perhaps some psychotic conditions.

OTHER BEHAVIOR THERAPIES. The theory behind *negative practice* is that practicing an undesirable habit, such as nailbiting, stuttering, or a tic, results in the extinction, or elimination, of the response in the absence of the unconditioned stimulus of anxiety and inhibition, or fatigue associated with making the response, so that performing it may be painful, and not performing it avoids an aversive situation and is, therefore, positively reinforcing. In addition, by being able to reproduce the habit upon desire, the patient gains a measure of control over it, leading to the ability to discontinue it upon desire as well.

Therapists who employ *assertion therapy* hypothesize that anxiety and the expression of resentment are incompatible, and if a person is able to assert himself, anxiety will be inhibited.

The therapist points out to the patient the irrationality of his fears and encourages him to assert his "rights." He may set up a series of progressively more difficult tasks for the patient to perform, may use practice or role playing in the therapy office situation, or may provide certain cues to which the patient must respond in the desired way, cues which the patient will actually encounter outside the therapy situation. In this last method, the patient comes to respond in a way that the desired behavior becomes a *conditioned reflex,* or an automatic response, elicited by the cue stimuli. Furthermore, increasing mastery of formerly anxiety-arousing situations is reinforcing to the patient.

In the use of *modeling,* the patient observes another individual making and being reinforced for the responses which he is to learn. This can be accomplished by having the patient view the other person through a one-way glass or by the therapist himself providing the appropriate model.

Psychotherapy as Alteration of Assumptions

A number of therapists conceive of psychotherapy as a process of helping the patient to change his faulty assumptions and plans. In this sense, psychotherapy is not so much a change of habits or of specific behaviors as it is a change of life style. Alfred Adler was the first, perhaps, to deal with an individual's life style as a relatively consistent means of achieving goals and coping with the problems of life.

He believed that, for the maladjusted person, the life style is likely to be interwoven with inaccurate assumptions which lead to neuroses or other difficulties. The task of the therapist then becomes one of understanding the patient's life style, discerning the mistaken assumptions which are producing the difficulty, and helping the patient to make changes which will lead to more effective interpersonal relationships and to a generally more fulfilling existence.

RATIONAL PSYCHOTHERAPY. Following a similar approach, rational, or rational-emotive psychotherapy, as developed by Albert Ellis, emphasizes the view that the patient's difficulties stem from certain inaccurate assumptions that are sustained by "self-talk," a kind of self-dialogue through which the patient continually affirms his own faulty assumptions. For example, the patient may tell himself that it is essential to be approved of by everyone, or that one should always be completely self-confident.

The task of the therapist becomes one of unmasking the patient's self-defeating verbalizations through the following:

1. Bringing them to the patient's attention, or into consciousness;
2. Showing the patient how they are causing and maintaining his difficulties;
3. Helping the patient to change his faulty assumptions and verbalize more constructive ones to himself; and
4. Encouraging the patient to put his new ideas into practice.

ASSERTION-STRUCTURED PSYCHOTHERAPY. This form of psychotherapy, as formulated by E. Lakin Phillips, analyzes the patient's difficulties in terms of a four-point model—assertion, disconfirmation, tension and redundancy.

In dealing with the problems of living and in attempting to meet his needs the individual makes certain assumptions or assertions. If these are correct he is likely to make an adequate adjustment. However, if they are *in*correct a vicious cycle begins. The assertion is disconfirmed. This leads to tension and a defensive tendency to reiterate the assertion more strongly than ever. Thus, there is further disconfirmation, additional tension, and this cycle becomes repetitious.

To break this cycle, Phillips has emphasized the importance of reducing the patient's negative feelings and fear of alternative solutions so that he has greater flexibility and can "move," psychologically, in any positive direction which he perceives as being open to him.

Client-Centered Psychotherapy

The client-centered, or non-directive approach, formulated by Carl Rogers, relies heavily upon the individual's drive toward personality integration, psychological health and self-actualization. In the maladjusted individual this drive has been blocked by faulty assumptions and emotional conflicts. Psychotherapy is aimed primarily at the removal of such blocks and the freeing of the person to accept his unique self and to grow and change in his own natural way. Much of the responsibility for the course and outcome of therapy is borne by the client. (Note: The client-centered psychotherapist does not use the term "patients," but instead prefers to refer to his counselees as "clients.")

There are five main steps in the non-directive therapeutic process.

1. THE CLIENT COMES FOR HELP. It is important that therapy be sought by the client because this is a sign that he has taken himself in hand and *on his own initiative* has taken the first step towards solving his problems.

2. EXPRESSION OF FEELING. By his accepting and permissive attitude the therapist encourages the free expression of feelings. By doing so he creates an atmosphere in which the emotions which have been blocked inside the client are permitted to be expressed freely. At this occurs, the therapist must recognize, accept and clarify these feelings and the assumptions underlying the client's difficulties.

When the client's feelings have been fully expressed, they are followed by faint, tentative expressions of positive regard which are also accepted and clarified by the therapist without praise or blame. Thus, the client can accept them as part of himself without the need to become defensive about them.

3. DEVELOPMENT OF INSIGHT. Gradually, increasing recognition and acceptance of the real self leads to the development of insight and understanding. Thus, at first, the client's perception of himself and his situation is distorted by emotional attitudes which keep him under stress but, as his feelings are released and clarified, he learns to view himself and his environment in a truer perspective.

4. POSITIVE STEPS. Following the development of insight, and intertwined with it, is the clarification of possible decisions and courses of action. At first, although the client sees himself more clearly, he is confused as to how to change his situation. As possible alternatives are seen, however, he begins to tentatively consider various steps which he must take.

5. ENDING THE CONTACTS. As the client graduates from fearful

and tentatively undertaken positive actions to an increasingly confident integration of positive and self-directed actions, there is a feeling of decreasing need for help and a recognition by the client that therapy must end. By terminating therapy under his own initiative, the client takes the final step towards independence and the assumption of a full measure of responsibility for his own life.

Psychoanalysis—The Classical Approach

Psychoanalysis, which was developed by Sigmund Freud, is an etiological type of psychotherapy. Its goal is the uncovering and modifying of unconscious psychological forces. Through analysis the patient discovers the influences which the unconscious forces have upon his life and behavior. Psychoanalysis attempts to explore the deeper layers of the patient's mind so that he may gain insight into his problems, and bring about a restructuring of personality by reorganizing the unfavorable patterns which were established during the early years of life. The psychoanalyst believes that the patient is motivated by unconscious drives and that the symptoms presented are, in fact, only signs of a deeply rooted problem. Successful treatment depends upon bringing the unconscious into conscious awareness.

There are several techniques employed in psychoanalysis. In *free association* the patient is directed to say whatever comes into his mind and to let his thoughts continue in uninterrupted sequence, withholding nothing. As material emerges, often in symbolic form, the consciously inaccessible portion of the mind becomes conscious. The patient explores early memories, reactivates relationships with other persons, relives significant events, etc. He is asked or advised to uncover for himself, or to interpret, the symbolism of his free associations.

Often an opposition is noted on the part of the patient to becoming aware of, and facing, the unconscious basis of a motive. This is called *resistance* and is manifested by sudden silences, denials, forgettings, evasions and the like. By observing the amount of resistance to a topic, the analyst gains information regarding its significance to the patient.

Transference is carrying over and attaching to the therapist of feelings and attitudes which the patient formerly had towards parents or other meaningful persons in his life. The patient behaves towards the therapist as if he, the therapist, were that other person. Thus, the therapist learns about the patient's relationships with others and helps him to work through associated problems.

Interpretation, the process whereby the therapist helps the patient to understand the meaning of his mental phenomena, involves interpreting the psychic behavior to the patient, penetrating personality defenses and bringing anxiety and conflict into consciousness so that they can be dealt with rationally and insight may be gained. The analyst interprets or explains the symbolism of free association, dreams, resistance and transference.

The analyst believes *dream interpretation* to be of great value in revealing unconscious thought processes, wishes, feelings and the like. The dream material, or content, is considered symbolic representation of the patient's inner tensions, childhood memories, repressed desires, etc.

Neo-Analytic Psychotherapy

The neo-analytic therapies, or non-Freudian, non-orthodox psychoanalytic methods stem from the thinking of several persons, but the term "neo-analytic" is usually associated with the therapies derived from the theories of Alfred Adler, Harry Stack Sullivan, Erich Fromm, Otto Rank and Karen Horney.

They differ in several aspects among themselves, but what makes this group of therapies stand apart is their departure from the classical psychoanalytic theories and approaches of Freud and the orthodox analysts. They tend to stress the experiential and the present rather than the historical, and the exploration of conscious processes rather than focussing on the unconscious drives and dream material. Interpersonal transactions are a major concern of therapy. Sex is denied the all-powerful role given it by traditional psychoanalysis. The importance of acting out is rejected and activity becomes a way of changing modes of thinking, feeling and doing. Resistance is not continuously worked with, but the mutual cooperation of patient and therapist is a center of concentration.

Since space does not permit a description of the techniques of all of the neo-analysts, one approach, the *interpersonal psychiatry* of Harry Stack Sullivan, has been selected as a representative example for discussion.

Sullivan felt the psychoanalyst to be a *participant observer,* a factor in the situation which confronts the patient. He tries to understand the anxiety which he observes in the patient and may comment upon it. He strives to understand the presuppositions held by the patient in seeking treatment. He is aware of his own emotional reactions to the patient because they may give him a clue to the patient's method of functioning and because his own feelings will produce shifts in the patient's interpersonal field.

Extensive *history taking* is considered part of the interpersonal experience for the patient. The analyst is formal, frank and direct, and informs the patient of what he knows of him from various sources. He also clarifies for the patient the reasons for which therapy has been sought.

In the history taking sessions free associations are tentatively used during memory lapses, the patient's relationship to the therapist is noted and particular attention is paid to periods of anxiety and the means of obtaining security experienced by the patient. The analyst then tries to clarify the issues which brought the patient to therapy.

In therapy, the analyst is sensitive to anxiety and to clues which indicate its presence, and to the kind of *security operation* which is employed by the patient to escape from the anxiety.

Much attention is focussed on the interactions between patient and therapist as an indication of the patient's general interpersonal behavior.

Supportive Psychotherapy

Supportive therapy is generally employed for brief periods of time to help a patient analyze and cope with a current problem. Through direct methods, in which the therapist takes an active role, patterns of behavior are modified, new roles or ways of behaving are taught to the patient, reassurance is provided and hopeful expectations are enhanced. Stressful, or anxiety-arousing terms and situations are calmly and matter-of-factly discussed by the therapist, thus lessening the patient's fears and apprehensions.

Some of the techniques of supportive psychotherapy include *re-assurance, suggestion* or *advice, reasoning* and *persuasion, ventilation,* in which the patient is given the opportunity to express his feelings openly and as emotionally as he wishes, *encouragement, communication of empathic understanding,* and *re-education.* These methods are employed for the immediate relief of an acute difficulty, or to "see a patient through" a particularly trying period of life, and for similar problems.

If the patient's family can be involved in the therapeutic process by extending the therapist's work into the home situation therapy may be made more effective.

Group Psychotherapy

Group psychotherapy is a flexible method which can employ a variety of techniques with both children and adults. Some groups operate on psychoanalytic priniciples, some use client-centered methods, some are supportive in nature.

Participants in a therapy group can number from two to twelve, or even more, although most groups have about four to seven members. Patients are usually grouped according to the similarity of their problems, needs, or other psychological variables, or they may be placed in a group on the basis of demographic variables, such as age, sex, or marital status. Groups can be used in conjunction with, or instead of individual therapy or as a special technique in their own right. Some group therapists are authoritarian and very active in the therapy sessions while others play a decidedly passive role and give free reign to discussion and acting out among the group members.

In the *supportive group* patients usually have similar problems and the therapist takes an active, directive, inspirational, or advice-giving role, emphasizing present reality. When the group members have learned how to handle their problems the group is discontinued.

In the *regressive-reconstructive group* patients are seen individually prior to their being placed in a group, depending upon their needs, difficulties and the therapist's evaluation. The goal of therapy is deep personality change of a permanent nature.

Therapy is continually ongoing, as is life. There are "births", as new members enter the group, and "deaths" as members leave for one or more reasons. The therapist promotes the expression of affect and encourages the re-enactment of events in the patients' histories, particularly intrafamilial relationships which are related to the behavior of the patients in the group. The immediate interaction of group members is analyzed as well as the fantasy life of each member.

The *repressive-inspirational group* is designed to foster a sense of group identification and the feeling of belonging. The enthusiasm of the therapist establishes the climate of the group. The emotional and actional factors in the members are emphasized. Mutual member support is strong, communal spirit is strengthened and social approval and acceptance are high among the participants.

The *directive-didactic group* relies upon pedagogy. A patient's problem may generally be discussed, with the therapist serving as leader and moderator. Sometimes the therapist enters into lecturing the group or has the group discuss printed material which has been distributed to them. Such a group is, obviously, highly structured with regard to its activities and interchanges. Psychotic patients and patients who have marked social distortion are most likely to benefit from participation is a group of this type.

Indications for Psychotherapy

While the previous section dealt with psychotherapy in general, and not specifically related to rehabilitation, this section will restrict itself to a discussion of psychotherapy with the physically disabled.

The decision as to when psychotherapy should be initiated with a rehabilitation patient is not always a clear one to make. The presence of a psychological difficulty is not a sufficient criterion in itself since other variables are involved, and the fact that a patient has a problem is only one variable. Another consideration is the patient's desire for psychotherapy. It is quite conceivable that a patient who, from the psychologist's viewpoint, requires therapeutic intervention, will refuse such help either because he feels it is not necessary or for any number of reasons. As is true of individuals in a non-disabled population, the rehabilitation patient cannot be coerced, against his will, to enter into a therapeutic relationship. Since psychotherapy is a cooperative endeavor for both therapist and patient, and without the willingness of either the effort will be fruitless, the patient must be motivated to seek help. Despite the apparent severity of a problem, if a patient does *not* want help *it cannot be forced upon him*.

There are times when a patient is not fully aware of the seriousness of his disorder, or of its implications, and then the psychologist may explain to him the importance of obtaining therapeutic assistance and may try to convince the patient of his need for therapy. However, if the patient is not persuaded by such dialogue the psychologist cannot proceed further at that time. He can try again, at a later date, to impress upon the patient that professional help should be sought, but he cannot order the patient to do so.

An important factor to consider is the severity of the psychological pathology. A patient may have a problem which the psychologist can help him work through, but if it is not of a magnitude which disrupts the patient's functioning, it may be decided by the psychologist not to intervene. It is always preferable for the patient to rely upon his own personal resources to work out his difficulties and, if the psychologist feels that this is possible, based upon his knowledge of the patient, he can choose to refrain from approaching the patient concerning therapy. If, after a given period of time, he observes that the patient has been unable to come to a solution, he may then offer his help.

Related to this last point is the effect of the patient's psychological disorder on others—on family, friends, hospital staff and other patients. If, because of the nature of one or more aspects of the disorder, the patient is having an adverse effect upon any of these persons, the psychologist may attempt to work out the difficulties with him after pointing out, if necessary, the need for such endeavor.

The matter of *timing* is essential to successful psychotherapy. If a patient is not psychologically "ready", or prepared for therapy, he is likely not to benefit from it. The patient must be aware that he has a problem, he must be somewhat aware of the nature of it, and he must be accepting of the fact that he needs help to solve it.

The question of when is the right time to initiate psychotherapy is a difficult one to answer, and there are diverse views on the subject. One cannot always wait for the patient to approach the psychologist. Often, the psychologist must decide when he should contact the patient. Sometimes, despite the apparent presence of a problem, the psychologist realizes that the patient should not be "picked up" for therapy at a particular time. One example of this situation is the young patient with a recent spinal cord injury which has left him quadriplegic or paraplegic, who is depressed. It may be considered psychologically healthy for this patient to be depressed at such a time because depression is a natural reaction to serious trauma and only after the initial depressive reaction, or "grief period", has abated to some degree should therapy be attempted. There are occasions when the patient has not yet accepted his disability or its consequences, as in the case of a paraplegic who refuses to believe his prognosis and fully expects to ambulate and resume his former activities. The psychologist may decide to wait until the patient does accept his status and is more realistic in his outlook. When such a change occurs, depression often results and the psychologist must then decide when to intervene. There are no strict rules or guidelines for the length of time which should take place between onset of disability and the initiation of psychotherapy. The psychologist makes a determination based upon his previous experiences and his knowledge of the patient.

The psychologist is often called upon to "do therapy" with a patient by the medical and paramedical staff. At that time he evaluates the patient's candidacy for therapy based upon discussions with the referring person, but primarily based upon interviews with the patient and consideration of the factors just discussed. The psychologist may or may not decide to attempt therapy with the patient, but this must be *his decision.*

In deciding whether or not a patient is a "good candidate" for psychotherapy, several considerations, in addition to the above, must be made. Two variables to take into account are the goals of psychotherapy, which vary from case to case, and the patient's medical condition. If a therapeutic goal is total restructuring of the patient's personality, an eighty-five year old man would be an unlikely candidate because by that advanced age a person's behavior patterns, habits, characteristics and ideas are well fixed and difficult to radically alter. If the goal of therapy is the modification of a negative behavior pattern and the patient is a recent CVA victim with mixed aphasia, therapy probably would not be attempted because there are certain aspects of behavior which are known concomitants of this disorder as a result of the brain damage, and also because the patient's communication disorder precludes meaningful participation in therapy.

A third consideration is the type of psychotherapy which will be employed. While theoretically the psychologist is knowledgable in all forms of therapy, most psychologists prefer a particular method or group of methods and are more effective with their preference and with the techniques with which they are most familiar. In addition, some therapies are more suited to certain psychological problems and to certain disorders than others, and some, by the very nature of their procedures, preclude certain individuals.

Both psychoanalysis and client-centered therapy, for example, require that the patient have a certain level of intelligence and a certain capacity for insight. Thus, the less intelligent, the brain-injured and the psychotic are not good candidates for these therapies. Orthodox psychoanalysts typically do not work with persons beyond their middle years, thereby precluding the geriatric population. Behavior therapy makes no distinctions based upon age, sex, disability, intelligence, capacity for insight, education, or any other variable, yet some patients may want to "talk out" their problems and learn more about themselves and would be unlikely to be seen by a therapist who applies specific techniques to manifest problems.

For those patients for whom it is clear that their difficulties lie in the fact that they are conducting their lives based upon incorrect assumptions about themselves or others, assertion-structured therapy, or rational-emotive psychotherapy would be the method of choice. There are patients who cannot, or will not, discuss their problems in front of others, and there group therapy would not be employed. On the other hand, for patients who require the social conditions of a group, such a procedure would be the main consideration.

When a patient has a marked communication disorder, such as aphasia or apraxia, obviously, a psychotherapy which relies upon verbal behavior cannot be utilized.

Many times, no single therapy, but rather a combination of approaches will be used by the psychologist. The therapy of choice depends upon the requirements of that approach for its patients and upon how well the individual in question meets those requirements.

PSYCHOPATHOLOGY OF REHABILITATION PATIENTS

The first thing to consider in a discussion of the psychological problems of the physically disabled is the fact that they are first and foremost, individuals. That is, they are not a special breed of people, psychologically—i.e. disabled persons—but are, instead, *persons with a disability*. They are subject to the same psychological conditions as the non-disabled, but have, in addition, a physical handicap.

The psychological disorders of the disabled may be a direct consequence of their disability, or they may be only directly or tangentially, related to the physical condition, or may have existed premorbidly and have been exacerbated by the disability, or they may bear no relationship to the disability at all. Some patients have had psychological problems for many years which first came to the attention of a psychologist when they entered a rehabilitation facility. Others may have undergone psychotherapy prior to their hospitalization.

This section will be concerned with those psychological disorders which are *a direct consequence* of physical disability.

Anxiety and Fear

Anxiety and fear are encountered very frequently in a rehabilitation population. They are seen in both the young and the aged, but are more prevalent among the former. They occur in patients who are disabled as a result of sudden trauma and in those whose disability is a consequence of progressive disease.

The physically disabled person is anxious about himself and his condition, often because of a lack of sufficient knowledge about the disorder. He wonders what has happened to him and why it has happened. He is concerned about his loss of function. He is anxious about the progression of the condition. He fears for his life and his future health. He fears for his family and how his absence from the home and loss of earning ability will affect them. These anxieties and fears may be considered "normal", although psychotherapeutic intervention is often necessary.

Depression

Depression is also a natural consequence of crippling injury or disease. Depression results from loss of function, from futility of action, from despair concerning the future, from feelings of loneliness, isolation and abandonment, and from estrangement from a former life and personal interactions. Most patients do not remain deeply depressed for long periods of time, although this does occur. The depressions accompanying acute injury may last for several weeks, but psychotherapy can be of much help, particularly once the severe depression lifts. In patients with progressive disease, each exacerbation of symptoms can result in renewed depression and thus, in chronic disorders, periods of depression can occur over many years.

Denial

Denial is more common in certain disability groups than in others. There are two main forms of denial. One is the denial, by the patient, that he has a disability because, due to brain damage, he is unaware of his condition. The second form, which the psychologist is more likely to deal with, is the psychological denial of a condition. Often seen, for example, in multiple sclerosis patients, is the refusal of the patient to admit to himslef that the diagnosis is correct, that he does, in fact, have the disease. He may admit it when questioned, but this is an intellectual admission which has not been accepted emotionally. The patient emotionally believes the diagnosis to be incorrect, and his symptoms are explained away to himself as manifestations of "something else".

Lack of Acceptance

Closely related to denial is lack of acceptance of a condition. The patient simply refuses to accept the fact that he can no longer function as he once did, and that he will not be able to resume his former activities once he is "better". This is a fairly common reaction among young patients with traumatic spinal cord injuries.

Dependence

Dependence, in this case, refers not to physical dependence, which is a natural result of many disabilities and is beyond the patient's control, but to psychological dependence. The dependent patient views himself as a hopeless cripple who can never be of use to himself or others. This attitude pervades his thinking and behavior so that he does not see the positive aspects and possibilities open to him, but comes to depend upon others for psychological support.

Loss of Self-Concept

A great many patients view their disability as something which has lessened them as a person. Since they often cannot resume work, or family responsibility, or sexual activities, they come to think of themselves as useless, worthless, "half a man", and the like.

Negativism

Some patients are so embittered by what has happened to them that they become negativistic, oppositional, angry and hostile, refusing help of any kind. They blame themselves for their condition, or others, and openly reject attempts at therapy or the advances of their family and friends.

Lack of Motivation

Contrary to popular expectation, not all disabled patients eagerly seek therapy and work hard towards improvement of their condition and towards ADL independence. Some are so depressed by their condition that they do not possess the energy, psychological and physical, to better themselves. Others feel that their case is hopeless and they will never improve regardless of effort. Still others believe their condition to be "God's will", or a fact of life to be accepted stoically or philosophically. The problem of motivating such patients is an ever-present one in rehabilitation.

PSYCHOLOGICAL PROBLEMS OF SOME SPECIFIC DISABILITY GROUPS

This section lists the kinds of psychological problems which are common to certain physical disabilities. Not all patients with a particular disability exhibit all of the difficulties included within each group and there may be patients with one of the disabilities who have problems which are not included therein. *Each patient is an individual, differing from all other individuals, regardless of the commonality of a medical diagnosis.* What is presented here is a general listing of those psychological conditions which are often associated with particular disabilities.

Amputations

Fear of loss of acceptance by peers and social rejection
Loss of positive self-concept
Depression
Inadequate control of tension
Resentment
General negative emotional reactions to situations
Anxiety
Defiance
Impulsivity
Inadequate compensatory ambition
Poor tolerance for stress
Shame and Guilt
Self-pity
Worry about family

Paranoid reactions
Indifference
Phobic reactions
Isolation
Somatization
Pessimism
Phantom pain
Unrealistic view of importance of the disability

Upper Extremity Amputation

Denial of consequences of the amputation
Unrealistic attitudes

Lower Extremity Amputation

Negative self-references
Non-acceptance of disability
Hostility
Dependency
Timidity
Superficial self-confidence
Variable motivation
Compulsive behavior
Rationalization of situations

Arthritis

Psychological tension
Hostility
Resentment
Immaturity
Feelings of inadequacy
Aggressive traits
Anxiety and fear
Passive dependence

Cardiac Disease

Fears, particularly of death
Anxiety
Depression
Denial
Negativism
Suspicion
Resentment

Irritability
Unrealistic attitudes

Hemiplegia

Distorted body perception
Perceptual and perceptual-motor deficits
Denial
Fear and anxiety
Depression
Unrealistic expectations
Disorientation and confusion
Memory impairments
Emotional lability
Irritability and anger
Difficulty with abstract reasoning
Difficulty in learning
Intellectual losses
Hostility
Negativism
Social withdrawal
Impaired judgement
Impulsivity
Fluctuating behavior
Reduced attention span and concentration ability

Cancer

Fear and anxiety
Denial
Guilt
Depression
Alteration of self-concept
Dependency
Hostility and anger
Mood changes
Irritability
Self-pity
Impaired logical reasoning ability

Multiple Sclerosis

Denial
Depression
Euphoria

Anxiety and fear
Dependency
Social withdrawal
Manipulativeness
Intolerance for stress
Anger and hostility
Despair and resultant motivational problems

Cerebral Palsy

Intellectual retardation
Depression
Anger and hostility
Negativism
Social immaturity
Motivational variability
Impaired self-concept
Dependency
Over-fantasizing
Excessive need for affection
Unrealistic attitudes and plans
Paranoid thinking

Spinal Cord Injuries

Anxiety
Depression
Resentment
Guilt
Hostility
Despair
Negative self-concept
Suspicion
Negativism
Lack of acceptance
Unrealistic thinking and planning
Dependence
Fluctuating motivation

A CONCLUDING NOTE ON REHABILITATION PSYCHOLOGY

Anyone who has ever worked in a rehabilitation medicine institution knows the necessity for having adequate psychological services. They are indispensable in determining which patients are to be admitted to the rehabilitation program, in deciding a patient's readiness for discharge, and for the total rehabilitation of a patient during his hospitalization. No hospital can claim to be providing complete patient care if it does not have a psychology staff, and, no rehabilitation team can truly be called a "team" without a psychologist.

Psychology services are rapidly growing and expanding in rehabilitation settings throughout the country and the future will see an even greater growth. As an increasing number of universities are providing graduate training in rehabilitation psychology as a specialized discipline, this branch of behavioral science is becoming recognized as one of the more important fields of psychological study and practice.

Rehabilitation psychology is a complex area of endeavor. Not only must the psychologist deal with the majority of problems which psychologists working in other clincal areas are confronted with, but he must additionally cope with the very unique problems which are consequential to physical disorder and disability. Sometimes, particularly when the psychological disorder is compounded by severe, overwhelming physical disability, the patient's problems seem almost insurmountable. But the psychologist's attitude is always that something *can* be done, help can be given, relief can be provided.

Since so much of a patient's total rehabilitation depends upon psychological variables, when a patient regains function and independence it is due, in large measure, to the psychologist who worked with him and for him during his rehabilitation period. And when a patient says, "Thank you, Doc. I couldn't have made it without you," the psychologist knows that he has done his job well.

Section V

References

1. American Psychiatric Association: *Diagnostic and Statistical Manual of Mental Disorders,* 2nd ed. Washington, American Psychiatric Association, 1968.
2. Anastasi, Anne: *Psychological Testing,* 3rd ed. New York, Macmillan, 1968.
3. Anderson, J. E. (Ed): *Psychological Aspects of Aging.* Washington, American Psychological Association, 1956.
4. Arieti, S. (Ed): *American Handbook of Psychiatry.* New York, Basic Books, 1959.
5. Baker, H. J.: *Introduction to Exceptional Children.* New York, Macmillan, 1959.
6. Beck, S. J.: *Rorschach's Test. II. A Variety of Personality Pictures.* New York, Grune and Stratton, 1949.
7. Bender, Lauretta: *Psychopathology of Children With Organic Brain Disorders.* Springfield, Thomas, 1956.
8. Bychowski, G. and Despert, J. Louise (Eds): *Specialized Techniques in Psychotherapy.* New York, Basic Books, 1952.
9. Coleman, J. C.: *Abnormal Psychology and Modern Life,* 3rd ed. Chicago, Scott, Foresman, 1964.
10. Cronbach, L. J.: *Essentials of Psychological Testing,* 2nd ed. New York, Harper and Row, 1960.
11. Cumming, Elaine and Henry, W. E.: *Growing Old: The Process of Disengagement.* New York, Basic Books, 1961.
12. Dunbar, F.: *Emotions and Bodily Changes,* 4th ed. New York, Columbia University Press, 1954.
13. English, H. B. and English, Ava C.: *A Comprehensive Dictionary of Psychological and Psychoanalytic Terms. A Guide to Usage.* New York, Longmans, Green, 1958.
14. Eysenck, H. J. (Ed): *Behaviour Therapy and the Neuroses,* New York, Pergamon, 1960.
15. Freeman, F. S.: *Theory and Practice of Psychological Testing,* Revised ed. New York, Holt, 1955.
16. Garrett, J. F.: *Applications of Clinical Psychology to Rehabilitation.* In *Progress in Clinical Psychology,* Vol. I. New York, Grune and Stratton, 1952.
17. Garrett, J. F. (Ed): *Psychological Aspects of Physical Disability* (Rehabilitation Service Series No. 210). Washington, Office of Vocational Rehabilitation, 1952.
18. Garrett, J. F. and Levine, Edna S. (Eds): *Psychological Practices With the Physically Disabled.* New York, Columbia University Press, 1962.
19. Geist, H.: *The Psychological Aspects of the Aging Process. With Sociological Implications.* St. Louis, Green, 1968.
20. Gilbert, J.: *Clinical Psychological Tests in Psychiatric and Medical Practice.* Springfield, Thomas, 1969.
21. Haley, J.: *Strategies of Psychotherapy.* New York, Grune and Stratton, 1963.
22. Harper, R. A.: *Psychoanalysis and Psychotherapy: 36 Systems.* Englewood Cliffs, Prentice–Hall, 1959.
23. Hinsie, L. E. and Campbell, R. J.: *Psychiatric Dictionary,* 3rd ed. New York, Oxford University Press, 1960.
24. Jones, A. and Freyberger, H. (Eds): *Advances in Psychosomatic Medicine* (Sym-

posium of the 4th European Conference on Psychosomatic Research) . New York, Brunner, 1961.

25. Klopfer, B., Ainsworth, Mary D., Klopfer, W. G., and Holt, R.: *Developments in the Rorschach Technique.* Vol. 1: *Technique and Theory.* New York, World, 1954.

26. Kolb, L. C.: Noyes' *Modern Clinical Psychiatry,* 7th ed. Philadelphia, Saunders, 1968.

27. London, P. and Rosenhan, D.: *Foundations of Abnormal Psychology.* New York, Holt, Rinehart, Winston, 1968.

28. Mowbray, R. M. and Rodger, T. F.: *Psychology in Relation to Medicine,* 2nd ed. Edinburgh, Livingstone, 1967.

29. Penfield, W. and Roberts, L.: *Speech and Brain Mechanisms.* Princeton, Princeton University Press, 1959.

30. Rickers–Ovsiankina, Marie A. (Ed) : *Rorschach Psychology.* New York, Wiley, 1960.

31. Rosenbaum, M. and Berger, M. (Eds) : *Group Therapy and Group Function.* New York, Basic Books, 1963.

32. Seidenfeld, M. A.: Progress in Rehabilitation of the Physically Handicapped. In *Progress in Clinical Psychology,* Vol. II. New York, Grune and Stratton, 1956.

33. Skinner, B. F.: *Science and Human Behavior.* New York, Macmillan, 1953.

34. Talland, G. A.: *Human Aging and Behavior. Recent Advances in Research and Theory.* New York, Academic, 1968.

35. Terman, L. M. and Merrill, Maude A.: *Stanford–Binet Intelligence Scale (Manual for the Third Revision. Form L-M).* Boston, Houghton–Mifflin, 1960.

36. Ullman, M.: *Behavioral Changes in Patients Following Strokes.* Springfield, Thomas, 1962.

37. Ullmann, L. P. and Krasner, L. (Eds) : *Case Studies in Behavior Modification.* New York, Holt, Rinehart, Winston, 1965.

38. Wechsler, D.: *The Measurement and Appraisal of Adult Intelligence,* 4th ed. Baltimore, Williams and Wilkins, 1958.

39. Weinstein, E. A. and Kahn, R. L.: *Denial of Illness: Symbolic and Physiological Aspects.* Springfield, Thomas, 1955.

40. Weiss, E. and English, O. S. (Eds) : *Psychosomatic Medicine,* 3rd ed. Philadelphia, Saunders, 1957.

41. Wolberg, L. R.: *The Technique of Psychotherapy.* New York, Grune and Stratton, 1954.

42. Wolman, B. B. (Ed) : *Handbook of Clinical Psychology.* New York, McGraw–Hill, 1965.

43. Wolpe, J. and Lazarus, A. H.: *Behavior Therapy Techniques: A Guide to the Treatment of Neuroses.* New York, Pergamon, 1966.

44. Wright, Beatrice A.: *Physical Disability—A Psychological Approach.* New York, Harper and Row, 1960.

45. Zinberg, N. E. and Kaufman, I.: *Normal Psychology and the Aging Process* (First Annual Scientific Meeting of the Boston Society for Gerontologic Psychiatry, Inc.) . New York, International Universities Press, 1963.

THE SOCIAL SERVICES

Chapter 17

THE SOCIAL WORK SERVICE

IT IS UNFORTUNATELY BELIEVED by some professionals in the rehabilitation field that the social worker is not a crucial member of the rehabilitation team. Nothing could be further from the truth. The services which the social worker brings to each patient, both while the patient is hospitalized and in providing for continuing care following discharge, are indispensable if the goals of a total rehabilitation program are to be realized.

It cannot be stressed too strongly or too often that a rehabilitation team which does not have as a member a competent, trained and dedicated social worker is doomed to failure in its efforts to restore the individual patient to as normal a life as possible. This truth is seen all too frequently in those cases where the social worker is not an integral part of the team. When inadequate staffing or incomplete planning does not permit or provide for a complete social service, the patient invariably suffers in one or more aspects of his rehabilitation. Any institution which does not furnish adequate social service coverage is failing in its obligation to its patients and cannot claim to be adhering to the true philosophy of rehabilitation.

BASIC PRINCIPLES OF SOCIAL CASEWORK

While certain distinct differences exist between social work in the health fields, such as rehabilitation medicine, and social work in other areas, there are many basic similarities which underlie all fields of social work practice. It is therefore worthwhile at this point to review the basic assumptions and techniques of social work before proceeding to some of its more specialized functions.

At the heart of social work practice is casework. *Social casework* may be defined as the process through which an individual, the caseworker, cooperates with another individual, the client, to achieve ends which benefit both the client and his society. While goals are achieved for, and with, the client, it is always borne in mind by the caseworker that a problem is essentially the client's and that it is the client who must basically be active and responsible for its solution.

The underlying assumption of social casework is that the individual and his society are interdependent. Social forces influence the behavior of individuals, and casework must always consider both the client and the society or subsociety within which he functions.

Many casework problems are interpersonal. The social worker employs the worker-client relationship to help define the problem at hand and to work it through to achieve the goals of treatment.

A social case is comprised of physical, psychological, economic and social variables interacting to various degrees. Fundamentally, all cases, regardless of their nature or of the setting in which they occur, have both the characteristics of the client and the situation involved. At times there may be a discrepancy between objective reality and reality as perceived by, and interpreted by the client, while at other times the client may perceive reality correctly but be unable to modify its effects on him. In the former case the social worker attempts to modify the client's views, while in the latter she either works with the client to achieve adjustment to a life situation or actually modifies the physical and/or social and/or economic environment itself.

There are certain attitudes which must prevail if the case worker is to work effectively with his or her clients. Perhaps of primary importance is the attitude of *acceptance*. This refers to a non-condemnatory attitude on the part of the caseworker towards the behavior of the client. Although the caseworker may hold opinions or make judgements, she must not allow these judgements to become condemnations, thereby interfering in her relationship with her client. The client is accepted as a human being and while his behavior may be illegal, immoral, unethical or antisocial, he himself is not rejected by the social worker. It has been said that only as the caseworker can feel the client's problem as a common human problem, which could possibly be hers as well, can real acceptance take place. A caseworker may question the client regarding the advisability of a course of behavior which he is pursuing, or she may disagree with certain acts or beliefs of the client, but the basic attitude of desiring the best for the client and actually believing in the worth of the individual must prevail.

It is permissible for the caseworker to disagree with statements which a client makes and it is also permissible for her to express disapproval at times since continual agreement and approval do not constitute acceptance, nor can the worker be sincere who always reacts in an approving manner. However, if the social worker is honest in her beliefs and if she truly feels that her client is a worthwhile person for whom time and effort should be expended to improve his life, she has accepted the client and can effectively work with him.

A second attitude which is found in the successful caseworker might best be termed *self-responsibility*. This describes the belief that persons have a choice in the conduct of their lives, and furthermore, that it is not only their right to exercise this choice but their obligation as well. It places the primary responsibility for behavior with the client. The caseworker promotes self-control and the development of wise behavioral choices, but does not interfere with the client's self-actualization unless extreme situations arise with which the client, for one or more reasons, is unable to cope. Such cases are typically those which involve overwhelming physical or psychological disability and the caseworker makes the judgement that self-determination must, at least temporarily, be superseded by the necessity of protection or direction for the welfare of the client. Only when other approaches have been demonstrated to be unsuccessful does the worker attempt to take full responsibility. At all other times she is constantly striving to aid the client in becoming a responsible and self-determined individual.

Caseworkers adhere to the theory that individuals are more likely to behave in their own and in others' best interests when they understand themselves and their fellows. Bearing this in mind, the caseworker attempts to develop the client's understanding of his own behavior, of the situations in which he lives, and of the behavior of others with whom he interacts. While such endeavors require lengthy worker-client relationships and achieve results less quickly than giving direct instructions, the caseworker assumes that this method achieves a longer lasting ability to become self-reliant and to gain self-understanding so that in the future the client will act more judiciously.

Social workers maintain that it is the *interpersonal relationships* between people upon which society is based. The lives of individuals are so related that one client can only be helped as he is viewed in his interactions with other people. This point of view is carried through in the belief that one individual bears the responsibility for improving the welfare of another. This responsibility is, in our society, shared by the various social agencies and institutions.

While social workers believe that all men are equal in terms of their essential value, they also hold the view that there is *importance in diversity*. Many life styles are possible and valuable, and each individual will, if given the proper opportunity, experiences and guidance, select his own solutions to his unique problems and develop his own pattern of behavior.

The social worker tries to free the client to find his life pattern and to establish his characteristic ways of dealing with situations and events rather than attempting to have the client model himself after her or another person.

Another fundamental premise upon which social work is based is that there is often *value in merely the relief of suffering*. Each caseworker sees many clients for whom "cure" or radical, positive change is not a feasible short-term, or even long-range goal. For such persons, the emphasis of social work shifts to the alleviation of suffering, to helping the person bear his misfortunes, to supporting him during hardship. This in itself is deemed worthwhile.

Recently, social casework has attempted to incorporate some of the principles of the *scientific method* into its framework. In theory, this means assuming that behavior is lawful and that, once the laws which govern behavior are understood, behavior will become modifiable and predictable. In practice, it means that the caseworker employs techniques of scientific observation, measurement, hypothesis formulation and testing, objective recording, and classifying in her daily work with her clients.

However, within the deterministic framework of science, social workers also believe that not all behavior is determined and inflexible as a consequence of past and present environmental and physical variables, but rather that constitutional factors, previous life experiences and the present environment permit a large measure of freedom. The social worker then, is not using science as proposed by the philosophies of Logical Positivism, Operationism and Behaviorism, but instead as proposed by the more "dynamically" oriented schools of thought. There is, of course, more than one approach to science and more than one way of incorporating scientific principles into one's work. The social worker's task is particularly difficult because of the nature of the variables which he deals with. The increasing use of a scientific approach will help him to function more effectively in serving his clients.

The caseworker also believes in the value of *intuition* as a method for correctly perceiving a client's feelings, and perhaps even as a technique for uncovering causes, and finding solutions to his problems.

Intuition is the primary means by which new insights are gained. It is the product of flashes of insight plus the social worker's knowledge of her client, combined with her general theoretical knowledge, which enables her to help him.

The caseworker is always careful not to become so lost in empathy for the client that she identifies with him and thus loses her objectivity and her ability to clearly perceive the realities of the situation. Empathy must be in the service of independent judgement, and the worker's feelings can be a source of further information about the client—i.e. the reactions he elicits from others.

The successful caseworker finds the proper balance between scientific objectivity and warm understanding and empathy, between guiding a client and guarding his freedom of choice, and between recognizing the commonality of human problems and the intrinsic worth and uniqueness of each individual. As equilibrium of these elements is achieved, the client is helped towards becoming a self-sufficient, more satisfied member of his society.

THE METHODS OF SOCIAL WORK

The number and diversity of problems which the social worker encounters each day are immense. They include problems of poverty and public assistance, unemployment and insurance benefits, transiency and substandard housing, broken homes and family maladjustment, physical and psychological disabilities and health services, geriatrics and economic aid, industrial injuries and workmen's compensation, antisocial behavior and legal services, recreation and child guidance, vocational rehabilitation and labor legislation, educational difficulties and delinquency, the culturally disadvantaged and resettlement, traveler's aid and immigration, and a multitude of others.

Not only must the caseworker know how to counsel individuals, families and groups with regard to these problem areas but she must be familiar with the many legal, social and health agencies and institutions which can assist in alleviating or solving the particular problem at hand. Not least of all, the caseworker must be aware of her limitations so that referrals are made to appropriate professionals when a particular issue arises which is beyond the pale of her own discipline.

There are several methods employed by social workers in dealing with the immense complexity of situations which they face.

The Worker-Client Relationship

Perhaps the most basic and most frequently utilized social work method is the worker-client relationship which is aimed at *helping people to help themselves.* The client brings to the relationship his attitudes and feelings about himself, other people, his work and his life situations. The caseworker contributes empathy and understanding, experience and a desire to help. The client makes use of the relationship to the extent that rapport has been achieved between the caseworker and himself, and it is incumbent upon the social worker to foster this rapport and use it effectively.

Not all relationships between caseworker and client are necessarily treatment relationships in the true therapeutic sense. An individual who is a self-directed person with no aberrant behaviors or serious problems may simply want information regarding public financial assistance, or housing, and, as such, does not require intensive counseling. When the information is provided he will be able to make effective use of it. On the other hand, the less mature person who may be confronted by legal difficulties, for example, may well require a strong worker-client relationship so that he will be able to cope with future problems in a more sophisticated way.

The counseling which is given by the caseworker revolves primarily about the presenting problems of the client. Thus, for example, if a hospitalized patient exhibits ambivalence regarding discharge to a foster home, the caseworker must help him to explore his feelings about such a plan so that it can be happily accepted by him or, if the plan is rejected by the client, alternatives can be discussed which are more satisfactory to him. In relation to such a case, which is not an uncommon one in a rehabilitation setting, the patient's feelings towards his own family and home, his views on leaving the hospital for a new environment, and his future plans may all be discussed, and in doing so the caseworker may come to understand the client's ambivalent attitudes concerning foster home placement. In this way, a placement can be effected which best meets the needs of the client. Were all relevant factors not thoroughly explored it is unlikely that such a discharge plan would be agreeable to anyone concerned, least of all to the most important person involved, the client.

If, during interviews with the client, problematic material arises which requires more intensive working through, as in psychotherapy, the caseworker refers her client to a psychologist and then both professionals may work as a team in bettering the client's adjustment in both the social and the psychological spheres.

The individual is never regarded as a problem, but rather as a person *with* a problem. Furthermore, the confidences of the client are always protected whenever possible, even though a particular case may involve several agencies. While the caseworker has a responsibility to her agency, to the community and to herself, primary consideration is always given to the client. The nature of the casework relationship is often such that a client must place himself unreservedly in the hands of the social worker. Once the worker betrays this trust the relationship may be so impaired as to be rendered ineffective.

Social Action

Social action involves techniques of public education, social legislation and cooperative and collective enterprises. When the social worker uses the resources and powers of the community and government to achieve her objectives rather than relying solely upon her initiative or on volunteer services or groups, this is termed social action. It implies utilizing the forces of health services, labor relations and legislation, industrial groups, public assistance agencies, recreational facilities, social education sources, agencies for the prevention of facilities, social education sources, agencies for the prevention of crime and juvenile delinquency, and intercultural integration committees.

A caseworker cannot always solve a problem through the worker-client relationship, nor can she always turn to others for solutions. Instead, a rapprochement between these methods may be the most effective, if often not the only way of meeting a client's needs. It is highly important that the caseworker be aware of the many helping sources in the community and know which ones to turn to when in need.

Community Organization

Community organization is related to social action. It is only recently that community organization has been concerned with public functions and their collaboration with voluntary and private agencies. Community organization is the study of human needs through surveys and research and the modification of society and societal aid to meet these needs in the present and in terms of future forecasts. Public programs of financial assistance, use of leisure time through recreational facilities, such as parks and playgrounds, and housing are some examples of community organization.

While certain functions, such as assistance and protection, are carried out by public, tax-supported agencies supported by voluntary efforts, others, as in the case of some health services, are within the domain of voluntary or private groups supported by public resources. It is believed that the consent and participation of citizens in all enterprises is necessary in welfare and community organization aims at securing this cooperation through social agencies. Social welfare

planning strives at representing the entire community, and this requires the efforts of labor unions, religious groups and other special
interest organizations, legal societies, and so on. It is the social work
profession which points the way to the study and treatment of social
needs.

Social Group Work

Social group work has been developed on the premise of a universal
need for group associations, and on the basis of the value which is
accorded such associations in our society. The fundamental purpose
of social group work is to assist people in developing emotionally and
socially through group experiences, and to help groups to contribute
to the greater social welfare.

The individual member of the group finds certain elements within
the group with which he can identify and invest his interests, while
simultaneously maintaining the particular individuality which he does
not wish to be absorbed into the larger whole. Thus, the main group
and the individuals of which it is comprised become interrelated and
also related in varying degrees to the agency and the larger community
of which they are a part. Social group work attempts to maintain an
equilibrium between the individual and the social forces which make
up the realities of life.

When a group participates in a program of social action its members gain the experience of interacting with society and learn of their
individual and shared responsibilities to it. Social participation contributes to individual growth and social group work is directed towards developing the group to meet socially desirable ends.

The social group worker strives, within the purposes of her profession and of the social agency of which she is an integral part, to contribute to the fulfillment of society's goals. The term *social agency*
refers to the institution which our society has developed through which
people are offered services which meet their economic and personal
needs. The *social group work agency* includes the administrative board
and executive staff who determine the agency's objectives and policies,
staff workers and the membership. Each agency, while sharing in the
common goal of developing individual growth through group experience, has specific purposes which have grown out of the needs of the
community and the clientele it serves, as well as from the objectives
of its administrative leaders and the national agency with which it may
be affiliated. National organizations, however, tend to express their
policies in relatively broad terms which leave local agencies fairly free
to develop programs that are geared specifically to the problems of
their own particular community.

Some groups are already formed and have clearly defined objectives in mind before they approach an agency with the hope that such an affiliation will help them to attain their goals. Other groups are formed by the social agency from nuclei of people with common interests, or of like ages. As the members gain group experience a collective sense of a goal develops and the group's purpose becomes more clearly defined. While individuals may join groups for friendship, recreation, leisure time activities, social action or other interest with varied hopes and plans, these reasons may have to be modified, or even abandoned, in terms of the group's emerging purposes. Although differences of opinion and thought are important, the group must be cohesive in acceptance of a common objective if progress is to be made. The group social worker is concerned with both the expressed and unexpressed purposes of groups. However, her purpose need not be identical with that of the group and her professional goal may even be contrary to it at times. She gives the group identification with professional and agency goals and directs it towards achievement.

Family Case Work

The worker is concerned here with the social dysfunction of a family or its members. In recent years social casework has come to accept the significance of cultural and sociological variables as etiological factors in social maladjustment. The worker dealing with a family in distress must be aware of the role that such factors play, not only in society at large, but with the individual family in particular.

Among the family problems which the caseworker faces are the following: personal and sexual difficulties, delinquent children, civil rights and liberties, property and inheritance rights, business and contractual obligations, legal processes, child neglect, divorce and settlement claims, separation, annulment, illegitimacy, school problems, health conditions and a host of other difficulties, most of which can be classified under the headings of child rearing, marital functions and financial conditions. The question is always how a social caseworker can better diagnose these problems and direct rehabilitative efforts in behalf of individuals and their families.

When family life becomes endangered by economic variables, such as loss of income, the maintenance of the family becomes the responsibilty of a tax-supported agency through some social security provisions. Casework services are also made available to those who request them in addition to the broader scheme of public assistance.

A chronically disturbed child is likely to reflect a disturbed family. Parents traditionally do not seek help for themselves but for their child, and the caseworker must diagnose where the crux of the problem lies and if, in fact, the child's behavior is a reaction to parental distress. In a case such as this the worker may see both the child and his parents in counseling, attempting to aid the family relationship of the latter and pointing out to them how their difficulties affect the child's behavior, while at the same time the worker will be teaching the child appropriate methods of coping with difficult situations.

From the time of the initial intake interview the parents are encouraged and, in fact, required to participate fully in the planning for, and continuous treatment of, their child. In addition to requiring the parents to make the appointments with the social worker, furnish necessary consents, provide documents and follow through on recommendations, the caseworker must evidence a genuine empathy with them. This is especially true in cases of separation, such as placement of the child in a foster home or institution, where parental anxiety and guilt are crucial factors to be dealt with. Warm and reliable support given to the parents during treatment and/or placement are indispensable aids in giving them the insight and the strength needed during such crisis periods.

A family is usually threatened in two major ways—lack of finances for the maintenance of the family unit and disruption by the handicaps and asocial behaviors of its members. The former difficulty is handled through assistance provided by various public agencies. The solution to the latter rests upon the skills of the caseworker as either a counselor or as a source of referral to other professional personnel. While services in both areas are far from complete, the social service profession has taken great strides forward in the last few decades.

MEDICAL SOCIAL WORK PRACTICE

In the medical setting the social worker is concerned with the physical health of her clients as one of several important elements of social living. Although it is true that such a general statement can also be made of the social worker in a non-medical setting, it is in the health field that the physical and medical features of each case become the focal point of study. The emphasis, however, is still always placed on social aspects.

In the medical field the social worker accepts the purposes and aims of the health professions and agencies and integrates them with those of her own profession. She must be familiar with the principles and methodology not only of social work practice in general, but of medical practice as well, and she must become knowledgeable in the areas of disease and disability which affect her clients.

While it is necessary to be concerned with psychological and social variables, it can never be forgotten that with the ill person it is medical and surgical treatment which is of paramount importance. The restoration to health and function is of the greatest concern to the patient and, hence, must be to the social worker as well. Other paramedical disciplines must view themselves as functioning together with the medical therapy team as integrated services but never as of greater importance to the patient. It is true that in many cases the rehabilitation of a patient is interfered with by social and psychosocial problems which must be resolved before progress can continue and, in such instances, the social worker's role takes on added significance. On the other hand, it has been frequently found that by the time a patient is restored to health and functioning satisfactorily once again, the social problems become more easily resolved by the patient himself. This is important in rehabilitation wherein independence is a primary goal for each patient.

There have been a great number of changes in hospital service within recent years which have affected the role and function of the medical social worker. The extension of economic support to patients through various insurance and public assistance programs is, in many ways, perhaps the most important social improvement which has come to shape modern hospital service. There may often be crosswinds between "Blue Cross", "Medicare", various state and city agencies, private insurance policies, and hospital patient funding, but the general trend is decidedly towards greater financial aid for the patient who is trying to meet rising medical costs.

As hospital financing has been strengthened, more hospital personnel have been added to staffs, including more medical social workers. Furthermore, these social workers have become freed from the tasks of seeking financial aid for their clients, in large part, and have become more able to render other necessary services. Economic assistance to hospitals has also served to decrease the number of indigent patients who come to these institutions, and the general effect of this change in patient population has been to further cast the social worker in the role of a colleague of the medical and other paramedical staffs in the total care of *all* patients in the hospital—not only those on "public" wards.

Another important movement in today's hospitals is seen in the increasingly systematic way in which they are organized and administrated. Hospitals have become elaborate complexes of personnel and equipment and, as such, cannot be administered in the informal manner of the past. It may be possible to complain of "red tape" or bureaucracy, but the overall advantages to the patients outweigh these considerations.

For the social worker who is an integral part of a diagnostic and treatment team, this means a greater need for her services and more appreciation of her functions. Social work has become a planned service as all other services are, and it is no longer the haphazard, catch-as-catch-can service left to the discretion of different practitioners with varying orientations it once was. In particular, in such a vast and complex organization as the modern hospital, where the individual tends to get "lost in the shuffle," it is the social worker, with her skills and knowledge of the patients and the institution's operations, who can prevent this.

A third phase of change in hospital service concerns the new modalities of therapy being required for the chronic care patient. As man's lifespan increases, a greater number of persons are requiring long-term medical and medico-social care in hospital and related institutional settings. Each new therapeutic regime, be it in a special wing of a hospital, a home-care program, a rehabilitation maintenance program, or a working relationship with a nursing home, requires the skills of the medical social service worker. She is the best equipped staff person to bridge the gap between the hospital bed, the patient's home, and the many health and welfare services of the institution and the community.

Concurrent with these tangible evidences of change is an increased attitude of sensitivity for the *total* needs of patients. There is a new patient-centered approach to illness which did not exist a few decades ago. In such a milieu, the role of the social worker takes on additional significance. She is the one who, on the front line of patient relations, interprets hospital policy and procedures to the patient. She is the one who must know about financial support, patients' rights, referral to different hospital professionals for help or advice, recreation facilities, health plans, legal matters, housing authorities, and an almost infinite list of other details which can answer the patient's questions and meet his needs.

Notable also in today's evolving hospital movement is the growing network of relationships between the hospital and other organizations. The hospital is no longer an isolated unit sufficient unto itself; it must work together with many other public and private agencies and institutions, such as the military, government bureaus, insurance companies, nursing homes, departments of public welfare, labor boards, sheltered workshops, community citizens' groups, and so on, if it is to provide totally for its patients. It is in the maintenance of many aspects of the inter-organizational liaisons that the social worker is an expert and the key staff person. Thus, the social worker must function not only within her own institution but within the total framework of providing all of the care and services a patient needs, both within the particular hospital and outside of it as well.

SOCIAL WORK PRACTICE IN REHABILITATION

The philosophy of social work in rehabilitation medicine is the same as that of the rehabilitation field in general: it affirms that individuals can accomplish a great deal despite limitations imposed upon them by a physical disability. The emphasis is shifted, however, from the disability itself to *the person* with the disability *and his family*. Social service helps the patient and the family in their adjustment to dysfunction produced by illness or accident. The service assists them in adjusting to hospital admission, aids them during the hospitalization period, and plans and augments discharge following termination of the rehabilitation program.

The social service worker is concerned with reaching the goal of improvement in the total social functioning of the individual within limitations presented by realistic boundaries. The social worker is both patient-oriented and family-oriented and hence, must understand not only the stresses placed on the disabled individual but also the consequent problems faced by his family, employer, work associates and the special groups within which he functioned; in addition she must know how all of these people have adapted to the patient. Since such understanding is dependent, to an extent, upon knowledge from other disciplines, the social worker needs to identify with and work closely with the other members of the rehabilitation team, such as the psychologist, vocational counselor, physician and physical therapy services. Furthermore, one of the major contributions which a social worker can make in a patient's total rehabilitation stems from her familiarity with community resources and the way these can provide assistance with various problems.

Through all of her work with and for the patient the social worker bears in mind the view that the patient has worth and the right to a basic essential dignity in his own eyes and in the eyes of others; that in him there is a drive towards the potential for progressive growth and change; that each human being has an important uniqueness; that social casework seeks to enhance the worth and dignity of the client through working with him towards self-understanding and acceptance, towards reasonable accomplishment within his means, and through the respect of his family, friends and the community.

Social casework is viewed by many as the core of rehabilitation efforts. This is the one-to-one relationship between the caseworker and the client by which a particular focus of a problem, such as economic assistance, housing, adjustment to an illness, effects of disability on a family, etc. is worked through. At times, the caseworker may act as a consultant on how a bill is to be paid, while at other times she may enter into a deeper relationship with her client. In many instances public relations becomes an important factor in a case and the caseworker must therefore be adept in this area. The team approach is the key to providing maximum service to the client and social services must dovetail with the other rehabilitation disciplines, contributing knowledge but also accepting the contributions of others.

Social caseworkers direct their professional skills toward understanding the individual client not only in relation to the problems which require solution, but also in relation to those which stand in the way of solution. This understanding derives from daily observation of the client in his rehabilitation activities, in his interactions with the caseworker and with the other members of the rehabilitation team. The social worker makes a contribution through her description and interpretation of her observations of the client and of her contacts with his family. She is interested in the client's attitudes and activities in relation to the reasons for his rehabilitation, and in his reactions to the professional opinions which he hears daily regarding his current status and course of progress. The ways in which the client recognizes and deals with various aspects of the rehabilitation process, such as prostheses, wheelchairs, braces and the like, are all important for the caseworker. Thus the overall attitudes of the patient towards himself at each stage of progress, are a prime focus of the caseworker's attention.

The Role of the Caseworker

The social caseworker's role in rehabilitation can be outlined under several broad topics.

Gaining Information

The obtaining of information from the client is achieved primarily through the initial evaluation which is conducted upon the client's admission to the hospital as a patient. During this session the social worker first gains knowledge about the client and his problems.

The first step in the evaluation process is the alerting of the social worker by the central coordinator of services and scheduling, that the client is arriving at the hospital and is to be interviewed by her. The social worker may then decide to go into the client's bed area prior to her interview with him and introduce herself. Thus, when he comes to see her for the initial evaluation he will not be seeing a stranger. In the case of a client's disability preventing him from going to her office, the social worker conducts the evaluation interview at bedside.

The case worker must have certain medical information prior to the actual evaluation session so that she can conduct the interview in accordance with the client's disability. If, for example, the client is brain-injured to the extent that he cannot understand language or respond appropriately to questions, the caseworker will need to interview the client with a family member present so that all pertinent data can be obtained correctly, If a client who has sustained a recent CVA has a severe expressive or receptive aphasia, a speech clinician may be requested to assist in the evaluation. While it is important, in terms of future work with the client, to establish rapport at this initial contact, it must be remembered that the evaluation session is mainly a fact-finding period and all pertinent information must be collected from as many sources as may be able to provide it.

The caseworker is interested in the client's explanation of the reasons for his rehabilitation hospitalization. She knows the medical facts but her inquiry revolves around *the client's* perception of his disability and need for therapeutic treatment. The realities of the situation may differ from the client's beliefs and expectations, and when these are in conflict rehabilitation can be seriously hampered. In such a case referral may be necessary and a psychologist will be called upon so that unrealistic perceptions are modified and progress advanced.

The vocational and recreational activities of the client prior to the onset of his disability are discussed. The social worker is interested in the client's work history, his hobbies and his interests. His desires and life goals are also considered highly important. It is often learned that a client's aspirations have remained unaltered by the fact of his disability which now makes such hopes unrealistic. Information which is gained in these areas can be relayed to the rehabilitation counselor who is engaged in helping the client plan for his future career. The closest member of the client's family usually is also interviewed with regard to these variables so that as complete a picture as possible of the client's premorbid behavior and goals may be obtained.

In addition, the caseworker wants information on family interrelationships. The strength of the family in adjusting to, and coping with, a disabled member plays a large role in the client's adjustment to the hospital and the rehabilitation program, and also in discharge plans which must be made upon completion of the therapeutic program.

In the case of a disabled child, it is important to learn how other children in the family have been affected by the disorder and by the situation of their parents having to devote a greater percentage of their time to the disabled sibling. In what way have family relationships been affected? This is the key question to be answered at this point since it may be demonstrated that some or all of the family members will require counseling as they attempt to adjust to the handicapped individual. Whether or not the child's schooling has been interfered with is determined in order for arrangements to be made for in-hospital education and, if necessary, placement in a special class or school upon discharge.

In the very practical matter of living arrangements the social worker learns of the client's present housing accommodations and the cost of such housing. She queries the client as to the existence of architectural barriers which might seriously handicap him and she determines the transportation facilities of the client's neighborhood.

The caseworker needs to become familiar with the financial resources of the client and his family, including medical payment plans, insurance policies, workmen's compensation, public assistance, and the like. Planning a return to the home and the community is necessarily different for each client and, unless all factors are known which might influence such planning, a satisfactory arrangement cannot be made. The client who comes from an upper socioeconomic background will be planned for quite differently than the indigent client. For example, while the indigent client may live on the third floor of a "walk-up" apartment building and cannot move because of financial circumstances, the economically well endowed client probably owns his own home or lives in an apartment house with an elevator, attended by doormen and other service staff members. Should a move prove necessary in the latter case, it would present no problems. Furthermore, in the present dwelling, architectural barriers can be removed; aids, such as guardrails on stairways, assist bars in bathrooms and kitchen modifications, can be added without many difficulties. In the case of the financially underprivileged client, however, even relatively minor changes can present problems which may, at times, prove unsurmountable.

Payment of long-term hospitalization and continuing medical and therapeutic care can be arranged easily for the client with private funds, while the same treatment can be provided for the welfare recipient only if certain medical insurance plans or public assistance funds are available and applicable to the individual case. The social worker must know the client's socioeconomic status in total if his needs are to be met adequately.

Discharge plans are begun from the day of the client's admission to the hospital. This is done to prevent them from becoming an "eleventh hour" problem which can force a client to remain in the institution beyond the termination of his rehabilitation program. Visits to the client's home are made whenever their necessity is indicated. This can occur when a family member is ill and cannot come to the institution for an interview. Home visits are also made to evaluate the architectural schema of the home. Such visits may be undertaken jointly by the social worker and an occupational therapist who is able to assess the adequacy of the home for the activities of daily living which the client engages in. Home visits may also be made following discharge to learn of the client's and his family's mutual adjustment, and to determine how satisfactorily the client is able to function in his environment. (Visits to the home are also often made by a visiting nurse who will report her findings to the rehabilitation team at the hospital.)

As stated earlier in this book, following a period of approximately four to six weeks after the patient's admission to the hospital, the rehabilitation team holds a re-evaluation conference at which each team member reports on his progress and current status in each area of therapy. Prior to this conference the caseworker typically conducts a re-evaluation interview with the client. This interview is also a fact-finding session. If, from the social worker's point of view, the client had no significant problems, she probably was not working with him on a regular basis and so the re-evaluation period consists largely of reviewing many of the same topics which were discussed during the initial evaluation. The caseworker will want to know of any changes which may have occurred in the client's self-perception and in his perception of rehabilitation. She will question the client regarding new interests he might have developed, new ideas which may have been formulated about vocational or educational pursuits, changes in family relationships that have emerged, changes in finances and new living arrangements which may have been made.

Clients are usually given the period of time until the first re-evaluation conference to become adjusted to themselves and the institution. It has been learned by social workers that to initiate contact for the purpose of assisting the client to make necessary life modifications prior to such an adjustment period is usually an error. Clients need time to come to know themselves as they are following the onset of a disability and they require time to familiarize themselves with hospital routine, administrative regulations, their rehabilitation program, the staff who works with them and their fellow patients. They are not ready to discuss their social situations, and time spent attempting to do so is often fruitless and may be viewed by the client as an unpleasant and wasteful experience. Furthermore, when the adjustment period is over, the social worker who has attempted to work with the client prematurely will find that the latter will recall his negative feelings at the time and be resistant to her efforts. It cannot be stated with certainty when the initial adjustment period has passed, for this differs with each patient. The caseworker must be sensitive to her client and be able to determine through observation the appropriate time to initiate a meaningful relationship.

During the re-evaluation session problems are discussed and plans are formulated for continued social counseling as it is indicated. At this time, the caseworker may broach the question of planning in the "what if" situation—i.e., *what if* the client does not recover complete function, *what if* he cannot return home? Discharge plans are often suggested at this time which are based upon the worker's knowledge of the client's medical and social status, and later sessions may be devoted to working through any difficulties which might be connected with these plans.

At each future re-evaluation conference the social worker will report on the client's status at that time. If there are problems in any area of social functioning, she will have been counseling the client regularly and will report on progress made towards their solutions.

Typically, a social caseworker's file on a client will include an initial report based upon the evaluation, progress reports and a closing summary written upon the client's discharge. The file is seldom completely closed, however, since the client is encouraged to report back periodically regarding his adjustment to his home and community. The social worker also makes follow-up telephone calls and/or visits to the client to assess his functioning outside of the hospital and to provide aid where needed.

Communicating With Other Team Members

A second area of activity which can be subsumed within the role of the social service worker is the interpretation and communication of her findings to other members of the rehabilitation team. Although, as pointed out above, the caseworker presents her data at staff meetings, much is also accomplished through individual contacts with professionals of other services and it is often these "behind the scenes" discussions which produce the most significant results. It is at these sessions, when the details of a problem can be discussed with staff members of related disciplines, that new insights are gained as each professional contributes his unique knowledge and skills towards solution of a problem.

Liaison Services

The third facet of the social worker's role concerns enabling and preparing the client to utilize services other than social casework. Preparatory services by the caseworker are frequently necessary before an ill person will be ready to make use of the other rehabilitation therapies.

In addition to working within her own prescribed area of competence, the caseworker is the most qualified person to serve as liaison between the client, the hospital administration and the other services which the hospital offers to its patients. The caseworker also bears the responsibility of helping the clients to avoid preparation for non-existent services. She must not only clarify what she and other staff members can do for the client, but she must also delineate what cannot be done, for various reasons, in the individual case.

A FINAL WORD

It is regrettable that some social workers consider the "small jobs" such as obtaining public economic assistance, or finding adequate housing, or advising on administrative policy, or insuring that a prosthesis or wheelchair is ordered promptly, or filling out a nursing home referral form, as being beneath them as a professional. This is far from true. It is these "small jobs" which are so meaningful to the client himself in terms of fulfillment of all of the aspects of his rehabilitation. This work can be as important, or in many cases, more important than the therapy he receives for his disability.

All too frequently observed is the case of the client who has completed a program of physical rehabilitation but cannot be discharged from the hospital because of delays in finding him a home, or in delivery of a brace, cane or wheelchair. These clients often regress in their physical condition, develop decubiti or other medical problems, and become frustrated and depressed, thus undoing all of the benefits of therapy.

The social worker performs some of the most vital services in the rehabilitation setting and often the "small jobs" hold the key to the health of the clients. As stated at the outset of this chapter, the rehabilitation center which does not provide adequate social services for its patients does not conform to the positive philosophy of rehabilitation and cannot be said to truly be meeting all of the needs of its patients.

Chapter 18

THE VOCATIONAL REHABILITATION SERVICE

I N FORMER YEARS, the procedure which guided the activities of the rehabilitation counselor was to first note the disability of his client and second, to try and locate a job which someone with that particular disability could be successful at. Such an approach was obviously often fruitless. Consider, for example, the case of a quadriplegic man, paralyzed in all four extremities, with remaining movement restricted to three fingers on one hand. If a vocational counselor were to attempt to find a work position for such a client his search would be long, frustrating, and likely to terminate in disappointment. Yet, only a few short years ago this was the method of vocational casework and placement.

Today, the emphasis in vocational rehabilitation counseling has shifted from the job to the individual. That is, no longer is the client being fitted for the job, but rather the vocation is selected *on the basis of the client's needs, wishes and abilities.* Instead of attempting to locate a position which a handicapped person might possibly be able to function in, the rehabilitation counselor asks the client what he, the client, would choose as employment and then both client and counselor work together towards the preferred goal. This approach is far more rewarding than previous methods and, as a consequence of this revised thinking, rehabilitation counselors are becoming increasingly successful in satisfactorily placing their disabled clients. As with all aspects of rehabilitation, the focus is always on what the client can do, rather than on what he cannot do.

(Note: The terms *vocational counselor, vocational rehabilitation counselor* and *rehabilitation counselor* will be used interchangeably in this chapter as they are so used in the profession itself. The counselor may have a different title depending upon the institution in which he works. However, the title *rehabilitation counselor* is coming to be the generally preferred one and thus will be employed more frequently herein.)

As a member of the rehabilitation team, the counselor plays a crucial role in the restoration of the disabled person to maximum capacity. He is one of the few team members who is concerned with the patient's functioning both within the hospital setting and following discharge and, in fact, perhaps the most important aspects of the counselor's work relate to the patient's life outside of the institutional environment.

It is to be remembered that the broad goal of all rehabilitation is the restoration of the individual to as normal a life as possible within the limitations imposed upon him by physical handicap. This goal, of necessity in our society, includes gainful employment. Since a large part of our attitudes and relationships with people are contingent upon our knowledge of their occupational status, the term "restoration to as normal a life as possible" must be interpreted to include enabling the individual patient to find his place in the world of work. It is the rehabilitation counselor who is concerned primarily with vocational guidance and placement, and so plays a very direct, concrete and important role in fulfilling the philosophy of rehabilitation.

There are seven major areas of activity which comprise the work of the rehabilitation counselor. These are as follows: vocational evaluation and investigation; vocational testing; vocational counseling and planning; vocational re-evaluation; vocational placement; job analysis and engineering; and the follow-up. In some instances a client's avocational interests may also be investigated and considered for future reference, but it is primarily the wage-paying job which is of interest to the counselor.

VOCATIONAL EVALUATION AND INVESTIGATION

All new admissions to the rehabilitation hospital are scheduled for an initial evaluation by the vocational counselor. The purpose of this interview is to determine the feasibility of the client's returning to work following his hospital discharge, and also to assess his motivation, or willingness to do so. It may be said that the prognosis for future employment is more favorable for the severely disabled person who is highly motivated than for the individual with a milder disability who does not exhibit such initiative.

In this initial session the counselor attempts to compile a profile of the client's previous work history as this has been found to be the most reliable predictor of future vocational performance. Of importance is the client's attitude towards employment. If he has enjoyed his work, has advanced in his vocational line and has a history of regular, steady employment, the indications for future vocational training and placement are favorable.

On a more formal level, the counselor notes the disability of the client, whether or not he possesses or requires prosthetic devices and how satisfactorily he is able to function with such aids. He also observes the physical limitations imposed upon the client by the disability.

With regard to prostheses, for example, the question is basically one of utilization. Is the artificial limb cosmetic or functional? Can the client ambulate with a prosthetic lower extremity as well, or nearly as well, as he did with his own leg? Is he restricted in some ways, such as being unable to climb stairs? Is the client confined to wheelchair travel or does he require the use of a wheelchair only occasionally? Must the wheelchair be propelled in a particular way, such as backwards, in order for the client to function with it? How imaginative or inventive is the client in surmounting obstacles which impede him as a consequence of his handicap? The answers to these questions are crucial in the planning and placement phases of the vocational rehabilitation counselor's work.

The basic issue at stake in the assessment of physical limitations in the ability of the client to compensate for his disadvantages. It is entirely possible that a severely disabled person will demonstrate greater compensation skills than an individual with a lesser handicap and thus be a more suitable candidate for vocational guidance.

Previous hospitalizations and their causes may be important for the counselor to determine. The client who has a history of frequent illness, particularly in recent years, must be considered an employment risk. This is especially true if the illnesses are related to, or stem from, the same chronic disease, as might be the case with recurrent urinary infection associated with quadriplegia or paraplegia. The length of each hospitalization must also be considered since frequent long periods of absence from work limit the type of employment which the client can seek.

The counselor obtains a record of the client's formal education. As is true of the non-disabled person, the farther an individual has advanced through school the greater are the number of opportunities available for his consideration. In the instance of a client with little education who has a job which primarily involved physical labor and who is able to return to that job following rehabilitation, lack of formal schooling presents no particular problems. However, if the disability is of a nature which makes returning to a previous position impossible, education deficiencies can impose serious limitations. This is because those vocations for which little education is necessary generally require a strong, sound body and it is for the very reason that the client no longer possesses physical strength that he cannot engage in this type of work. The vocational potential of the uneducated, disabled person is, in fact, low. Many employers will not accept a client who has not completed high school or obtained a high school equivalency diploma. It is possible, however, for education to be obtained within the hospital setting through the cooperation of local school authorities and state organizations, thus making possible remediation of deficiencies. This will be discussed in detail in a later section of this chapter.

Specific details of the client's employment history are recorded by the rehabilitation counselor. These include the kinds of jobs which the client has held in the past and the tasks involved in each job, the length of time spent in each occupation, the salaries earned and the client's reasons for leaving each position. Beyond the factual data the counselor is interested in which jobs the client found most rewarding and which aspects of them were interesting and satisfying to him.

The question is often posed to the client: If you had a choice, disregarding your education and training, what would you have liked to do? The answers to such a question can provide the vocational counselor with many clues which can serve as an aid in future placement. Education can be provided or supplemented and training can be given which may qualify the client for a new occupation in accord with his needs and wishes. It may have been the case that a client originally became involved with a certain kind of employment because of social or situational factors which prevented other work, but now that he is unable to return to his former job action can be taken to help him reach the goals he has always really aspired to.

There are, of course, those individuals who have never been truly committed to any particular field of work and their occupational choices have been guided primarily by convenience or through following a course of least resistance. The types of positions which they held were generally fairly structured and not of the kind which generate a special interest commitment on the part of an employee. Work, then, is seen by them mainly as a source of financial support, and satisfaction is gained through the pursuit of avocational interests.

Job changes are frequent since adherence and dedication are uncommon.

In gaining a vocational picture of the client the counselor will note whether the individual has varied work experience or a substantial work history with regular progressions up the position ladder of his particular field. The client with little or no employment experience must also be considered seriously. People choose occupations largely because of experiences which they have had. Therefore, the rehabilitation counselor needs to know the variety and extent of these experiences so that he and the client can make productive use of future counseling sessions. A different kind of guidance is needed for the man who has no work experience than for the one who has a varied or a steady employment background.

The age of the client is often highly important, particularly if the counselor is confronted with an elderly person. Social and employer acceptance are an inverse function of increasing age. This is even more apparent when the older worker is physically disabled. However, the reductions of function which accompany advancing age can often be compensated for by responsibility, knowledge gained through experience, and stability, and there are many occupations where these factors are of greater importance than either speed or vitality.

Social factors are thoroughly investigated in each case. While attitudes of dependency on the part of the client may be fostered by familial overprotection thus impeding vocational planning, a family's desire to help and work with the client and the vocational counselor, plus the existence of other financial resources of the family can be great assets both in motivating the client and in sustaining him through difficult periods.

Once it is decided by the counselor that the client is a feasible candidate for vocational rehabilitation and is motivated towards that end, the client is assigned to a rehabilitation counselor who then assumes primary responsibility for guidance and placement.

VOCATIONAL TESTING

In no vocational guidance and counseling program are tests employed in an indiscriminate and automatic manner. Testing is never considered to be an end in itself but only a means to an end. The test is one step along the route to a successful vocational placement which serves to both help the client become more aware of his interests and abilities and to help the counselor learn more about the particular individual he is working with. It has been said that there is a difference between *knowing about* someone and *knowing* someone. Testing is one aid which is employed to help the rehabilitation counselor know the client, but primarily, it is used to assist the client in knowing himself.

There are several areas in which vocational testing is used and the tests are selected for administration depending upon the age, interests, needs, goals, experiences and wishes of the individual client. If the client is uncertain regarding the fields of endeavor in which his interests may lie, he may be requested to take one or more of the following: the Kuder Preference Record; the Strong Vocational Interest Blank; the Brainard Occupational Interest Inventory; or the Minnesota Vocational Interest Inventory.

Should he indicate an interest in mechanics, testing might include these: the Bennett Mechanical Comprehension Test; the Crawford Small Parts Test; the Purdue Pegboard Manual Profile; the Stromberg Dexterity Test; or the SRA Mechanical Aptitude Test.

For those clients who are considering work in the general secretarial line the appropriate instruments can be as follows: the General Clerical Test; the SRA Clerical Test; or the Stenographic Aptitude Test.

There are also specific tests for many occupations, such as the Data Processing Aptitude Test and the Maitland-Graves Design Judgement Test.

These are but a few of the many measurement tools which the vocational rehabilitation counselor has at his disposal to help the client to make a wise decision regarding his future employment.

Some clients initially refuse testing, only to request it themselves at a later date. Others may never show a willingness to be tested. There are those individuals who have certain preconceived, negative ideas about testing, or who are afraid of being tested, or who feel that testing infringes upon their personal rights or is an invasion of privacy. For such persons the counselor omits testing from his procedures. He may encourage reticent clients and explain his reasons for suggesting a formal measurement procedure, but he never imposes his will upon anyone who is opposed to being evaluated in this way.

There are also clients who are fully cognizant of their abilities and interests, and vocational testing is then considered unnecessary. Counseling and placement can proceed smoothly without it. Testing is not always considered to be a necessary prerequisite to vocational guidance and job placement. When it is useful and applicable it is employed, but the counselor is aware of contraindications to testing and proceeds accordingly.

Testing procedures in a rehabilitation setting frequently need to be modified for the disability of the individual client. Thus, tests which require responses to be written may be administered and answered orally in the case of a quadriplegic patient who does not have the use of his hands; or special consideration may be given to the hemiplegic who must take the test with his non-dominant hand; or a test will be scored as a power function only, rather than as a test of power and speed for the arthritic patient whose limited range of motion and/or pain prevents rapid responding. On the other hand, there is no reason to give special consideration to the lower extremity amputee on a timed test when testing for college aptitude is involved. His particular disability is not of a nature which would interfere with his possessing those traits which are measured by the test and which are relevant to his objectives.

In interpreting the test performance of rehabilitation patients, the counselor is aware that despite their limitations most handicapped people will be competing in the labor market with able-bodied individuals. Therefore, the testing methods, scoring and interpretation of scores should remain as close to the prescribed standards as possible, including using the norms on which the tests were developed. As pointed out above, whenever necessary, the counselor departs from standard methodology, but wherever possible, the client must be evaluated in terms of the people with whom he will be competing in the future.

It should also be remembered that while an individual may be penalized by his disability on a test, he may be an effective worker on a job as a result of the mechanical or other compensations he has made. In addition, machinery and tools can often be modified for use by handicapped people. The experienced rehabilitation counselor is knowledgable in these facts and hence, considers test performance as only one facet of a client's overall employment potential.

VOCATIONAL COUNSELING AND PLANNING

Vocational planning generally is not begun immediately following the evaluation period. A patient requires time to adjust to his disability and to the hospital and to a new way of life before he is considered "ready" for such pursuits. He must have reached some degree of health and a level of rehabilitation before discussions of future employment can be realistic and meaningful to him. Once this stage has been achieved, the counselor may initiate a relationship, although it is frequently found that the first step in vocational guidance is taken by the client.

Some Basic Viewpoints

There are several theoretical models of counseling which the rehabilitation counselor may follow in his interaction with his clients. These include those of Rogers, Thorne, Williamson, and Pepinsky, to name but a few. We are concerned here, however, not with generally applicable philosophical positions but rather with vocational selection, and in this area of specialization there are also several theories. These will now be discussed in turn.

Hoppock states that occupations are selected on the basis of how well they meet our needs, and occupational choice begins when we first become aware that an occupation can meet those needs. The choice of a job is facilitated by having information about ourselves and about occupations. We are satisfied with a job to the extent that it meets the needs which we felt it should meet, or promises to meet them in the future. An occupational choice always remains subject to change if we feel that another job will better meet our needs.

Brill, speaking from a psychoanalytic background, claims that "normal" individuals require no guidance in the selection of an occupation since they can "sense" the wisest course to follow. There is always an underlying psychic determinant which lays the foundation for a later vocational choice. Those individuals who are "sensible" neither want nor need guidance, while those who do not possess such sense will fail despite the best advice.

Caplow feels that, while we do not like to admit it, error and accident play a large role in selection of an occupation. Our choice is often dependent upon such environmental factors as a school curriculum, which is both impersonal and remote from the realities of an employment situation. It is typical for old aspirations to be abandoned in favor of more realistic choices and more limited goals. Only late in the average individual's career can he compare his expectations, aspirations and achievements and arrive at a permanent sense of complacency or frustration, or irregular fluctuations between these extremes.

Maslow postulates a hierarchy of needs which is related to the choice of an occupation. There are physiological needs, safety needs, belongingness needs, esteem needs and the need for self-actualization. An individual will select a vocation which is commensurate with his own personal need structure. When environmental conditions are such that the person cannot choose an occupation which meets his needs, he will become dissatisfied with his work and seek avocational interests which will satisfy them.

Ginzberg believes occupational choice to be an ongoing process which takes place over a period of several years. The fantasy period is one in which the child considers an occupation in terms of his wish to be an adult. The tentative period brings about the realization that he has a problem of occupational choice and must begin to consider factors of reality. The realistic period is based heavily upon reality and the individual realizes that he must work out a compromise. Each decision made during adolescence is related to prior experiences and influences the next decision, but the process of arriving at decisions is essentially irreversible. Occupational choice is the end product of combining elements of subjectivity with the limitations or reality and is, inevitably, a compromise.

Super proposes a theory of vocational development. People differ in their interests and abilities, and each person is qualified for a number of occupations. Occupations also permit some variety among the individuals who enter them. Vocational choice and adjustment is a continuous process. This process is basically one of developing and implementing a self-concept. It can be explained in a series of life stages—growth, exploration, establishment, maintenance and decline.

While a rehabilitation counselor may feel that one or another of these theories of occupational choice is "correct", and may choose to work within such a framework, he obviously cannot adhere dogmatically to any one of them. This is simply because none mention, or attempt in any way to deal with, the physically disabled; and yet in rehabilitation it is frequently the case that the disability of the client is the major factor in the selection of an occupation. Even where it may not be the only, or even the primary consideration, the disability always plays a large role in any decision-making in which the client engages. The rehabilitation counselor, therefore, must modify his theoretical approach to include those variables which are not considered by existing viewpoints.

Steps in Pre-Vocational Planning

Prior to beginning counseling with a client the counselor reviews all of the data which has been collected up to that point. This material will include the information gained from the initial evaluation, testing and social history, plus information about the client's disability, physical limitations, education, motivation, self-concept and attitudes towards work. Assuming that the client is considered to be a feasible candidate for vocational guidance, planning is initiated through active participation of both client and counselor.

It has been learned that unless a client actively engages in his own vocational planning, the likelihood of successful placement is small. It is true that a client can remain passive while the counselor decides on an occupation for him and places him in a job, but in such a case the client has no "stake" in the selection and determination of a highly important part of his future life. Unless there is a personal involvement, a commitment on the part of the client, work satisfaction will probably be slight and frequent job changes can be expected. Every counselor is aware of this and therefore encourages as much active participation as possible by the client.

It is usually a wise procedure for the rehabilitation counselor to begin vocational planning by listening to the client's ideas and his thoughts about occupations. What the client is interested in doing provides the first stepping stone to further exploration and discussion. It not only gives the counselor leads as to the client's interests and aspirations, but also provides him with insight into possible difficulties which might arise in attempting to meet those wishes and permits him to judge how realistically the client views himself in relation to the world of work.

Once the client has expressed his views the vocational counselor is able to discuss them with him. They may be rational and realistic, and planning can then progress relatively smoothly. Educational and vocational training programs may have to be utilized before the final goal is reached, but decisions of occupational choice and resolution of obstacles in the path of such decisions do not play a predominant role in the counseling sessions. The counselor may produce data obtained from tests, interviews and the reports of the other rehabilitation services which confirm the soundness of selection. He may also employ occupational information as found in the *Dictionary of Occupational Titles (DOT)* or the *Occupational Outlook Handbook (OOH)* as aids in learning more about the client's particular choices. When such information further supports the client's thoughts, planning moves ahead in a meaningful way.

However, it is often the case that clients are uncertain about their interests or have unrealistic ideas concerning the type of vocation which they should enter. The counselor will discuss their views to learn the reasons for a particular choice and to find possible alternatives in the client's thinking. Should the client feel strongly about his preference, having considered no alternative possibilities, the counselor may wish to discuss his test results and other reports with him. For the client who has no firm conception of employment the counselor can point out where he scored highly on interest tests and on tests of specific abilities. Then, through the use of the *DOT* or the *OOH*, the details of jobs related to the client's interests and abilities are explained to him, and possibilities for entry into such occupations are explored.

In the instance of a client who has made an unrealistic vocational choice, the test results can be used to point out to him reasons for altering his decision and considering other areas suggested by the counselor. The *DOT* and the *OOH* are employed to assist the client towards a wiser selection. Counseling is a slow, gradual process of learning and achieving insight, but as every counselor knows, the satisfaction which is gained from helping an individual to return to a productive life is great.

Assistance in Training for Future Placement

An integral part of the planning phase is training. Training can be either educational or vocational in nature, or both, and it is often related to the kinds of goals which the client has set for himself. Let us now examine two possible long-range plans, one involving education and the other involving vocational training.

If a client wishes to attend college and test results indicate that he possesses the intellectual capacity for such an undertaking, a plan can be devised whereby he can attend school while still an in-patient at the rehabilitation hospital. Funds are available from state or federal government agencies for the cost of tuition, textbooks and other school-related expenses. The hospital can provide transportation to and from classes, again financed by government sources or occasionally by the hospital itself, and often, in addition, a "guide" can be provided who will aid the client in navigating stairs, corridors, etc., should the client be handicapped by a wheelchair or other device, will assist him in carrying materials, and may even take notes for him in class, since there are some instructors who do not permit the use of a tape recorder in the classroom regardless of the circumstances. It should be added parenthetically that the supplying of such a guiding person to a client is very rare and may only be seen in very special cases.

When there is some doubt as to the ability of a client to succeed in college, a curriculum consisting of only one or two courses can be arranged with the school as a "trial period" before the client assumes a full program of study.

If the educational goal is a high school diploma, local schools are contacted and most will make certain concessions regarding course or credit hour requirements. Often teachers or guidance counselors are willing to work closely with the disabled student to help him to overcome difficulties, many of which cannot be anticipated before the student actually enters the academic setting. For the client who, because of the nature of his disability, must remain bedridden within the hospital, many cities have local television stations which broadcast high school courses that are accredited towards a diploma. There is, in addition, a device known as Executone®, manufactured by the Bell Telephone Company, which permits the hospitalized student to listen to what is occurring in the classroom and to also ask questions of the teacher and participate in class discussion directly from special booths in the hospital. This apparatus can be used for high school and college study and enables the severely disabled individual, such as a respirator-bound, post-poliomyelitis patient, to actually be a participating member of his class.

When an individual is not able to participate in or benefit from higher academic instruction, but test results and other data indicate that he can profit from long-term vocational training, both hospital services and outside industry can cooperate to assist him. For example, some large corporations, such as the Bulova Watch Company, will accept disabled persons for a one-year, on-the-job training program, and will then, upon successful completion of this program, employ these individuals.

Should the client and his vocational counselor be uncertain regarding the exact type of employment which would be most suited to the client's needs and abilities, a general vocational evaluation program can be arranged through the hospital's own facilities or through various city and state agencies.

Many rehabilitation institutions have a pre-vocational shop which is usually under the aegis of either the Occupational Therapy Service or the Vocational Rehabilitation Service. Here, the client can be evaluated as to his skills in operating a key-punch machine, telephone switchboard, typewriter and other office equipment, computer programming apparatus, photographic equipment and the like. Arrangements are often made between the client's hospital and other hospitals and agencies which will evaluate his abilities and train him for future employment.

One such institution which provides these services in the ICD Rehabilitation and Research Center in New York City. Some of the areas in which a client's skills can be assessed at ICD include optics, jewelry making, leather craft, clerical work, sewing, machine and lathe operation, and tool and die work. These assessments are not made for the purpose of specific employment, but rather to learn what skills a client possesses. Once a client demonstrates abilities in an area he may be given a period of training in that field and then re-evaluated following the training to determine what he has learned, how interesting the work was to him, and how motivated he is to remain in that line of work.

Assistance in training and placing the physically disabled can frequently be obtained from federal or state funding agencies. The Vocational Rehabilitation Administration in Washington, D.C. is the federal office which provides economic aid, either through direct funding or through local agencies which are under the national administration. These sources arrange for training, education, placement, transportation and, in fact, any aspect of vocational rehabilitation may be covered by their policies. They are typically supported in part by the state and in part by the federal government, but are under local administration. Placement is often made through the local State Employment Service's special section for placement of the handicapped.

The Developing Role of the Government

It may be of interest to the reader to learn how government support for the handicapped evolved.

In 1911, ten states enacted workmen's compensation statutes which survived various constitutional tests. This occurred on the heels of failures of similar attempts by Montana in 1909 and New York in 1910.

A section to provide for the rehabilitation of civilian employees of the United States government, who had become permanently disabled in the course of their employment, was initially included in a bill establishing rehabilitation services for disabled veterans of World War I. This section was later removed and a separate bill was introduced which encompassed rehabilitation for all disabled civilians. It became law in 1920 as the Federal Vocational Rehabilitation Act, although even prior to the enactment of this federal legislation several states already had their own vocational rehabilitation laws, with most of them being restricted to benefits for the industrially injured.

It was from these concepts of rehabilitating veterans and compensating workers injured on the job, that the philosophy of rehabilitation services for all disabled persons who needed them emerged.

Congress, however, did not vote such policy into permanent legislation for many years, and so this first federal law had to be reviewed every three years for fifteen years until the Social Security Act of 1935 established a public vocational rehabilitation program on a permanent basis.

The next significant advance came with the passage of the Barden-LaFollette Act of 1943 which authorized rehabilitation services for the mentally handicapped, use of federal funds by state agencies for rehabilitation of the blind, and additional rehabilitation services to those previously available through the public agencies.

Perhaps the greatest step forward has resulted from the Vocational Rehabilitation Amendments of 1954. What amounted to essentially a totally new program was established. Measures now made it possible to establish a research demonstration grant program, to institute a training program designed to increase the number of qualified rehabilitation personnel, to encourage the expansion of rehabilitation facilities, to improve the administrative structure of the program, and to facilitate cooperative activity between state agencies and nonprofit, voluntary organizations.

There are, today, vocational rehabilitation agencies in all fifty states, the District of Columbia, Puerto Rico, Guam and the Virgin Islands, which provide the services necessary for returning the disabled individual to work. The federal government's responsibilities are centered in the Vocational Rehabilitation Administration which is under the auspices of the United States Department of Health, Education and Welfare.

In order for an individual to be eligible for such services he must have a mental or physical disability which substantially interferes with suitable employment, and he must offer a reasonable expectation that, once he is provided with rehabilitation services, he will be capable of employment. To determine this eligibility the state agency must obtain all relevant information concerning the client's current medical status, psychological adjustment, social history, educational and vocational background, functional limitations, employment prospects, and availability of vocational rehabilitation services. This information is gained from the client's rehabilitation institution and the agencies where he may have been evaluated for skill assessment and training. Contact is initiated by the rehabilitation counselor, and the state then works together with the counselor to provide needed services and funds.

VOCATIONAL RE-EVALUATION

The rehabilitation counselor is expected to report at the periodic re-evaluation conferences with regard to the advances his clients are making. The counselor who is working with a client on a regular basis is familiar with all aspects of the client's course of progression and he informs the rehabilitation team as to the way vocational planning is proceeding. This report will include the various assessments which have been made in a workshop or other agency of the client's skills, the nature of the training or education which the client may be involved in, learning ability which the client is demonstrating, the client's initiative, his current level of motivation and tentative future plans.

If the client has been dissatisfied with his original plans regarding an occupational choice, he may have been re-tested so as to learn of other interests or abilities which he possesses, or further testing may have been indicated to ascertain what he has learned *since* being in a training program. In either case, the test findings are reported at the re-evaluation conference and are interpreted to the rehabilitation staff members in terms of their meaning for the client's future. It is not unusual for therapeutic programs and discharge plans to be largely dependent upon vocational plans, and it is through the medium of the re-evaluation conference that the rehabilitation team learns of the client's status and progress, and can plan his future program accordingly.

VOCATIONAL PLACEMENT

The rehabilitation counselor accepts the responsibility for the placement of his clients. In vocational counseling it is *the final outcome* which is important. The disabled client who has completed his rehabilitation program, who has come to accept a handicap, who is aware of his limitations and abilities, and who is adequately trained, but yet who has not achieved a reasonable level of vocational adjustment, has not been rehabilitated in the full sense of the word.

Any plan for the vocational placement of disabled persons is based upon the same principles as those which are involved in the effective employment of able-bodied workers. In essence, this means matching people with the jobs for which they are suited by virtue of age, education, experience, interests, skills and physical abilities. In some instances finding employment for the handicapped may appear to be a relatively simple matter. An individual with a unilateral below-knee amputation might easily be placed in a lower level job, such as an elevator operator, for example, but in such a case, while the problem has been solved in one sense, this placement has missed the mark of true rehabilitation. It has not considered the skills and interest of the client and therefore must be termed unsatisfactory.

Vocational planning and placement can take place on a relatively short-term basis. That is, there are schools which provide six-week to six-month training periods for jobs requiring minimal skill or which retrain and/or review previous skills. Following this brief training the counselor initiates placement procedures. In an even more rapid fashion the client may be placed in a job immediately following the initial investigation and evaluation period if the nature of his disability and therapeutic requirements are such that they permit it. However the majority of cases which are encountered in a physical medicine and rehabilitation institution require more intensive placement work.

Obtaining a Job

In order for the rehabilitation counselor to function successfully he must constantly be aware of job opportunities in the community and he must be familiar with the steps which are necessary to secure vacant positions for his clients. There are several sources which provide the counselor with information regarding employment opportunities. These are described below.

The Client

It has been learned that in recent years almost one-half of all rehabilitation clients who were candidates for work were able to find their own jobs without placement assistance from their counselor. Clients typically learn of opportunities from friends and relatives, former co-workers, and from knowledge based upon their past experience. Information frequently comes from the counselor's former clients who keep him informed as to their progress and to vacancies which become available in their own place of employment.

The Counselor's List of Employer Contacts

The effective counselor is one who knows employers and, in turn, is known to them. Over the years, counselors develop a list of businessmen who are willing to hire disabled persons.

It is considered advantageous for the counselor to speak with a prospective employer about a client and inform him specifically of the client's disability and limitations so as to avoid "surprising" him, thus preventing future biases against hiring the handicapped. Some counselors make a practice of first referring several clients who are excellent vocational prospects to an employer before asking him to accept a greater risk with a client whose potential is perhaps not as high. If the employer has had satisfactory experiences in the past with disabled workers, he will be more willing to "take a chance" with a client regarding whom the counselor may have certain reservations. The relationships which a rehabilitation counselor develops with private employers, are invaluable in helping his clients to obtain the positions they seek.

The State Employment Services

As mentioned previously, state employment services maintain a section for placement of the handicapped. It provides testing, counseling and placement services, as well as supplying information on job opportunities within the state and in other states, and the rehabilitation counselor often takes advantage of these facilities.

The Vocational Rehabilitation Act of 1965, Public Law 89–33, states that the State Plan shall provide for cooperation with public employment offices in the state and should make maximum use of job placement, vocational counseling services and other services and facilities provided by these offices. The responsibility for the utilization of these services rests with the counselor.

Since both public employment offices and vocational rehabilitation agencies offer placement assistance, there often appears to be duplication of function. However, the important fact to know is that it is the counselor who is ultimately responsible for placement of each client accepted for service. This is true even though the client may secure his own job or may actually be placed by a training agency or rehired by a former employer.

Obligation for successful placement is the counselor's. It should also be realized that when a vocational counselor in a rehabilitation hospital refers a client to the state employment services this does not end his responsibility to that individual. The state services are utilized in addition to, not in lieu of, other community resources and only supplement the counselor's continuing efforts to locate employment for his clients. It is frequently a combination of the endeavors of both the rehabilitation counselor and the state agency which results in suitable occupational placement.

Former Employers

One of the sources which is first contacted by the rehabilitation counselor upon the client's completion of his rehabilitation program and, in fact, usually prior to such time, is the client's former employer. If the client was a skillful, reliable employee prior to the onset of his disability, and if the counselor can convince the employer that the client is still able to satisfactorily function on the job, this can be an extremely fruitful source to tap.

Many counselors feel that if the client sustained his injury while on the job the employer *may* rehire him from a sense of responsibility. While this can be true it is more gratifying for a client to be rehired because he can still be an able worker and also because his success can pave the way for other disabled individuals with that employer. The rehabilitation counselor is primarily concerned with the client of the hour, but he is also greatly interested in overcoming employers' prejudices regarding the handicapped so that there will be more opportunities for his future clients.

Classified Advertisements

Some counselors believe that the "help wanted" columns of the daily newspapers are a good source for locating positions. Through pursuing these advertisements they come into direct contact with employers who have an immediate need for workers. Many counselors who use the newspapers in this way prefer to let the client contact the prospective employer. Often, this approach will make a better impression than if the counselor called on behalf of the client. Furthermore, it gives the client experience in obtaining his own employment.

Business Reports

Newspaper accounts, industrial reports and surveys conducted by a chamber of commerce can be sources of information for the counselor regarding business and industrial relocations in the community, expansions of existing facilities and job trends which might provide leads which the counselor can take advantage of in assisting his clients. There are occupations which are seasonal, cyclic in nature, or fluctuate due to changes in supply and demand which, if the counselor maintains his awareness, can yield opportunities for the qualified client.

New Enterprises

When the rehabilitation counselor becomes familiar with his territory he can find leads to jobs in the construction of new enterprises, such as service stations, factories and franchised operations. By knowing of such new or forthcoming ventures he may be able to "get in on the ground floor". If he waits until they are completed and engaged in business it may be too late to place a disabled client. This points out the need for the counselor to have his "finger on the pulse" of the community which he services.

Training Agencies

The various training agencies in the community, such as colleges, technical, trade and vocational schools, high schools, workshops, etc., have their own lists of employer contacts. They can often supply the rehabilitation counselor with leads to employment openings. Most of these agencies will furnish leads even to those clients who are not a part of their program if they do not have a trainee who is qualified for a particular vacancy.

Key Worker Contacts

Interestingly, it is often not the employer in a company who is the best source of occupational information, but the worker. Vocational counselors know certain key employees in business and industry who are aware of openings due to dismissal, retirement, resignation, operation changes and the like even before the administrative office does. He can speak with these workers on a more informal basis than he can to their administration, and via the "grapevine" can get an early start on position openings.

Civil Service and Merit System Examinations and Employment Announcements

One large field of employment, regardless of the type of work which a client is skilled at, is the goverment—federal, state, county and local. Federal agencies and many state and some local governments have adopted the policy that an individual cannot be denied employment because of a disability, as long as he is qualified, can perform the duties of the job without risk to himself and co-workers, and can pass the necessary civil service examination. Announcements of these examinations and job opportunities with specifications regarding qualifications, pay scales, duties and locations are posted regularly in post offices and other public buildings, and are published in public media. If the client is interested in a government position and is qualified for the work, the counselor can investigate such announcements and assist the client with making the necessary preparations.

The Labor Unions

Business managers, stewards and their union personnel are usually quite familiar with local and national events which affect the employment of the union members and hence, can prove to be an important fund of information. Direct job referrals are generally reserved for union members only, but a disabled person may have been a member prior to the onset of his disability and therefore can utilize his union's resources. Even if the client is not a member, the union may be called upon by the counselor for job leads in different fields of work.

Trade Associations

Many kinds of businesses organize associations to promote their mutual interests. This often include the recruitment of qualified personnel. In metropolitan areas some trade associations maintain employment offices for their members, and officials of these groups can provide occupational information which is current and local and can be of assistance to the rehabilitation counselor.

Client Advisory Committees

A counselor may organize a temporary committee of people drawn from the community to advise and assist him with placement of a particular client. The committee members participate on a voluntary basis and are selected from the community because of their interest in rehabilitation and in the client involved. They are citizens of recognized leadership and status who are familiar with local resources and as such can be of much value in solving a counselor's problem. Once the client for whom the committee was formed is successfully placed in a job, the committee is disbanded.

Civic and Religious Organizations

Civic and service clubs in the community are usually prepared to meet requests for assistance to the handicapped. Religious organizations will aid in the rehabilitation of their members. Special interest groups, such as the United Heart Association, United Cerebral Palsy, and Multiple Sclerosis Societies can be of great help in obtaining information for the placement of individuals with particular disabilities.

JOB Committees

JOB (Just One Break) committees function in a manner similar to that of the client advisory committee, with the exception that they are continuing groups working on the problems of *many* individuals rather than temporary ones concerned with placing one particular individual. JOB functions to coordinate the work of the rehabilitation agencies with various private and public employment services. Its members are drawn from industry and labor and are involved in a continuous program of community relations. If a client qualifies for JOB consideration and assistance, placement is usually relatively rapid.

The Client and the Employer

Once the rehabilitation counselor has located a potential employer he must then arrange for him to meet with the client. It is assumed that at this time the position for which the client is applying is one which meets his needs and is commensurate with his abilities.

It is incumbent upon the counselor to present as clear and as accurate a picture of his client as possible to the prospective employer. Naturally, confidences are not revealed and it is always the best interests of the client which the counselor has in mind. Nonetheless, the counselor must be fair with the employer. Medical information, psychological and social data and vocational facts are presented wherever applicable, and the employer is made aware of the client's physical limitations. Not only is honesty the best policy for a particular client's welfare, but also to prevent future prospective clients from being discriminated against in hiring procedures.

It may be up to the counselor to arrange for an interview between his client and the prospective employer, but it is the client himself who must speak with the latter alone. This is the practice with non-disabled workers and there is no reason for the physically handicapped to follow a different procedure. After the interview the client and the counselor will discuss what transpired and together they can arrive at certain conclusions regarding the advisability of the client's accepting the available position. The employer may also call the counselor to inform him of impressions of the client or to request additional information. Perhaps a second meeting between the employer and the client will be deemed necessary.

If the employer decides against hiring the client it is the counselor's obligation to learn the reasons for the decision. If it was based solely on the fact that the client was disabled, the counselor will want to correct misconceptions which the employer may have regarding the handicapped. If the client was not hired because of a lack of education or certain basic skills the counselor will try to ascertain if further training will later make the client eligible for the position. If the client simply did not "fit" the expectations of the employer for the particular job in question, the counselor can attempt to obtain leads to other openings in the same field of work. It is often what the counselor learns from the client and the employer subsequent to the job interview, that is most helpful in future placement.

JOB ANALYSIS AND ENGINEERING

While there may be jobs available which appear suitable for a disabled person and although the client in question might indicate a high level of motivation for a vacant position, placement can still present certain difficulties. It is therefore obligatory for the vocational rehabilitation counselor to make an analysis of the job prior to the client's entry into it.

A job analysis is a thorough study of the physical and psychological qualifications required for the occupation, the amount of responsibility to be assumed, and the initiative, judgement and adaptability necessary for success. It takes into account the environmental working conditions, the hours of labor involved and the characteristics of the administration and the other employees. Such a study usually only can be made in the actual setting in which the client will work— the shop, store, factory or office where his working time will be spent. Only by undertaking such research can the counselor be assured of the suitability of his client for the position and vice versa.

It is highly important for the rehabilitation counselor to communicate to the employer that his client is ready and able to compete, without any special considerations, for employment in his chosen occupational field. However, it may be learned from a job analysis, or from a visit to the plant, or from a conversation with the client that he would be able to perform at an even higher level of competence if some minor modifications were made in the work situation.

These changes might include seating arrangements, placement of tools, redirection of lighting, re-arrangement of some equipment controls, and so on. While requesting such changes of an employer can result in extra expenditures for the company, or possible prejudice on the part of the other workers, or reluctance by the company to hire additional disabled personnel, they also can produce better functioning on the job for the client and, at times, for all of the workers in a particular industry. When the latter is the case, production is increased, money is saved and better relations are secured betwen the counselor, the client and the company.

THE FOLLOW-UP

The obligation of the rehabilitation counselor to his client does not end with the placement of the client in a job. It is the counselor's responsibility to follow up such placement to determine if the client is employed according to his potential, if he is happy with his work, and if the employer is satisfied with him. With some cases the counselor may follow up within only one week of placement, while with others he may wait several months. Such consideration is dictated by the circumstances of the individual case. The usual period of follow-up is initiated from fifteen to thirty days post-placement. This gives the client the opportunity to adjust to the job situation and to formulate some opinions about his work. It also permits the employer and the co-workers to judge the client's acceptability, both as a worker and as a person.

Additional follow-ups can be scheduled at sixty-day and ninety-day intervals for a period of several months. The counselor prepares a schedule for visits so that he can speak with his client and confer with the employer regarding satisfactions and problems which have arisen. Without a suitable follow-up period the counselor cannot be certain of the success of his client's placement.

SOME PROBLEMS

The rehabilitation counselor's row is a difficult one to hoe. There are numerous difficulties to be faced at every step, from the initial interview to the final follow-up after a client has been placed on a job. Most of these cannot be entirely anticipated and provided for. There are, however, some obstacles which are frequently encountered by the counselor and are therefore important to discuss at this time.

The attitudes of employers are a frequent stumbling block to placement of the disabled. Despite current information on how well the handicapped perform on a job if they are given the opportunity, and despite the encouragement and urging given to employers via public media messages, a large percentage of companies are reluctant to hire a physically disabled person. Much of the uphill battle of placing a disabled worker is spent trying to overcome the prejudices of prospective employers and convincing them that the hiring of the disabled is good business practice.

The counselor can point out to the employer the results of a survey taken by the Civil Service Commission which found that disabled workers perform as well or better than able-bodied employees in both quantity and quality of work produced; that handicapped workers have a far lower rate of attrition; that handicapped workers have fewer time-lost accidents than the non-handicapped; and that handicapped workers' absentee records compare favorably with the records of able-bodied employees. He can also point out that a company's insurance rates are not affected by hiring the disabled, as many employers erroneously believe. The counselor can add that the employer is performing a much needed public service by giving work to a disabled person. The most persuasive argument, however, is the successful performance of the client himself. If a counselor can get his "foot in the door" with a firm, and if the client who is placed there works out satisfactorily on the job, this provides the best reason for hiring more disabled individuals in the future.

Architectural barriers often present a major difficulty for the disabled individual. At present, the majority of homes, apartment buildings, shops, factories, industrial plants, office buildings, colleges and universities do not provide special access for the disabled person, particularly those who must travel in a wheelchair. Doorways are too narrow, particularly in bathrooms, the only entrances to buildings are staircases, and no provisions are made for avoiding "rush hour" periods. It is true that this situation is being slowly corrected, most notably in colleges and universities, and that such architectural changes as are necessary are quite costly, but as a consequence of present inadequacies many handicapped persons are being denied the right to attend the school of their choice or to work at the job for which they are suited. They simply cannot get into the buildings.

It is hoped that the needed changes will come about more rapidly and be more encompassing as the public learns how vital these people are to the nation's growth.

Transportation of the disabled is a very great problem. At this time, in New York City, for example, only private companies engage in such work. They are quite expensive, the usual rate being from one dollar to $1.25 per mile. Furthermore, there are no regulations governing the safety of these vehicles for the passengers. Wheelchairs frequently tip over or crash into other passengers presenting a real hazard. In addition, such transportation is often unreliable, arriving late, too early, and sometimes, not at all.

Another undesirable feature is the fact that a private car may pick up several passengers before depositing one. Thus, a man who must get to his place of employment only five miles away from his home will be picked up, driven ten miles in a different direction to pick up a second person, then driven another five miles for a third, and finally, be taken to work. A five mile trip has turned into a thirty-five mile one.

What is needed in the area of transportation is legislation on fares, safety, and obligation to the disabled person who is dependent upon private companies, and the establishment of much needed public conveyances for the handicapped.

IN CONCLUSION

Vocational counseling is the newest of the rehabilitation services. The work is arduous, fraught with difficulties and frustrations, and often tedious. The counselor must operate not only within a medical setting but he must work with clients who have some of the severest disabilities known to Man. He must consistently interact with a community which is reluctant to accept his efforts and recommendations. Yet, his is a most rewarding kind of work. He is rehabilitating an individual in the full sense of the word. He is not only providing a job and its financial rewards, but he is giving his clients dignity. He is restoring self-confidence, a feeling of worthiness, a sense of belonging to society, and of being truly needed by that society. He is giving his clients a reason to live. He is giving them back a part of their soul.

Chapter 19

THE RECREATION SERVICE

ALL OF THE SCHEDULED SERVICES which are offered by a rehabilitation institution are geared directly towards improving the medico-physical and psychological functioning of the patients. This is also true of the Recreation Service, for although the activities which it provides are primarily diversional, it is unquestionably the case that there is measurable improvement in the general health of the patients who engage in these activities.

The Recreation Service, however, is unique among the rehabilitation services in that it is not typically a scheduled part of a patient's therapy program. This might be considered unfortunate since recreation curricula undoubtedly contribute to the patients' total rehabilitation, but the fact remains that patients usually are only seen in recreation when they have available time following completion of their daily therapeutic regimen. This situation probably exists because of the relative newness of reacreation to the field of rehabilitation medicine and because many physicians have not yet come to realize the importance of leisure time activity. As the values of such activity continue to be domonstrated, recreation will become an increasingly integral part of each patient's total rehabilitation program.

It is the philosophy of the Recreation Service that each patient is a person, an individual—and not merely an amputee, or a cardiovascular disorder, or a neuromuscular disease—and as such has many needs which should be met in addition to those which are treated by the medical and behavioral sciences. Thus, recreation attempts to bridge the gap which exists between the hospital and the life which the patient led prior to his hospitalization.

Since the nature of the disabilities which necessitate rehabilitation institutionalization are such that the hospitalization period is a comparatively lengthy one, effort is expended to make hospital life resemble premorbid life as closely as possible. Thus, the patients are provided with opportunities to engage in as many activities which they formerly enjoyed as is feasible within the institutional setting. Furthermore, since hospitalization is rarely a pleasant existence, the Recreation Service plays an important role in making this period of a patient's life more bearable. The activities in which the patient takes part help to make the time seem to pass more rapidly and provide a measure of enjoyment in an otherwise dull, and often unpleasant, day. These activities enable the patient to eagerly anticipate at least some portion of his waking hours and often serve as a "reward" for strenuous participation on a therapy program, although, of course, they are not so intended.

In addition, the very existence of certain recreational activities, such as out-trips from the hospital, can serve as motivating events for the patient to progress in his physical therapies. Such outings are more enjoyable for a patient when he is able to ambulate independently rather than being confined to a wheelchair. Improvement in the tasks of occupational therapy may enable a patient to participate in certain games and events which he would be unable to engage in if he were in a less functional condition. Therefore, the patient becomes more motivated to do well in the occupational therapy area.

The purposes, therefore, of the Recreation Service are to provide opportunities for the patients to voluntarily participate in activities during leisure time which are socially acceptable and constructive in nature, and which offer immediate and direct satisfaction. This service presents a variety of activities of a diversional nature from which the patients derive enjoyment and attain a greater deegree of health. The patients are additionally helped to develop proper attitudes towards the effective use of leisure time and many learn skills which permit them to pursue an activity of interest upon their return to their home and the community.

A BRIEF HISTORY OF HOSPITAL RECREATION

Although the history of recreation as a form of medical therapeutics can be traced back to ancient Egypt when the Egyptians recognized the importance of games and music for the relief of depression, recreation has only expanded into the hospital milieu since World War I. Hospital administrators were alerted to the values of recreational diversions for patients by the American Red Cross which provided incidental recreation services to the servicement who were hospitalized during the war. Until 1931, recreation leaders and activity therapy services were furnished by the Red Cross to military and veterans' hospitals. In that year, the recreation programs in veterans' hospitals were encompassed within the United States Veterans' Bureau.

During the 1920's and 1930's, recreation programs began to appear in some of the state-operated psychiatric hospitals and in schools for the intellectually retarded. Most of the programs were conducted by untrained personnel and were of a purely diversional nature, yet they did make a contribution to the hospitals' treatment programs.

It was not until 1960 that recreation in veterans' hospitals came under the supervision of the Department of Physical Medicine and Rehabilitation. Recreation programs became available to patients on general medical and surgery units, tuberculosis wards, orthopedic wards and neuropsychiatric units. The types of activities programmed for each unit were as different as the diverse patient populations, with each type of patient receiving a unique form of recreation program. When the recreation activities were developed and programmed to meet the needs of specific individuals or groups of individuals, the concept of recreation in a medical setting began to change and to take on the pattern of true medical and therapeutic recreation.

Today, almost all rehabilitation institutions have a recreation department within the department of rehabilitation medicine. The 1960's have been the time for the entry and expansion of recreation services into the physical rehabilitation field, and the contributions of these services are becoming increasingly important for the welfare of the disabled patients.

THE RECREATION STAFF

Although the Recreation Service of a rehabilitation hospital can design a complete program of many diverse activities, it cannot guarantee that patients will attend scheduled events or participate in the activity programs. Patients typically are preoccupied with their medical problems and physical status and often are apathetic regarding extracurricular activities. It is one matter to plan a recreation program and quite another to gain patient involvement, particularly when it is difficult for the patients to participate because of an overrriding physical disability.

Patients frequently do not initially understand the values of such participation. It is therefore incumbent upon the recreation workers to not only plan a curriculum, but also to assure patient attendance. Such a task requires the skills of a dedicated and qualified staff who enjoy working with people and who are willing to expend much effort to achieve their goals.

There must be a constant flow of communication between the recreation worker who is assigned to a particular patient floor or ward, and the patients on the unit. Only when the worker and the patients have come to know each other well and good rapport between them has been established, will the worker be able to involve the patients in the recreation programs.

The number and kind of staff which comprises the Recreation Service varies between institutions. There are, however, many basic similarities, particularly with regard to the qualifications of the recreation workers and the job responsibilities of each staff member. The following description may be considered to be "typical" of a recreation department in a rehabilitation hospital where a well developed recreation program has become a part of the services which are offered to the patients.

The Director of the department is an individual who has obtained at least an M.A. degree in therapeutic recreation or in an associated social science from a recognized college or university. He has had at least five years of experience at the level of Assistant Director or Recreation Supervisor in addition to other professional experience.

The Director's role is essentially an administrative one. He plans a recreation program based upon his knowledge of the individual needs and interests of the patients in the institution, and thus bears the primary responsibility for scheduling events and activities. In addition, he prepares reports on the program's progress which are presented at staff meetings over which he presides. The Director maintains records and reports of the patients' responses to the recreation programs.

It is his duty to prepare budget requests and to obtain the authorization of the hospital administration on expenditures for recreation services and supplies. Interpretations of the goals and procedures of the recreation programs are made by the Director to the hospital staff and volunteer workers, to the relatives of patients and to the public at large.

He directs volunteer activities and provides training, supervision and placement services for volunteers and for students who are in training to become recreation workers. The Director represents his department and the hospital at local, regional and national meetings and conferences which deal with therapeutic recreation.

The Director is also the person who advises and counsels families of patients as to the proper activities to initiate upon the patients' discharge to the home, and he is the primary source of information on community recreation facilities to which the patients can be referred once they leave the hospital setting.

The Recreation Supervisor possesses either a Master's degree in therapeutic recreation for the ill and handicapped and has completed one year of work experience, or has a Master's degree in therapeutic recreation plus at least two years of experience in working with the sick and disabled, or has earned a B.A. degree with a major in therapeutic recreation and has been working with the disabled for at least four years. He works under the general supervision of the Director and is responsible for the conduct of the total recreation program. He acts as the Assistant Director of the Recreation Service.

Among the numerous job responsibilities of the Recreation Supervisor is the supervision of the Recreation Leaders and Assistants in the planning, organizing and conducting of the various hospital programs. It is his responsibility to schedule staff and program assignments. In addition, the Supervisor orders supplies, keeps inventory records, reviews and evaluates reports submitted by staff members, keeps progress records of patients on the different recreation programs, assists in assigning patients to activities, arranges for workshops, plans social events and out-trips, and bears the responsibility for the safety of equipment and facilities which are used in the recreation programs.

The Recreation Supervisor conducts periodic supervisory conferences with the Recreation Leaders and other members of the staff, makes decisions which involve the recreation program and its relationship to the administrative policy of the institution, assists with the training of aides and volunteer workers, and assumes the duties and leadership role of the Director in the latter's absence.

The Recreation Leader is a recreation therapist who has earned a B.A. or B.S. degree in therapeutic recreation or in a discipline which emphasizes psychology, sociology, music, arts, crafts or dramatics. It is his role to plan and execute recreation activities under the direction of his immediate Recreation Supervisor.

The Recreation Leader must secure medical approval for patients to participate in the activity programs. Under the direction of the Supervisor he schedules events and diversions for the patients. He instructs and moderates special interest groups, games, arts and crafts activities, hobby club meetings, newspaper activities, musical programs and parties, and he schedules the showing of motion pictures to the patients.

The Leader assists in the movement of patients to and from recreation areas, works with volunteers in their own activities, reports on the budget and on the progress of the programs under his jurisdiction, attends patient council meetings and maintains the supply of equipment which is utilized by his programs.

The Recreation Leaders, together with the Assistants, form the "backbone" of the department, without whose efforts such services would be greatly curtailed, and in all likelihood might not be able to exist at all.

The **Recreation Specialist** functions much as the title of his position implies. He is a specialist in *one* particular facet of recreation, such as music, art, dramatics or crafts, and when programs are offered in these areas it is his duty to plan, organize and lead them. He also performs, as in the case of a musician or an actor, for patients' special interest groups and at patient and hospital social functions. His job includes instructing interested patients in the performing arts or in creative media when these special activities are scheduled.

A **music therapist** must have a B.A. degree in music or music therapy, plus several years of experience on the professional level. At least two years of college training with art as a major field of concentration, or a certificate of course completion from an accredited art school is required of an **art therapist**. In order to function as a **crafts specialist**, an individual must possess a college degree and be able to work in all of the craft areas which are encountered on a hospital recreation crafts program. The **dramatics specialist** has achieved a college degree in dramatics or has had at least ten years of active dramatic experience.

The Recreation Specialists perform not only a needed service in the rehabilitation hospital, but add many unique and enjoyable activities to the recreation program for which the patients are always grateful.

Forming the core of the department are the **Recreation Assistants**, the workers on the patient floors and wards. These are the staff members who establish rapport with the patients, who involve the patients in the recreation programs, who conduct recreation activities at bedside for those patients who cannot otherwise participate, who bear the brunt of working with the patients on the various programs, and who transport patients and supplies to and from the floors, wards and recreation areas. When the patient thinks of a recreation worker, it is the Recreation Assistant of whom he is thinking.

Recreation Assistants have had at least two years of college education and undergo a minimum of six months of training in the recreation field prior to joining the department's staff.

RECREATION ACTIVITIES AND PROGRAMS

The designing of a recreation program does not mean merely providing a series of activities which are conducted in a particular area of the hospital and enticing the patients to come to that area and participate in them. As pointed out above, many patients do not eagerly seek out recreation services. The staff of the department must establish a measure of rapport and encourage patient attendance at activities because of the inherent values of such involvement. Furthermore, it is conceivable that many recreational events and activities can be offered, yet patients do not participate in them because these diversions do not meet their current needs. It is therefore necessary for the recreation staff to become familiar with the patient population of their particular institution, to know the individuals who comprise this population and to schedule a recreation curriculum which is appropriate for them. This requires consideration of the ages, disabilities, and educational, vocational and social backgrounds of the patients each time a decision is made concerning which activities are to be offered to them.

The following description of recreation activities is not intended to be typical of any particular rehabilitation institution. Rather, these are listed so as to provide the reader with knowledge of the variety of activities which can be offered by a recreation service. Programs will, of course, vary between institutions. Thus, for example, in a nursing home, where the population in primarily geriatric, the emphasis would be placed on providing the activities which are described in the section dealing with recreation for the aged. In a rehabilitation hospital setting, where a younger group of patients may be in the majority, the Recreation Service will schedule more social events such as parties and out-trips than sedentary activities. The reader can review the listed items presented herein and determine which kinds of recreational events are most suited for the population with which he works.

Activities for the Aged

For purposes of discussion, the term "aged" refers to individuals who are past the age of sixty-five.

Music Appreciation

This feature of a recreation program is conducted by a music specialist. He may lead community sings on the patient floors or wards or in a designated recreation area. Patients are led in song, or sing along with a phonograph record or "live" music, such as a piano. Many patients only keep time to the music with instruments such as a tambourine or cymbals, or by clapping their hands. It is often helpful to employ slides on which the words to the songs are printed so that every patient can join in the singing.

Choral groups of patients may be formed and they then travel about the hospital entertaining other patients. Patients who are able to play a musical instrument are encouraged to do so and the recreation department will provide the necessary instruments if the patients do not have their own. If there are enough of these talented patients the music therapist will often help them to form a small band, lead practice sessions and encourage them to play at patient and hospital social gatherings.

There are many phonograph records available of old, familiar songs which may remind patients of people and events in their lives when these songs were popular. The recreation specialist can play such tunes and then ask the patients to recall those times and discuss what they were doing then, which fashions were in style, what was happening in the news of the day and so on. Much active discussion can be generated through listening to music.

Classical, semi-classical and theatrical music may be played and the music therapist can inform the patients of the significant themes and movements of the selections they hear. The lives of the composers are also frequently discussed.

There are few patients who do not like music, and activities of this kind are among the most enjoyable that can be offered in a hospital.

Discussion Groups

A discussion group may be composed of patients with either similar or diverse backgrounds and interests. The moderator of a discussion group must be skilled in such work to insure that each patient in the group is given an opportunity to participate, thus not permitting the group to become dominated by one or two outspoken individuals. He must be able to lead the group from one topic to another, sensing when a change of discussion material is warranted.

The primary focus of such groups is on events which occurred in the previous years of the patients' lives. It has been learned through experience that elderly people prefer to talk of times when they were healthy and led useful, productive lives. True, many patients will speak of their current medical and physical problems and of difficulties encountered within the hospital, but the skilled group leader does not permit this kind of discussion to become prolonged. Patients will often speak about these matters for want of other topics, and at such times the leader will furnish discussion material which takes their minds off present discomforts and which are of more general interest to the group.

Current events are also brought under discussion but these too are related to similar events with which the patients were familiar in their premorbid and more youthful lives. Comparisons are made between news occurrences in the present and what happened in the past, thereby enabling the patients to more easily relate to today's world.

Quiz Sessions

Most patients enjoy quizzes and the value of such sessions lies in both social group participation and in dissemination of information. Interested patients are organized into small groups of three or four patients each, and usually two or three groups compete simultaneously. The recreation worker who moderates such quiz sessions will ask questions pertaining to past and current events, famous people, proverbs, show business, sporting events, etc., and the quiz groups compete for prizes and certificates.

Games

Although all hospitalized patients can play and enjoy some games, it is the elderly who particularly require such activities. Games for a rehabilitation population are generally of a sedentary nature, such as chess, checkers, bingo, cards, dominoes and Scrabble.® The aged patient not only has a disability which prevents him from engaging in many activities, but advancing years have made him even less capable. Therefore, a recreation department always maintains a large supply of table games.

To further interest the patients, tournaments are held in which patients compete for prizes and "championships". These games are often the very diversions which the patients would engage in outside of the institution and so, the Recreation Service bridges the gap between hospital and extra-hospital life, attempting to make the former resemble the latter as closely as possible.

There are certain sports which the elderly are able to play even if they are wheelchair-bound. Among these are table tennis, bowling and shuffleboard. For those patients whose physical abilities permit of these athletics the Recreation Service sets up tables and equipment in designated playing areas.

General Recreation Activities

Although the activities described in the preceding section are persented as examples of recreation for a geriatric population, they are also appropriate for younger patients. Thus, music appreciation, for example, is enjoyed by patients other than the elderly. Discussion groups are of value for teenagers as well as oldsters, although the topics will be more closely related to today's living than to past experiences. Games are also played by the more youthful patients, but they are of a more active and energetic type than those scheduled for the elderly.

Films

The showing of motion pcitures is another popular recreation feature which can be enjoyed by young and old alike. There are several companies which supply hospitals with free films. Among them are the Canadian Travel Film Library of New York City, Barbre Productions, Inc. of Denver, Colorado, and the American and National Leagues of Professional Baseball Clubs, Motion Picture Division of Chicago, Illinois. The major motion picture studios of Hollywood will also provide films at no charge for hospitalized patients upon request.

Most recreation departments in large cities will occasionally call upon professional entertainers to come to the hospital and perform for the patients. People in show business are always ready and willing to donate their services wherever their schedules permit and hospital shows with professional, "name" entertainers are extremely popular with all age patient groups.

Social Recreation

The activities which are included within this category are parties, picnics and barbecues, and out-trips to ballgames, the theater, parks and amusement areas. In addition to providing enjoyment, such events foster leadership since the patients are asked to become involved with the planning, organizing and scheduling of these events. They select the type of trip, the kind of place to eat in, the date of travel, the theme of a party, the site for a picnic, and so on.

By arranging events in this way the Recreation Service permits patients to "have a say" in their own programs. Such activities are more enjoyed by the patients than if the recreation staff did all of the work and then merely informed them of what was planned. Patients are given a sense of responsibility, a role of leadership, a feeling of being needed, and the knowledge that their efforts are serving a useful purpose.

Art Therapy

Art therapy is a specialty area and classes are conducted by a qualified art major. All media which are feasible for patient utilization are employed, including oil and water color paints, charcoal, pen and ink, and finger paints and crayons. The therapist instructs the patients in the use of the various media, provides all supplies and supervises the work of the patients. The artistic creations of the patients are frequently displayed throughout the hospital and usually there is an annual art show at which time the paintings, drawings and sculptures are exhibited and often sold.

Art therapy is quite popular among rehabilitation patients. Even the severely disabled are usually able to participate to some extent. Many fine paintings have been created by patients whose only way of holding a brush was by mouth or foot. Art work enables the handicapped individual to be creative and productive despite limitations which prevent other activity and therefore is a valuable asset to any recreation program.

Crafts

As another specialty, crafts work requires the skills and knowledge of an experienced recreation staff member who can instruct patients on the qualities and uses of tools and materials required for creative handiwork.

Copper and ceramic tiles are employed in making such items as ashtrays, plaques, bookmarks, letter openers and bookends. Leatherwork includes producing belts, wallets, pocketbooks, purses, checkbook holders, bookmarks and watch bands. Wood is used for bookends, small articles of furniture, and trays. Modeling with clay, salt clay and papier mache provides many hours of relaxation and enjoyment in addition to aiding the patient in increasing strength, manual dexterity and range of motion in the wrists, hands and fingers. Most women are proficient in sewing, knitting, embroidery and crewel work, but the recreation therapist can demonstrate new techniques and additional ways of being creative with these skills.

One advantage to a crafts program is that patients are able to engage in many of the activities in their bed areas since the materials are usually easily portable. Thus, idle hours, when patients are not actively engaged in rehabilitative therapy, can be pleasurably spent. Even bedridden patients can participate, and many craft instruction and supervision sessions are conducted at bedside for these people.

Periodic crafts exhibits are held by the recreation staff where the patients' work is displayed. Most institutions permit the patients to sell or keep the articles which they have made.

Dramatics

Dramatics provides patients with an opportunity to express themselves, to join with others in a cooperative venture and to provide entertainment for other patients. As a specialty field it requires the leadership of a qualified staff member. It serves to foster leadership qualities and to promote interrelationships among patients and staff.

The patients select a play, rehearse it and present it, generally to the entire hospital, in one or more performances. Those patients who are not interested in performing but who wish to have a part in the production can, if they are physically able, design costumes and scenery, help with lighting and do other backstage work. A post-show party for cast and crew usually follows. Dramatics is a rewarding activity for those involved in the production and for the patients who see the show.

Re-Motivation

Although many recreation departments do not yet offer a re-motivation program, this is rapidly becoming an accepted part of the recreation curriculum. It is designed primarily for the socially isolated patient.

One observation which is often made in may rehabilitation hospitals is that patients are frequently unfamiliar with other patients, even those who reside in adjoining beds or who sit across the mealtime table from them. The patient who is an outgoing individual will voluntarily meet others, initiate conversation and make friends. However, the more reticent patient may spend his entire hospitalization period aloof from his fellows. Since companionship often helps to make hospitalization more pleasant, a number of recreation departments have taken steps to correct this situation. These programs are termed *re-motivation,* or *re-socialization,* or have a similar title, but the goal is always the same: to bring the socially isolated and withdrawn patients into contact with others.

A typical re-motivation program consists of five steps, or phases.

Phase One involves creating *a climate of acceptance* for the patients. Once a group of isolated patients has been selected, the recreation staff member places their seats or wheelchairs in a circular or semi-circular arrangement. He then addresses himself to the group, introducing himself and explaining the rationale for such a gathering. Next, he calls upon each member of the patient group to give his name and relate a little information about his personal background. He will encourage hesitant patients or allow them to "pass" until the others have spoken. Then he will return to them and request that they participate. This is the introductory phase of re-motivation and patients begin to learn about their fellows.

Phase Two revolves around structuring *a bridge to reality,* as it is frequently termed. The group leader may read a poem, or an article from a magazine or newspaper to the group, or show them a photograph or a painting, or some artistic or mechanical object. By describing what he has exhibited, or by relating additional information about the poem or narrative he begins to promote discussion among the patients. They may ask questions or relate what they have heard to something personal in their own lives. Thus, patients hear others' opinions and come to know about today's world and its activities.

The second step of re-motivation leads into Phase Three, *sharing the world we live in.* The group leader has a pre-planned discussion topic which is related to current events. He also has a set of prepared questions which he will ask the individuals in the group to respond to. This leads patients to deal with a more structured situation and to speak of matters which might previously have been unfamiliar to them. It is also an educational experience. Futhermore, it guides the patients away from free discussion, which they most often engage in, to a more direct type of dialogue.

Phase Four is directed towards giving the patients *an appreciation of the work of the world.* They are encouraged to regard work in relation to themselves. Each group member describes the type of occupation he was engaged in, and all members gain an appreciation of work for its own sake and rewards regardless of the particular kind of job in question. Many patients learn that they worked at the same, or similar jobs prior to their hospitalization and many friendships have been formed on this basis.

Finally, in Phase Five, *a climate of appreciation* is created. The recreation therapist expresses his pleasure and gratitude to the patients for their attendance and participation. He lets them know that it is they who are the important people in the group and that it is their involvement which makes such a venture meaningful. It is not unusual for members of re-motivation groups to become volunteer assistants to the Recreation Service in planning and conducting such groups for other socially isolated patients, thus effectively demonstrating the worth of the program which they have experienced.

Additional Activities

Musical activities, such as glee clubs, poetry reading and analysis, and pottery are also frequently part of a recreation curriculum.

Some rehabilitation institutions have kitchens which can be used for recreation activities, and in those cases the Recreation Service conducts cooking and baking classes.

Most hospitals have a patients' library which, although usually staffed by volunteer workers and hospital auxilians, can be used by patients who act as assistants to the librarians. A well-stocked library, of course, also affords patients many hours of enjoyable and well-spent time.

One activity which is becoming increasingly popular, expecially among younger patients, in sensitivity training. Briefly, this involves learning, or re-learning to become aware of one's self and one's fellows through utilizing touch and other sensory modalities. It is geared towards helping one to experience the world we live in.

For those patients who are physically able to participate, some isometric and isotonic exercise classes are held, upon approval of the medical staff.

The preceding list of recreation activities is far from complete. Space does not permit a description of all of the possible events, activities and diversions which can be offered by a recreation department. Furthermore, each new day, creative recreation therapists are discovering new ways of making prolonged rehabilitation hospitalization more pleasant for the patients. As one Recreation Leader remarked, ". . . possibilities are almost unlimited. All we have to do is think of them and then try them out. If we only keep the patients' interests in mind we will be successful."

THE RECREATION THERAPIST
AS A MEMBER OF THE REHABILITATION TEAM

It was mentioned previously that recreation activities are not haphazardly scheduled, but are designed to meet the needs of the individual patients. One way in which the recreation staff learns of these needs is by attending the periodic evaluation and re-evaluation conferences which are held by the medical and paramedical staffs of the hospital.

When a new patient is evaluated for admission to the rehabilitation program, all disciplines report on the various aspects of his functioning. The recreation worker listens to the reports, takes notes, and asks questions about data which are of importance and interest to him.

He is concerned with the patient's strength, range of motion, independence in ADL, and medical problems, such as a cardiac condition, for example, which might preclude the patient's participating in certain activities. The worker wants to know about the patient's ability to attend to, and concentrate on a task, his memory, affect, motivation and general psychological status. Speech, language and hearing problems are noted. The social worker's report on the patient's social and educational history are important, as is the rehabilitation counselor's report concerning the patient's work background.

On the basis of what he learns at the evaluation conference, the recreation therapist formulates a picture of each patient, gains ideas regarding which activities might interest the patient, and he learns how to best approach him to gain his participation and involvement.

At the re-evaluation conferences the recreation worker takes a more active part by reporting on what the patient is doing on the reccreation program, how rapidly he learns new tasks, how well he is enjoying the activities and on whether or not changes have been observed in the patient's bahavior or physical condition. The worker hears what the other team members report and on the basis of their findings may modify the patient's recreation schedule.

Many times another rehabilitation team member will come to the Recreation Service with new information which can help that staff to plan a program for a particular patient or group of patients. For example, a social worker might relate that a patient was a mechanic, or an electronics repairman prior to the onset of his disability. The recreation worker assigned to that patient may then enlist his aid in repairing equipment in the department or in other areas of the hospital, or he may teach the patient to operate the projector for the motion pictures that are shown and give him primary responsibility for its proper maintenance and operation. Attempts are always made to relate the patient's hospital activities to his own background and experiences.

A psychologist might point out a withdrawn or socially isolated patient to a recreation therapist, suggesting that this individual be placed on a therapeutic recreation program, such as re-motivation. The therapist will then try and involve that patient in such a group or in other suitable activities, thus contributing to his psychological health.

If a recreation program is to be effective in achieving its goals, the Recreation Service must be an active member of the rehabilitation team. In a great many institutions the amount of contact which the recreation staff has with the patients is second only to that of the nursing staff. Furthermore, the recreation worker sees the patients in a way which is different from that of the other disciplines and, therefore, can make highly important contributions to the patient's rehabilitation.

THE HOSPITAL AUXILIARY

The auxiliary is an integral part of the hospital. It is a voluntary association which is organized solely to serve the hospital. It is created with the approval of the hospital's governing board and operates under the guidance of the hospital administration. It works directly, and in close coordination with, the Recreation Service.

Hospital auxiliaries usually serve four main functions.

1. The auxiliary raises funds through various programs, such as sales, entertainments, community fund-raising drives, public appeals, advertising campaigns, etc.

2. It enlists essential community support. This is achieved primarily through recruitment of in-service volunteers. Auxilians present talks to groups regarding recruitment, prepare and distribute recruitment literature, prepare publicity for public news media, and contact individuals and groups for service and donations.

3. Another basic function of the auxiliary is to develop the channels of communication between the institution and the community so that wider and deeper mutual understanding is gained.

4. Lastly, auxiliary members seek and test new projects. In the past, they have rolled bandages and sewed garments for hospital patients. These services are now, of course, obsolete, but social service work, which was once pioneered by the auxiliaries, has continued and become an independent service. Auxilians are currently investigating how they can be of assistance in programs of professional education, hospital careers and research.

Hospital auxiliaries are staffed by volunteers from the community who donate their time to serve others. Its members are of all races, religions, national origins and socioeconomic statuses. Some auxiliaries charge nominal dues to help support their activities, while others have no dues requirements. Auxilians typically follow a policy of rotation of officers and committee chairmen so that each member has the opportunity to serve in a different capacity.

There are three basic forms which a hospital auxiliary can assume: (1) an integrated part of the hospital corporate organization which functions primarily within the hospital, as is typically the case in a rehabilitation institution; (2) an unincorporated association of the individuals within the community; and (3) a separately incorporated non-profit membership corporation.

In order for auxiliaries to successfully discharge their responsibilities they rely upon several well coordinated committees. These may include a finance committee, which is responsible for planning ways of meeting the budgetary requirements of the auxiliary; a membership committee, through which men and women of all ages are drawn from the community to serve and support the hospital; a nominating committee, which proposes members for elective office; a by-laws committee, which has the responsibility of assuring that the auxiliary is operating in conformity with its regulations; a coffee shop committee; a gift shop committee; and fund-raising committee.

Auxilians also frequently staff patient libraries, serve patients at bedside with a rolling magazine and book cart, run thrift shops and hold rummage sales. Suffice it to say that a great deal of patient service is provided by the hospital auxiliary. Together with the Recreation Service, the auxiliary meets the needs of the patients in many important ways. Auxilians have a long and proud history of service and, as hospital and patient needs grow in the future, the role of the auxiliary will be seen as an increasingly vital one.

FINANCING OF RECREATION SERVICES

The funds for recreation services can come from three primary sources. One is the hospital auxiliary. Through its rummage sales, coffee shop and thrift shop incomes and fund-raising programs, money is obtained which is used to finance many recreational activities and events.

A second source of income is private donations. Citizens and private organizations which are aware of, and are sympathetic to, the needs of the hospital donate funds for use by the Recreation Service. Perhaps the most active and generous organization in this regard is the National Council of Jewish Women.

The third method of obtaining working capital is directly from the institution in which the Recreation Service operates. The department is recognized as a part of the rehabilitation service and is allocated funds on the regular hospital budget.

CONCLUSION

Recreation, as a therapeutic activity, has a long history. Its values have been recognized for thousands of years; yet only within the last half century has it been employed with hospitalized patients and, even more recently, within the rehabilitation hospital. It still needs to gain the recognition and status which it deserves.

Any service which brings isolated patients into communicative contact with others, which increases muscle strength and range of motion of the trunk and extremities, which motivates patients to succeed on rehabilitation therapy programs and which makes long hospitalization a more pleasant experience, cannot be denied its importance. The Recreation Service is such a service.

Section VI

References

A. *The Social Work Service (Chapter 17)*

1. Bartlett, Harriet M.: *Analyzing Social Work Practice by Fields.* New York, National Association of Social Workers, 1961.
2. Bartlett, Harriet M.: *Social Work Practice in the Health Field.* New York, National Association of Social Workers, 1961.
3. Bartlett, Harriet M.: Toward classification and improvement of social work practice. *Social Work, 3:* 3, 1958.
4. Benney, Celia: The role of the caseworker in rehabilitation. *Social Casework, 36:* 1, 1955.
5. Goldstine, Dora (Ed): *Readings in the Theory and Practice of Medical Social Work.* Chicago, University of Chicago Press, 1965.
6. Hamilton, G.: *Theory and Practice of Social Case Work.* New York, Columbia University Press, 1952.
7. Hamilton, K.: *Counseling the Handicapped in the Rehabilitation Process.* New York, Ronald, 1950.
8. Hollis, Florence: *Casework: A Psychosocial Therapy.* New York, Random House, 1966.
9. Phillips, Helen U.: *Essentials of Social Group Work Skill.* New York, Association, 1965.
10. Roemer, M. I.: Current developments in hospital service and their significance for medical social work. In *Casework Papers, 1960. National Conference on Social Welfare.* New York, Family Service Association of America, 1960.
11. Tibbitts, C. and Donahue, W. (Eds): *Social and Psychological Aspects of Aging.* New York, Columbia University Press, 1962.
12. Voiland, Alice L.: *Family Casework Diagnosis.* New York, Columbia University Press, 1962.
13. Younghusband, Eileen (Ed): *Social Work and Social Values.* London, Allen and Unwin, 1967.

B. *The Vocational Rehabilitation Service (Chapter 18)*

1. Anderson, R. P.: The rehabilitation counselor as counselor. *Journal of Rehabilitation, 24:* 4, 1958.
2. Berkowitz, M. (Ed): *Rehabilitation for the Disabled Worker. A Platform for Action.* Washington, U.S. Department of Health, Education and Welfare, 1963.
3. Dawis, R. V., England, G. W. and Lofquist, L. H.: A theory of work adjustment. *Minnesota Studies in Vocational Rehabilitation: XV* (Bulletin 38). Minneapolis, University of Minnesota Press, 1964.
4. Felton, Jean S., Perkins, Dorothy C. and Lewin, Molly: *A Survey of Medicine and Medical Practice for the Rehabilitation Counselor.* Washington, Vocational Rehabilitation Administration, 1966.
5. Hamilton, K. W.: *Counseling the Handicapped in the Rehabilitation Process.* New York, Ronald, 1950.
6. Jacobs, A., Jordaan, J. P. and DiMichael, S. C. (Eds): *Counseling and the*

Rehabilitation Process. New York, Columbia University Bureau of Publications, 1961.

7. Jaffe, A. J., Day, L. and Adonis, W.: *Disabled Workers in the Labor Market.* Totowa, Bedminster, 1964.

8. Krusen, F. H.: Relationships between the medical and vocational aspects of rehabilitation. *Rehabilitation Record, 1:* 30, 1960.

9. Krusen, F. H., Kottke, F. J. and Ellwood, P. M.: *Handbook of Physical Medicine and Rehabilitation.* Philadelphia, Saunders, 1966.

10. Lofquist, L. H.: An operational definition of rehabilitation counseling. *Journal of Rehabilitation, 25:* 7, 1959.

11. McGowan, J. F. and Porter, T. L.: *An Introduction to the Vocational Rehabilitation Process.* Washington, Vocational Rehabilitation Administration, 1967.

12. Muthard, J. E. and Morris, W. W. (Eds): *Counseling the Older Disabled Worker.* Washington, Office of Vocational Rehabilitation, 1961.

13. Nosow, S. and Form, W. H. (Eds): *Man, Work and Society. The Sociology of Occupations.* New York, Basic Books, 1962.

14. Ogg, Elizabeth: *Rehabilitation Counselor: Helper of the Handicapped.* Washington, Public Affairs Committee, 1967.

15. Rusalem, H.: *Guiding the Physically Handicapped College Student.* New York, Columbia University Bureau of Publications, 1962.

16. Scott, R. A.: Rehabilitation counseling in medical settings. *Rehabilitation Counseling Bulletin, 5:* 183, 1962.

17. *Selective Placement. Hiring the Handicapped According to Their Abilities* (Personnel Methods, Series 9). Washington, U.S. Civil Service Commission, 1963.

18. Thomason, B. and Barrett, A. M.: Casework performance in vocational rehabilitation. In *Proceedings of Guidance, Training and Placement Workshops.* Washington, Office of Vocational Rehabilitation Administration, 1959.

19. Thomason, B. and Barrett, A. M. (Eds): The placement process in vocational rehabilitation counseling. In *Proceedings of Guidance, Training and Placement Workshops.* Washington, Office of Vocational Rehabilitation Administration, 1964.

20. *Training Guides in the Evaluation of Vocational Potential for Vocational Rehabilitation Staff* (Rehabilitation Service Series 66–23). Washington, Office of Vocational Rehabilitation Administration, 1965.

C. The Recreational Service (Chapter 19)

1. *Basic Concepts of Hospital Recreation.* Washington, American Recreation Society, Hospital Recreation Section, 1962.

2. Chapman, F. M.: *Recreation Activities for the Handicapped.* New York, Ronald, 1960.

3. *Essentials for Hospital Auxilliaries. A Guide.* New York, United Hospital Fund, 1963.

4. Haun, P., Krauss, R. G. and Avedon, E. M. (Eds): *Recreation: A Medical Viewpoint.* New York, Columbia University Press, Teachers College Bureau of Publications, 1965.

5. Hunt, Valerie V.: *Recreation for the Handicapped.* New York, Prentice-Hall, 1955.

6. Merrill, Toni: *Activities for the Aged and Infirm.* Springfield, Thomas, 1967.

7. O'Morrow, G. S. (Ed): *Administration of Activity Therapy Service.* Springfield, Thomas, 1966.

8. Rathbone, Josephine L. and Lucas, Carol: *Recreation and Total Rehabilitation.* Springfield, Thomas, 1959.

PATIENT CARE

Chapter 20

THE REHABILITATION NURSING SERVICE

WERE A SURVEY TO BE CONDUCTED among rehabilitation patients (and perhaps it has already been done) regarding which hospital staff members they considered most important for their day-to-day living, it would be the nursing services, the nurses and nurse's aides, which would emerge at the top of the list. By sheer number of hours of patient contact, nurses assume a formidable role in the rehabilitation process. Furthermore, the great number and variety of services which they provide, many of which are vital to patient care and health, places nursing personnel in the position of being, in many ways, the most crucial staff members for the patient. By their treatment and handling of patients and by their attitudes in both the medical and psychosocial spheres, nurses can either contribute towards a patient's rehabilitation and independence or they can significantly retard progress. This is well known to the other members of the rehabilitation team and is most obvious to the patients.

Rehabilitation nursing is a specialty which shares common features with other nursing specialties, but which also is different in many respects. It is not the purpose of the present chapter to deal with medical-surgical nursing in general, since there are many fine texts covering the field and the interested reader will find a number of them listed at the end of the chapter. There are, naturally, certain routine duties which the rehabilitation nurse performs which other nursing specialists also carry out, and these will be described, but discussion will focus primarily on the services which make rehabilitation nursing a unique discipline.

OBSERVATION AND CHARTING

Observation of the patient is of the utmost importance. The physician and paramedical staff members rely upon the nurse's observations

535

in both diagnosing and treating a patient, and at the evaluation and re-evaluation conferences the nurse's report is attended to very carefully. Often the nurse, because of her intimate daily contact with the patient, is in the best position to detect early signs of medical or psychological difficulty. She may also be the first to observe generalization of what the patient is taught in therapy classes to the activities of daily living. She may be able to assist the social service worker in planning for home visits or discharge of the patient because she is the one who sees the patient's family and other visitors and can observe the frequency of visits and the type of relationship which the patient has with his family members. Through conversations with the patient, the nurse can gain information regarding his skills, interests and occupational attitudes and goals, which is important for the rehabilitation counselor. Therefore, in many ways, the nurse can be the *central* figure in the total rehabilitation of the patient.

Among the important clinical observations which the nursing staff can make, that will be of interest to the physician, are the following: color and condition of skin, fingernails, toenails, mucous membranes, eyes, hair and teeth; contour and positioning of body parts; moisture or dryness of body areas; rashes, bruises and wounds; the presence of decubitous ulcers; dressings on wounds; swellings; drainage and discharge from sores and body cavities; temperature changes; condition of body cavities and tongue; changes in weight; changes in sleeping and eating habits; unusual odors; chills or perspiration; convulsions; coughing and expectoration; condition of urine and fecal matter; incontinence; diarrhea; *oliguria,* or small urine excretion; and *polyuria,* or large urine excretion; presence of edema; tremors; reactions to medication; changes in respiration; pain; bleeding; and emergency conditions.

There are also important signs that the nurse can detect which are useful for the psychologist. These include: changes in alertness; lethargy; apathy; disorientation; memory losses; confusion, emotional changes, such as mood swings; acting out; refusal to take medication or cooperate with other procedures; hallucinations, delusions or illusions; inability to relate to staff or other patients; level of activity and interests; motivational variables; depression; suicidal varbalizations or attempts; hostility; passivity; clearing or clouding of general psychological status; negativism; sexual behavior; phobias and anxieties; dependence; euphoria and grandiosity; chronic complaints; psychotic behavior; and acute distress.

The observations of the nursing staff member can be of considerable value for the therapists on the rehabilitation team. She can report to them on the following: the patient's attempts to ambulate; his pattern and type of gait; his posture during standing and walking; pain in upper and lower extremities; ability of the patient to transfer and his need for assistance; independence or dependence in ADL; his ability to grasp and use utensils; wheelchair mobility; the patient's ability in putting on and taking off prostheses and orthotic devices; changes in muscle strength; changes in range of motion; attempts at speech; voice quality; hearing ability; ability to understand language and nonverbal commands; and the patient's interest in and motivation for the various activities of rehabilitation.

The nurse's task is not completed when she has made her observations. She must both report them to the charge, or head nurse and to the appropriate staff professional, and record them in the patient's chart. The medical chart is the written record of the patient as he progresses from day to day in all areas of rehabilitation during his hospitalization.

Charting, by the nurse, consists of entering her observations in brief statements. Each nursing shift records the patient's general condition, complaints offered by the patient, and conversations between the patient and the nurse which have bearing and relevance for his case. It is the nurse's responsibility to maintain the chart, which includes data obtained upon admission, reports from all of the disciplines which are concerned with the patient, referrals for special consultations and the consultant's reports, demographic data, special dietetic considerations, records of medications and prescriptions, reports of conferences concerning the patient, the patient's therapy schedule, and, in fact, all information about the patient which is pertinent to his diagnosis, treatment and hospital stay.

As reports arrive at the nurse's desk she adds them to the chart in chronological order and by subject matter. It is the nurse's job to become familiar with the chart of each patient assigned to her care so that she can administer correct management and be able to provide staff members with the documents and information which they may request.

THE MAINTENANCE OF ASEPSIS

The major responsibility for asepsis of patient quarters and ward or floor facilities rests with the nursing staff.

Asepsis is the term used to designate complete absence of bacteria. There are two categories of asepsis, medical asepsis and surgical asepsis. *Medical asepsis* is aimed at confining agents of contamination to a given area and preventing the escape of organisms from that area.

Surgical asepsis requires that any object which comes into contact with a wound must be free of pathogenic organisms.

Medical asepsis involves the use of the methods of disinfection and sterilization. Surgical asepsis is accomplished through sterilization. The rehabilitation nurse must be concerned with both. The development of central supply units in hospitals and the use of disposable equipment has greatly aided the nursing staff in their work but there is still much which the nurse must do to maintain the health of her patients.

Chemical Means of Disinfection

There are a large number of chemical agents on the market, appearing under various trade names. None are effective for all purposes and those which have been found to be effective during laboratory testing may be ineffective under conditions of actual clinical usage.

Generally, the greater the strength of the solution, the greater its disinfecting power. A very weak solution may have antiseptic value, but many microorganisms are highly resistant to disinfection and require very strong solutions in order to be eliminated. Most disinfectants do not act quickly. Usually, the greater the strength of the solution, the more rapid is its effectiveness. Furthermore, although bacteria are often eliminated when the solution is heated, it may not be possible or desirable to heat some solutions, further compounding the problem.

There are some widely employed chemical disinfectants. Two emollient detergent soaps are *pHisoderm®* and *pHisoHex,®* which is pHisoderm®with hexachlorophene added. Regular washing of the skin with pHisoHex® reduces the number of resident skin bacteria.

Chlorine compounds can be used for disinfecting urine and feces.

Ammonium compounds may be used as a skin disinfectant and for disinfecting instruments. The standard solution for skin disinfection is 1:1,000, but this can vary depending upon the purpose to which the solution will be put.

Ethyl alcohol and isopropyl alcohol, in seventy per cent to ninety-nine per cent by weight solutions, are used as skin disinfectants but have limited value for disinfecting instruments because of corrosive effects, and they are relatively useless against spores.

Iodophors combine iodine with another agent, such as a detergent, and can be used as skin disinfectants, disinfection in medical asepsis and as sanitizers for floors.

For many years, chemical solutions were almost the only means of sterilization and disinfection. There are now more effective ways of destroying microorganisms through physical methods, and chemical sterilization has largely been discredited. Chemical disinfection, although less popular than it has been in the past, is still extensively employed.

Physical Methods of Sterilization
and Disinfection

Physical sterilization and disinfection are typically accomplished through using heat. They occur when the heat is of sufficient intensity to destroy microorganisms and thus, the higher the temperature, the more quickly the organisms are killed. The nurse must load and pack the sterilizer in such a way that equipment is properly exposed to the heat.

Steam Under Pressure

Moist heat in the form of steam under pressure is the most dependable means of destroying all forms of microbial life. The higher temperature which results from higher pressure is the effective force.

The *autoclave* is a pressure steam sterilizer. During sterilization it is maintained at a temperature of 121° C. to 123° C. (250° F. to 254° F.) and at fifteen to seventeen pounds of pressure for a specified period of time. The length of time for sterilization depends upon the article being exposed, and can vary from ten minutes to fifteen minutes for instruments in trays with muslin covers, to forty-five minutes for dressing drums with muslin liners.

Dry Heat

Dry heat sterilization utilizes circulating hot air provided by an electric oven sterilizer. It is effective in sterilizing glassware, sharp instruments, syringes and needles, but is undesirable for textile materials. For most articles, sterilization occurs at about one to two hours at a temperature of 160° C. (320° F.)

Boiling Water

Boiling is one of the oldest methods of sterilization. Equipment to be sterilized is immersed completely in the water and timing begins when the water begins to boil.

Clean equipment can be sterilized within several minutes. Equipment which is contaminated with vegetative forms of bacteria can be sterilized if submerged in boiling water for ten to twenty minutes.

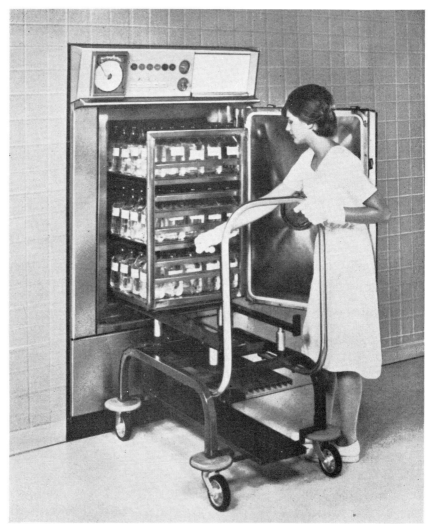

FIGURE 95. Floor loading steam sterilizer. (*Courtesy of Amsco Marketing, Division of American Sterilizer Co.*)

Sometimes, trisodium phosphate or sodium carbonate is added to the water, helping to remove grease which may harbor organisms and reducing the time required for sterilization and disinfection by increasing the "wetting power" of the water. When an alkali is added to the water, the boiling time can be of fifteen minutes duration.

If spores are present on equipment, boiling water is not a satisfactory method of sterilization. Water temperature cannot rise above 100° C. (212° F.). Some spores are highly resistant and the time re-

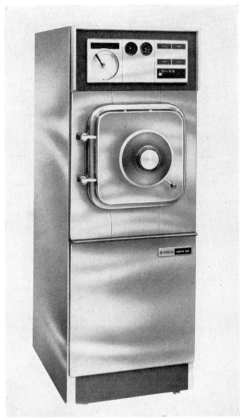

FIGURE 96. Steam sterilizer, straightline type. (*Courtesy of Castle Co., Division of Sybron Corp., Rochester, N. Y.*)

quired to kill susceptible spores is too long or too unspecific. In addition, some viruses are resistant to boiling.

Free-Flowing Steam

Free-flowing steam is used for sterilization at a temperature of 100°C (212° F.) and thus is employed for the same length of time as boiling water. Since it is difficult to load a free-flowing steam sterilizer so that all equipment is fully exposed to the steam, this method is of limited practical value.

Ethylene Oxide Gas

There are articles which cannot be subjected to steam or soaked in a disinfecting solution. For such items, ethylene oxide gas is an effective germicidal agent. It is effective against all forms of vegetative

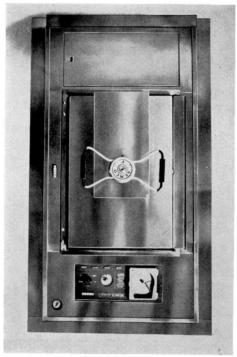

FIGURE 97. Bulk sterilizer. *(Courtesy of Vernitron Medical Products, Inc., Carlstadt, N. J.)*

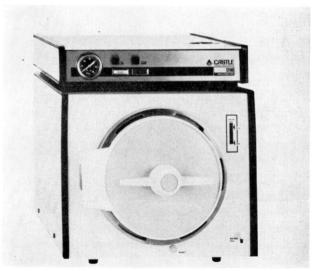

FIGURE 98. Steam sterilizer, table top model. *(Courtesy of Castle Co., Division of Sybron Corp., Rochester, N. Y.)*

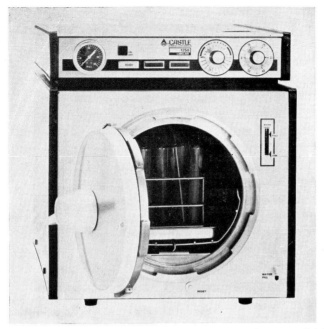

FIGURE 99. A table top model autoclave. (*Courtesy of Castle Co., Division of Sybron Corp., Rochester, N. Y.*)

bacteria, spore-bearing bacteria, fungus and some viruses. It is also used by manufacturers to sterilize pre-packaged materials. It is of value in sterilizing rubber, polyethylene tubing, uretal catheters, cycstoscopy instruments, lenses of examining apparatus and delicate machine components.

Ethylene oxide sterilization requires more time than autoclaving. There are several types of sterilizers available, including one which combines the gas with steam, and one which can sterilize large objects, such as pillows, blankets and mattresses.

One disadvantage of ethylene oxide is that it is slightly toxic and may cause nausea, vomiting, dizziness and irritation to mucous membranes if it is inhaled. Items sterilized by this method must remain unused until the gas dissipates.

Ultraviolet Light

Ultraviolet light is used more as a disinfectant for the home than it is for the hospital. Objects are placed where the sun's rays can fall directly on them for a period of from six to eight hours.

Cleansing

It is important to cleanse items properly prior to their sterilization since bacteria which are imbedded in organic material or under fat or grease are resistant to disinfection. Cleansing also reduces the number of bacteria present, thus making sterilization easier.

Cleansing of objects is performed as soon after they have been used as possible for ease of cleansing and prevention of transfer of bacteria by air currents. Articles are cleansed by the nurse, wearing rubber gloves, with a brush having stiff bristles, in water with a soap or detergent. Warm water is more effective than cold water, except for equipment contaminated by organisms in body secretions containing protein which are coagulated by heat. Following cleansing, the gloves, brush and basin in which the objects have been cleansed are disposed of or sterilized.

Various kinds of materials require different cleansing and disinfecting techniques. Bedpans and urinals are usually made of Monel® or enamelware. Monel® and enamelware are cleansed with soap or detergent solutions. Abrasives can be used for removing soilage. A brush, cloth or sponge may be used and discarded or disinfected following usage. Steam under pressure is the preferred sterilization method, but dry heat may also be used and boiling water is satisfactory.

Glassware is washed in soap or detergents. Brushes especially designed for lumens and barrels are employed. Non-disposable syringes are disassembled after use to prevent their barrels and plungers from locking. They are thoroughly soaked and rinsed so that the contents will not dry in the barrel, hampering cleaning efforts. Steam under pressure is the preferred sterilization technique.

Instruments are scrubbed with a brush in a soap or detergent solution and are thoroughly dried. Instruments without a cutting edge are sterilized in an autoclave. Those with a cutting edge are sterilized by dry heat. Chemicals may be employed for certain purposes.

Needles present a cleaning problem because of their small lumen. Immediately after its use, cold water is forced through the needle with a syringe. Alcohol or ether, forced through the lumen will help to remove fatty or oily substances. Needles are sterilized by dry heat or steam under pressure. Boiling is used when other methods are not available.

Rubber and plastic items are washed in a soap or detergent solution. Catheters are rinsed immediately after use and are soaked for short periods of time to help clean them. A soap or detergent is forced through the lumen until it is clean. Tubing which has contained blood is disposed of. Autoclaving is the desired method of sterilizing rubber goods. Dry heat can be employed for certain types. Boiling is also used and chemicals are sometimes utilized.

Thorough laundering is usually sufficiently safe for linen materials.

As it is essential for all equipment to be aseptic, it is equally important for the individual using this equipment to be free of harmful bacteria.

There are two types of bacteria which are found on the hands. *Transient bacteria* are relatively few on clean and exposed skin areas. They are picked up by the hands in normal daily activities. They are attached loosely to the skin, usually in grease, fats and dirt, and are found in greater abundance under the fingernails. Frequent, thorough handwashing can remove this type of bacteria easily. *Resident bacteria* are relatively stable in both type and number. They are located in the creases and crevices of the skin and cling by adhesion and adsorption. Considerable friction must be applied with a brush during washing to remove them. In general, they are less susceptible to antiseptic action than are transient bacteria, and some are so deeply imbedded in the skin that they cannot be removed until scrubbing has continued for fifteen minutes or longer. It is not practically possible to cleanse the skin completely of all bacteria.

Soaps and detergents, by lowering the surface tension of water and acting as emulsifiers, are good cleansing agents. Soap used in hard water, however, is an ineffective cleaner. Detergents, such as the sulfonated detergents and the quarternary detergents are effective in hard water, and the latter have been found to have disinfectant action.

In the practice of medical asepsis, the nurse washes her hands for a period of thirty seconds to one minute to remove transient bacteria. If her hands have been contaminated by blood, purulent matter, mucous, saliva or secretions, washing is carried out from two to three minutes. (Gross contamination requires the careful use of a sterile brush. Subungual areas are cleansed with a sterile nail file or orange stick.)

Hands are washed preferably under running water at a sink having foot-controlled faucets. Liquid soap or detergent, dispensed by a foot pedal is simple to use and avoids problems arising from the use of soap bars. Following washing and rinsing, hands are dried with either a disposable paper towel, which may also be used for opening and closing hand-operated faucets, or an individual towel which is then deposited for sanitizing. A lotion or cream, applied to the skin following washing, keeps it soft and pliable and avoids chapping which can lead to skin breaks with repeated washings.

Practicing surgical asepsis means eliminating all microbial life. Hence, all items which are brought into contact with broken skin surfaces, or which are used to penetrate the skin or enter body cavities, must be sterile. The nurse's hands which come into contact with these items must be encased in sterile gloves.

THE MAINTENANCE OF PATIENT SAFETY AND COMFORT

It is the nurse's responsibility to insure both the safety and the comfort of the patients in her charge. On a rehabilitation service these conditions are of utmost importance. A broken tile can lead an amputee to trip, fall, and possibly suffer a hip fracture. Discomfort in a paraplegic may be an early sign of a skin lesion leading to a decubitous ulcer.

Safety Measures

There are several types of injuries which may befall patients, to which the nursing staff must be alert.

Mechanical injury can be the result of a broken or defective siderail on a bed, an open or loose window, cords, wires or tubing lying tangled on the floor, equipment, such as wheelchairs or stretchers, out of place, a defective lifter, a broken handrail in a bathroom or corridor, a loose or broken tile on the floor, a floor which has been waxed too smoothly, absence of a rubber mat in a bathtub or shower, a wheelchair with defective brakes, and many more possible sources.

Thermal injury may be caused by fires, such as from the cigarette of a patient who lacks sensation, or from frayed electrical cords or overloaded electrical sockets, by applications of heat in the form of electrical heating pads and hot water bottles, expecially with patients who have sensory losses, by steam inhalers and by solutions used in treatment which are too hot. The nurse must know her patients and maintain constant vigil or her floor or ward.

Chemical injury is produced externally by the use of too-strong chemicals on the skin, and internally by ingestion of incorrect drugs or an overdose of prescribed medication. The nurse must adhere to the physician's prescription of medication and must insure that other drugs are not placed or left within reach of patients. The solutions that are used to treat wounds and infections must be supervised by the nurse to guarantee correct proportions and applications.

Injury from allergens can be a consequence of insect bites, feathers, pillow and mattress ticking, food, cosmetics, lotions, powders, soap and dust. The nurse must be alert for signs of allergy, such as sneezing, coughing, rashes, watery eyes and stertorous respiration. Prevention of allergic reactions includes measures such as using allergy-free bedding, placing plastic covers on pillows and mattresses, using dustless cleaning methods, watching patients' reactions to foods and substances applied to the skin, and making certain that window screens are tightly placed and in good condition.

The nurse also periodically checks electrical equipment in the patient areas as a precaution against **electrical injury** resulting from defective wiring or equipment.

Maintaining Patient Comfort

For the rehabilitation patient, as well as for the acutely ill patient, comfort while in the hospital is an important variable. Sometimes, because of the nature of the institution or the physical design of the hospital, certain factors, such as attractive paint, curtains, carpeting, etc. cannot be controlled. Within such limits, however, there is a great deal which can be done towards making the patient comfortable and thus making his hospitalization more pleasant, towards improving morale and attitudes and generally towards contributing to the patient's emotional and motivational drives for active participation on a rehabilitation program.

Since the largest part of the hospital environment which is amenable to manipulation for comfort purposes is the patient's bed area, and since much of his time is spent there, the majority of the efforts to maintain patient comfort become the responsibility of the nursing service.

Very few patients desire total elimination of noise, but noise in excess can be very disturbing and at certain levels, harmful. Sounds above fifty decibels are usually found to be disturbing. A loud radio produces approximately eighty decibels. Soft speech produces twenty decibels and a whisper, about ten decibels. Sensitivity to, and tolerance of, noise varies with each patient from day to day, depending upon his state of health, fatigue, emotional status and personal desires.

Not all noise can be reduced, but much can be done to make sound levels tolerable. Metal carts and carriers can be made relatively soundproof by adding rubber wheels and bumpers. Wheels of stretchers can be periodically lubricated. Radios and television sets can be maintained at a comfortable level of sound. Care can be taken to avoid noise-creating damage, such as glass breakage and dropping of trays and instruments. Conversation between staff members can be kept within tolerable limits and shouting from distances can be completely eliminated.

Disagreeable tactile sensations, resulting from a rough and/or heavy blanket, wrinkled and rough bedclothes, hardness or roughness or a bedpan or other equipment, sharpness of a nurse's fingernails, and rough handling of patients can and should be reduced as far as possible.

Unpleasant odors can inhibit gastric reflexes and produce nausea. Most disagreeable odors emanate from soiled dressings, soiled sheets and bedclothes, bedpans, drainage from patients' bodies, bodily perspiration, garbage, disinfecting solutions and decaying food.

Odors are best eliminated by removing the source of the smells, by proper ventilation and by the use of fragrant and non-fragrant deodorizers.

Atmospheric conditions which contribute to, or detract from, patient comfort include temperature, humidity and ventilation.

Most individuals are comfortable with an indoor temperature which varies between sixty-five and seventy-five degrees Fahrenheit. A high environmental temperature will increase pulse rate and perspiration. A room temperature which is too low can cause chills. With patients who lack proper sensation, the nurse must be alert to temperature factors since these people are unable to accurately report climate conditions.

Temperature, however, is less important than humidity. Low humidity requires a higher room temperature than does an average humidity of sixty-six per cent.

When humidity is high, less moisture is evaporated from the skin and sensations of heat and cold are magnified because of the conductive properties of water. When humidity is low, evaporation from the skin is more rapid, resulting in the individual feeling "chilly".

Ventilation is movement in the air. The velocity of this movement should be at a rate of approximately fifteen to forty-five feet per minute. Proper ventilation supplies fresh air, maintains air movement and controls humidity. Fresh air is relatively free of bacteria and dust. Air motion increases radiation of heat from the skin and improves respiration and circulation. Cool moving air stimulates the superficial capillaries.

An air-conditioner is, by far, the most desirable means of maintaining proper ventilation. When this is not available, other means, such as electric fans and open windows and doors must be employed.

Good lighting in the patient's environment provides both safety and comfort. Sunlight should be utilized wherever possible. Artificial light should be strong enough to avoid eyestrain and to illuminate the area, and diffused enough to prevent glare. The patient who is able to manipulate his own light controls should have a lamp within his reach at bedside. Stairways, bathrooms, fire exits, corridors and ward areas must be well lighted.

It is also important for the nurse to bear in mind that with increased age, most patients require greater levels of illumination. She must also know of any visual deficiencies in her patients so that accommodations can be made for them.

Bedmaking is a part of the routine of the nursing staff of every hospital. There are various types of bedmaking procedures, some of which are not applicable in the rehabilitation hospital. Those which are employed are described below.

A *closed bed* is a bed which is made following the discharge of a patient and prior to the admission of a new patient. The spread covers the top linens and extends to the head of the mattress. It may also cover the pillow, depending upon the policy of the individual institution.

The *open bed* is the type employed when the bed has been assigned to a new patient, or for any bed occupied by a patient. This then, is the bedmaking most often used from day to day on a rehabilitation nursing service. The spread is turned under the top of the blanket and the top sheet is turned back over the blanket and the spread.

The *occupied bed* is used when a patient must remain constantly in bed, or in bed for a prolonged period of time, such as might be the case with acute infections, some decubiti, certain respiratory diseases or cardiac conditions and the like. Here, the nurse must make the bed and change the linens while the patient is in bed. The top cover are made in a fold similar to the open bed upon completion of bedmaking.

A *cradle bed* contains a device for holding the top covers off the patient's feet and/legs. It is used to avoid pressure on body parts which may lead to pain or decubiti. An enlarged cradle may be used to keep the top sheets off the legs and/or trunk. The cradles are made of wood or metal.

THE MAINTENANCE OF PATIENT HYGIENE

There are patients who are of the opinion that being disabled exempts them from continuing their personal care and cleanliness. In addition, the sociocultural and environmental background of some patients are such that personal hygiene is not important. Furthermore, individual patients have particular habits and idiosyncracies involving hygienic practices. However, regardless of personal habits, cultural and economic backgrounds, and feelings related to a disability and hospitalization, personal cleanliness must be maintained for good health, general physiologic functioning and comfort for as long as the patient is on the rehabilitation service. The practice of patient hygiene is within the province of nursing.

The Skin

The primary purpose of cleansing the skin is to remove dirt, oils and perspiration, and transient bacteria. Soap or detergent and water are the most commonly used materials for skin care and are, perhaps, the best. It makes little, if any, difference which commercial soap is used. If the water is hard or cold, soaps will not lather well and detergents are then the best to use. If a patient exhibits sensitivity to bath soap and detergent, cleansing creams are employed but these are a less effective substitute and cannot cleanse the skin thoroughly of dirt and oils.

Ethyl or grain alcohol in a fifty to seventy-five per cent concentration is an effective cleanser and its rapid evaporation cools and refreshes the skin. However, alcohol, as well as witch hazel, tends to harden the skin. The skin may be softened with oil of thebroma, cold cream or petrolatum.

Powders, such as zinc stearate powder, are useful skin antiseptics and are, therefore, healing, but should not be used on a moist or exuding skin surface that is infected since they prevent proper drainage. Two mild liquid antiseptics which are in wide use are gentian violet and tincture of benzoin.

After the skin has been cleansed a deodorant may be applied. Most deodorants are based upon the principle that an astringent will constrict skin pores and decrease the flow of perspiration. Deodorants which perform this function usually contain aluminum chloride, aluminum sulfate, tannic acid or zinc sulfate. Deodorants which only eliminate odor typically contain zinc stearate or boric acid.

The nurse must be on the alert for adverse skin reactions to all of these chemical substances.

Bathing

Bathing of patients is done routinely by the nursing staff. The frequency of bathing varies with the individual's general health, skin condition and cleanliness needs. Baths may be given to all patients on a ward or floor at a predesignated time, or on a staggered time schedule, or on individual patient needs and/or demands.

Because of the physical status of the majority of rehabilitation patients, shower baths are given infrequently and the tub bath is the most often employed method of bathing.

In addition to cleansing the skin, the bath also has physiological benefits. The friction of washing stimulates peripheral nerve endings and circulation. Firm stroking movements stimulate muscles and aid circulation, often increasing kidney function. The nurse can assist the physical and occupational therapists by providing range of motion exercises in the tub and by helping to teach the patient transfer activities.

Bath temperatures vary depending upon the individual's desires, tolerance and needs. A hot bath is usually maintained at a temperature of from 40.5° C. to 48.8° C. (105° F. to 120° F.). A warm bath varies between 35.0° C. and 40.5° C. (95° F. and 105° F.). A tepid bath can range between temperatures of 31.1° C. and 35.0° C. (88° F. and 95° F.).

Patients who must remain in bed but can bathe themselves are permitted to do so. The nurse removes the top linen and replaces it with a bath blanket to prevent the patient's bedding from getting wet. She places the basin, soap, washcloths and towels within easy reach of the patient and puts clothing, shaving articles and cosmetics in a convenient location. Body areas which the patient's disability prevents him from reaching are washed by the nurse or nurse's aides. For those bedridden patients who are unable to bathe themselves, the nursing staff assumes all of the responsibility for the bath and the after-bath care.

Water for a bed bath is drawn into the basin at a temperature of from 44° C. to 46° C. (110° F. to 115° F.). Room temperature for bathing is kept near 22.2° C. (72°F.).

On a rehabilitation service it is a formidable responsibility of the nursing staff to insure the safety of the patients during these procedures. Many patients need to be lifted in and out of the tub. Their extremities, if paralyzed or paretic, must be moved for them. Washing skin which lacks sensation must be done with extreme caution regarding water temperature, soap or detergent employed, and friction of washing and drying. Those patients who are able to transfer independently still require careful supervision since the tub room can be a slippery and hazardous place. Those who need assistance in tranfers must receive it.

The bath also provides the nurse with the opportunity to instruct the patients on general skin cleanliness and care.

The Hair

The hair is exposed to the same dirt and oils as is the skin, in addition to receiving more oil from the sebaceous glands, and therefore should be washed as often. Dry hair may be treated with oils, such as pure castor oil, olive oil or mineral oil. Oily hair requires more frequent shampooing.

Various shampoos which are commercially available are satisfactory. Liquid and cream shampoos are more easily rinsed from the hair than bar soap. Detergents are more effective than soap when used with hard water. If there is any infestation by lice, such as *pediculus capitis,* a *pediculicide,* or *paraciticide,* may be used. Vinegar is employed for the removal of nits. In extreme cases, the hair may have to be shaved off.

Grooming, both daily and following washing, is important, particularly to female patients. The nursing staff on a rehabilitation service may have to comb, brush and set the hair of many of their patients who are unable to do so because of limitations imposed by their disability. Many hospitals have the services of a professional beautician and a barber for the male patients. Good grooming is not only a matter of health, but promotes feelings of well-being, self-worth and motivation in the patients.

The Nails

The rate of nail growth varies with the season of the year, the patient's age, and, in the case of an outpatient, his occupation. It also varies between families and sexes. The average rate of growth is approximately one millimeter per week. Fingernails grow more rapidly than do toenails, and nails of the right hand grow faster than those of the left.

The fingernails are trimmed by cutting or filing them in an oval shape. They are not trimmed too far down on the sides because of the possibility of injury to the cuticle or the skin around the nail. Hangnails are cut close to the skin and treated with an antiseptic if they leave a bleeding point. Toenails are cut straight to prevent them from becoming ingrown. Ingrown toenails are often caused by hosiery or shoes which are too tight. When they are trimmed, the lateral margins of the nail should lie beyond the distal part of the nail fold.

Since dirt which accumulates under the nails provides a medium for bacterial growth, this should be removed with a blunt instrument. Creams and oils may be applied to the nails to prevent dryness.

The Mouth

Mouthcare is provided for patient comfort as well as to prevent infection and the spread of disease. Treatment is given to maintain the mouth and teeth in a healthy condition, to prevent the gums from becoming dry and cracked, to prevent ulcerations and to prevent bacteria from resulting in oral infections.

Patients who are able to brush their teeth, rinse their mouths and provide general oral care for themselves can maintain their own cleanliness, although the nurse often must supervise these activities to insure regularity and correctness of procedure. Severely disabled patients who are unable to care for themselves must be cared for by the nursing staff. It is the nurse's responsibility to make certain that their teeth are brushed regularly, their mouths rinsed when needed, and their oral cavity, gums, lips, etc. kept moist, and that, in the case of children, fluoride is topically applied. Unusual odor and signs of decay are reported to the attending physician and/or the dentist.

For the disabled patient who can manage some dental care activities with orthotic devices, including electric toothbrushes, assistance is provided with such apparatus.

Many patients, particularly the elderly, wear dentures made of vulcanite or more expensive plastics. If the patient is unable to care for his own dentures, the nurse must do so for him.

The Eyes, Ears and Nose

The nurse can remove secretions from the eyes or discharge from the mucous membranes with water or a physiologic solution, and a clean washcloth or disposable tissues.

Wiping of the eyes is done from the inner canthus, or nasal corner, to the outer canthus, or temporal corner, to reduce the possibility of forcing the discharge into the area drained by the nasolacrimal duct.

The ears are washed and dried with a soft towel. Cotton swabs may be used to remove excess wax. An overexcess of wax should be reported to the physician.

Irrigation of the nose is contraindicated unless prescribed by a physician and gentle blowing through the nostrils by the patient is recommended as the best cleansing method. If the external nares, or nostrils, are encrusted with discharge, mineral oil can be applied for softening and removing of the crusts.

Elimination

Nurses are aware of the fact that effective physiologic functioning is partially dependent upon the excretion of body wastes. Patterns of defecation, or elimination from the bowels, and micturition, or voiding from the urinary bladder, vary between individuals. Most people defecate once per day when healthy, although twice and three times per day, or even per week is considered normal. Normality is more closely related to regularity and type of stool than to frequency of elimination.

The nurse should become familiar with her patients and maintain them on their regular schedule. Impacted fecal matter can present a variety of problems and should be avoided. The nurse is also alert to color, odor, consistency, shape, frequency, amount and the presence of blood, pus, mucous and parasites, and reports her observations to the physician. Patients who lack bowel control as a result of their disability must be given the opportunity to eliminate at regular intervals to prevent soiling. Pain during elimination, or excess, or little or no passing of gas may be important signs which the nurse reports to the medical staff.

Healthy adults excrete approximately one thousand to 1800 cc. of urine each twenty-four hour period, but this may vary depending upon activity, fluid intake, diet, climate and, in children, body weight. The more urine being produced, the more frequent will be the voiding. Nursing personnel observe the frequency, color, odor, amount and general appearance of the urine and report abnormalities to the physician. For those patients who lack sensation, or the ability to control their elimination, a habit pattern of regular voiding should be established by the nurse.

If a patient is able to ambulate he may use the bathrooms of his sleeping area, but should still be supervised by the nurse because of the possibility of falling on the hard surfaces in the room. If the patient needs assistance in transferring from wheelchair to toilet and back to the wheelchair, the nursing personnel provides such aid. Most rehabilitation patients require either assistance or supervision in toilet activities. For the patient who must remain in bed for an extended length of time, the use of a bedpan is essential. Bedpans are made of enamelware, Monel, plastic or nylon resin. The nurse or nurse's aide lifts the patient and places him on the bedpan and then folds the top linen back over him. She leaves bathroom tissue within convenient reach and following elimination removes the bedpan and provides the patient with soap and water to wash his hands. The contents of the bedpan are noted carefully for abnormalities. Some patients use commode chairs which are wheelchairs with open seats and a shelf, or holder under the seat on which the bedpan is placed.

For certain diseases, or as part of hospital routine, or as a periodic inspection, the physician requests that a patient's fluid intake and output be measured. This is the nurse's responsibility. She must record both variables in the patient's medical chart. In addition, when the laboratory requests samples of uring or feces the nurse must obtain them and forward them directly to the technicians for study.

Another responsibility of the rehabilitation nurse is *catheterization*.

This is the introduction of a catheter, or tube, into the bladder for purposes of removal of urine.

In a general hospital, catheterization may be performed to obtain a sterile sample for laboratory study, to remove urine following surgery because the patient cannot void due to lack of muscle tone resulting from sedation or manipulation, to remove urine when it is inadvisable for the patient to void, to insure complete emptying of the bladder prior to surgery or delivery, to prevent bed-wetting in the incontinent pateint, or to remove urine from a greatly distended bladder.

The catheter is made of rubber, glass, metal, woven silk or synthetic fiber. The size depends upon the patient and the purpose (s) to which the catheter will be put. The most frequently employed catheters are made of rubber or synthetic material.

In rehabilitation, many patients with hemiplegia secondary to a cerebrovascular accident, paraplegia and quadriplegia due to spinal cord lesions, multiple sclerosis and other disabilities and diseases cannot void properly and require the use of an *indwelling,* or *retention catheter* which remains in the bladder for long periods of time to keep it empty. The most frequently employed indwelling catheter is probably the *Foley catheter* which empties the bladder into a recepticle such as a glass bottle or plastic bag.

The nurse must constantly make certain that the catheter is in place, is not leaking and is not blocked by any matter. She also checks the collecting device frequently and empties or changes it when it is full if the patient cannot do this for himself. Part of her duties involves teaching the able patient to insert, remove, clean and generally manage his own catheter.

PREVENTIVE NURSING

Prevention of Deformities

The rehabilitation of any patient must begin with the utilization of methods designed to prevent contracture deformities, since these can seriously hinder progress. The nurse must apply effective posture technics and the principles of body alignment to correct positioning of the patients. Mechanical aids, such as slings, bedboards, footboards, pillows and sandbags are used to position the patient properly and to prevent foot drop, wrist drop, "claw" hand, "frozen" shoulder, and other deformities. The nurse can initiate simple preventive exercises for the maintenance of muscle tone as well as programs of self-care activities.

Prevention of Decubitous Ulcers

Constant vigilance is required on the part of the nursing staff if decubiti, or pressure sores, are to be prevented. Once a decubitus occurs, a long period of treatment and inactivity may follow which can prevent a patient from participating on a rehabilitation program. Efforts must be directed towards relieving pressure on body areas, particularly those which lack normal sensation and which are common sites of pressure, such as the back, buttocks, hips, heels and elbows.

Patients who cannot turn themselves in bed must be turned by the nurse from side to side and from pronation to supination every two hours in each twenty-four hour period. In addition, daily bathing, application of alcohol and powder, use of foam rubber or liquid-filled pillows, pads and mattresses, inspection of braces for areas of friction against the body, proper amounts of protein in the diet, washing and changing of urinary devices, changing of bedclothes, prevention of moisture on the skin and daily observation of patients are all employed by the nursing staff in their efforts to prevent decubiti.

The Use of the Tiltboard

Placing a patient in the upright position has several values. It enables a paralyzed patient to assume the erect position, prevents contracture deformities and prevents deconditioning effects due to prolonged bed rest, such as loss of muscle tone, calculi, urinary infection, interference of peripheral vascular circulation and decubiti. The nurse bears the primary responsibility for use of the tiltboard on the patient floors.

ASSISTING THE REHABILITATION TEAM
Assisting the Physician

The nurse has many responsibilities connected with her role as an aide to the physician. In the physical examination of the patients, she prepares them, assists the physician in his procedures, positions the patients and cares for the apparatus which is used during the examination.

As an extension of the physician on the floor or ward, the nurse takes each patient's temperature daily, as well as periodically measuring pulse rate, blood pressure and weight, and observing respiration. Her measurements are recorded in the medical charts, and abnormalities or changes are promptly reported to the physician. Upon receiving a prescription for medication, the nurse must obtain the drug (s) and make certain that the medication is administered exactly as prescribed. Adverse side reactions are charted and reported to the physician prior to further drug administration.

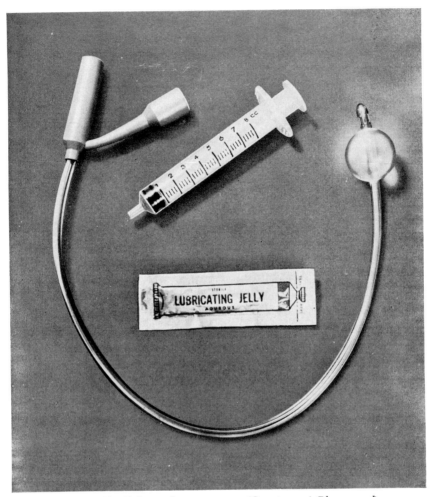

FIGURE 100. Foley catheter system. (*Courtesy of Pharmaseal*)

Several patients on a rehabilitation service may have a special diet prescribed for them because of particular disease which they have—e.g., diabetes mellitus. The nurse is responsible for checking each patient's food tray to ascertain that the hospital's dietary service has followed the physician's orders and that each patient receives the food prescribed for him. Not only is proper diet essential to good health, but, in many cases, eating the incorrect foods can be harmful and even dangerous for the patient.

Assisting the Physical Therapist

A physical therapist often may believe it desirable for a patient to practice ambulation outside of the actual physical therapy gymnasium. The best place for this activity to be performed is on the patient's own

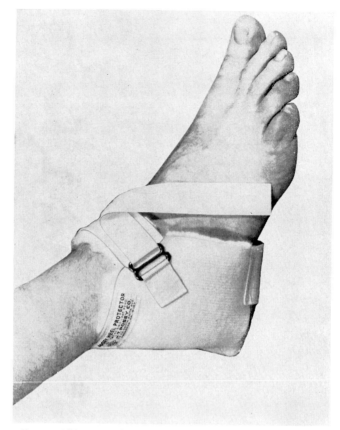

Figure 101. Foam heel protector. (*Courtesy of Posey Co.*)

floor or ward where he can be supervised and assisted by nursing personnel. Upon order from the physical therapist and attending physician, the nurse will arrange a schedule of ambulation for the patient. She will walk with him, either only observing, or actually assisting him, and will follow the therapist's instructions regarding rate, distance, length of ambulation time and correction of gait pattern abnormalities.

In addition, the nurse will help patients put on and take off protheses, stump socks, bandages and braces, while following the therapist's directions concerning training the patients to become independent in these tasks.

Assisting the Occupational Therapist

Since one problem which is often met with among rehabilitation patients is failure to generalize what they have learned in therapy to other situations, the nurse can be a vital extension of therapy. A great many of the activities of daily living are performed in the patient's bed area, such as transferring, eating, grooming, washing and dressing. The nurse assists the occupational therapist by following her instructions regarding supervising or assisting the patients in these activities. She also aids the patient in the use of orthotic devices and in generally encouraging independence.

One important way in which the nurse assists other members of the rehabilitation team is by making certain that patients arrive at their therapy sessions on time and ready for treatment. On a rehabilitation service many patients must be either assisted, or lifted out of bed, and placed in a wheelchair or on a stretcher. Usually, one, or at most, two staff members can help the patient, but in the case of a patient who is unable to move himself and must be totally lifted, two, three and sometimes, four persons, depending upon the size and weight of the patient, must work in getting him out of bed. The use of a mechanical or hydraulic lifter greatly simplifies the task, but great care must be taken to avoid injury to the patient in placing him in the lifter, raising him up, positioning him over the wheelchair seat and gently settling him down into the chair.

In addition to getting the patient out of bed, the nursing staff must see to it that the patient is properly dressed, has completed his necessary toilet activities, has with him the orthotic and/or prosthetic devices he will need in therapy, and goes to his treatment classes at the correct time. If a patient is physically or psychologically unable to get to his therapy sessions, one of the nursing personnel must take him and, upon completion of therapy, retrieve him and bring him back to his bed area or take him to his next class. Nurses have their patients' therapy schedules at the nurse's station and must adhere to them if the patients in their charge are to receive full benefit from a rehabilitation program.

The nurse reports at team conferences, such as the initial evaluation conference and the periodic re-evaluation meetings. Her report on the patient's physical condition, complaints, eating and sleeping habits, independence in daily activities, motivation, relationships with staff and other patients, unusual behaviors, cooperation, ambulation, communication skills and apparent family relationships has much meaning for all of the rehabilitation professionals. Since the nursing staff sees the patient for more time than do the other team members, she is able to impart a great deal of valuable information which others are not in a position to observe.

THE NURSE AND THE PATIENT'S FAMILY

One of the most important functions which the rehabilitation nurse performs is that of providing the patient and his family with information which is pertinent to the patient's condition, progress and continuing care.

While the initial explanation of a patient's disability and its probable, or known, etiology and prognosis is provided to the family by the physician, it is the responsibility of the nurse to ascertain if they are aware of what to expect when they first visit the patient in the hospital. In rehabilitation medicine, where the disabilities of patients are often severe, fear becomes a variable in the attitude of the patient's family which the nurse must deal with. Aside from the fear engendered by a diagnostic report, families can be frightened by seeing wheelchairs, stretchers, braces, Stryker frames, water mattresses, prosthetic limbs, orthotic devices and assistive breathing apparatus. They may experience fear upon first seeing the patient himself. The loss of one or more limbs in the amputee, drooling and obvious paralysis in the stroke patient, spasms in the patient with a spinal cord injury and tremors in the patient with multiple sclerosis, to give but a few examples, all arouse emotional feelings. Many questions may arise during an initial visit with a patient which the physician did not answer and it is the nurse's duty to meet with the family prior to their visit to prepare them for what they will see, and again, following their visit, to answer the questions which have developed from their experience.

With additional visits, the nurse informs the family regarding the patient's progress. Telling them that the patient is "doing well", or is "just fine" will not suffice. The family's questions must be answered and their anxieties allayed as much as possible. Just as the patient needs support, so does his family. The nurse must be realistic without being pessimistic. She must be positive without giving false hope. She must also know when to refer the family to the physician when questions arise which are beyond her scope or responsibility to answer.

The nurse's station is the central repository for information about the patient. The nurse, therefore, is in the best position to provide the family with information regarding other hospital services and other professionals they might consult or speak with in order to gain a complete picture of the treatment their family member is receiving. She can also refer the family to literature which can explain to them changes in behavior patterns of the patient which may have resulted as a consequence of his disability, so that they can gain a fuller understanding of him in his present stage of rehabilitation.

Prior to the discharge of a patient who will require additional care at home, the nurse explains to the members of the family the procedures which must be carried out by them. Techniques for preventing decubiti and contractures, for changing and irrigating catheters, for assisting the patient in ADL, etc. are all described carefully and in detail, and questions regarding these procedures are answered accurately and thoroughly.

The nurse, then, eases the transition for the family from the home to the rehabilitation hospital and then to the home again.

A LAST WORD ON REHABILITATION NURSING

There is more to good nursing care than the mechanics of the daily routine. There is also compassion, empathy and understanding. While these intangibles hold true for all hospitalized patients, they are particularly important in rehabilitation where a great many of the patients are totally or partially dependent for personal care, or lack the ability to communicate their needs and wants.

The nurse must never permit the patients to see that she feels her work is a chore, or that she is put upon, or annoyed by having to do so much for them. No one dislikes the patients' forced dependence more than the patients themselves, and they are usually very willing to do whatever they can for themselves without having to constantly rely upon others. The good rehabilitation nurse is aware of this and responds promptly, maintaining a cheerful manner and an empathic attitude.

Patients do not want pity, but they do need understanding. By permitting the aphasic patient to take time to express himself, by not complaining when she must help a paraplegic patient to dress himself, by showing a real willingness to comb the hair of a quadriplegic patient, by exhibiting graciousness with the hemiplegic who is incontinent, by having patience when teaching an amputee to put on his stump sock, or a patient with a hip fracture to ambulate, by being pleasant with the family of a child with a neuromuscular disease—these are the ways in which a rehabilitation nurse truly fulfills her role as a helper of the disabled. This is how she can be of most service to those who are in such need.

Section VII

References

1. Barbata, Jean C., Jensen, Deborah M. and Patterson, W. G.: *A Textbook of Medical–Surgical Nursing.* New York, Putnam. 1964.
2. Beland, Irene L.: *Clinical Nursing. Pathophysiological and Psychosocial Approaches,* 2nd ed. New York, Macmillan, 1970.
3. Brown, Esther L.: *New Dimensions of Patient Care.* Part III: *Patients as People.* New York, Russell Sage Foundation, 1964.
4. Brunner, Lillian S., Emerson, C. P. Jr., Ferguson, L. K. and Suddarth, Doris S.: *Textbook of Medical–Surgical Nursing,* 2nd ed. New York, Lippincott, 1970.
5. Dison, Norma G.: *An Atlas of Nursing Techniques.* St. Louis, Mosby, 1967.
6. Fuerst, Elinor V. and Wolff, LeeVerne: *Fundamentals of Nursing. The Humanities and the Sciences in Nursing,* 3rd ed. Philadelphia, Lippincott, 1964.
7. Gragg, Shirley H. and Rees, Olive M.: *Scientific Principles of Nursing,* 6th ed. St. Louis, Mosby, 1970.
8. Isler, Charlotte: *The Nurse's Aide in the Hospital.* New York, Springer, 1968.
9. Jensen, Deborah M. (Ed): *Principles and Technics of Rehabilitation Nursing,* 2nd ed. St. Louis, Mosby, 1961.
10. Johnston, Dorothy, F.: *Total Patient Care. Foundations and Practice,* 2nd ed. St. Louis, Mosby, 1967.
11. Jokl, E.: *The Scope of Exercise in Rehabilitation.* Springfield, Thomas, 1964.
12. Kelly, Cordelia: *Dimensions of Professional Nursing.* New York, Macmillan, 1962.
13. Larson, Carroll B. and Gould, Marjorie: *Calderwood's Orthopedic Nursing,* 6th ed. St. Louis, Mosby, 1965.
14. Mead, S.: Rehabilitation. In Cowdry, E. V. (Ed): *The Care of the Geriatric Patient,* 2nd ed. St. Louis, Mosby, 1963.
15. Morrissey, Alice B.: *Rehabilitation Nursing.* New York, Putnam, 1951.
16. *Mosby's Comprehensive Review of Nursing,* 7th ed. St. Louis, Mosby, 1969.
17. Nordmark, Marilyn T. and Rohweder, Anne W.: *Science Principles Applied to Nursing.* Philadelphia, Lippincott, 1959.
18. Rinehart, Elna L.: *Management of Nursing Care.* New York, Macmillan, 1969.
19. Roper, Nancy: *Principles of Nursing.* London, Livingstone, 1967.
20. Rusk, H.: *Rehabilitation Medicine. A Textbook of Physical Medicine and Rehabilitation,* 2nd ed. St. Louis, Mosby, 1964.
21. Shafer, Kathleen N., Sawyer, Janet R., McCluskey, Audrey M. and Beck, Edna L.: *Medical–Surgical Nursing,* 4th ed. St. Louis, Mosby, 1967.
22. Smith, Dorothy W. and Gips, Claudia D.: *Care of the Adult Patient. Medical–Surgical Nursing,* 2nd ed. Philadelphia, Lippincott, 1966.
23. Smith, Genevieve: *Care of the Patient With a Stroke.* New York, Springer, 1959.
24. Sutton, Audrey L.: *Bedside Nursing Techniques in Medicine and Surgery.* Philadelphia, Saunders, 1964.

INDEX

A

topographic involvement, 49
 hemiplegia, 49
 paraplegia, 49
 quadriplegia, 49
 triplegia, 49
course of, 50, 51
hearing loss in, 49, 50
intellectual deterioration in, 50
kernicterus in, 50
learning difficulties in, 50
problems in, 47
seizures in, 49
sensory losses in, 50
speech defects in, 50
types of, 47
 acquired, 47
 congenital, 47
visual impairment in, 50
Cerebral palsy speech and language disorders, 339–347
 evaluation of, 343, 344
 breathing, 343, 344
 oral language development, 344
 speech, 343
 voice, 344
 of articulation, 340, 341
 of language development, 340
 of respiration, 341, 342
 therapy for, 344–347
 breath control, 345
 language, 346, 347
 relaxation, 345
 phonation and articulation, 345, 346
 voice, 346
Cerebrovascular accident (Stroke), 7, 8
Character disorders (*see* Personality disorders)
Childhood aphasia, 324–326, 331–337
 accompanying handicaps, 325
 characteristics of, 325, 326
 congenital *vs* acquired, 325
 diagnosis of, 325
 etiology of, 324
 therapy for, 331–337
 general principles of, 331, 332
 techniques of, 335–337
 for auditory verbal recognition, 336
 for formulation, 336, 337
 for naming, 335
 for visual verbal recognition, 335, 336
Childhood dysarthria, 326, 327, 337–339
 definition of, 326
 etiology of, 326, 327
 exercises, 337–339
 goals of, 337

speech in, 327
symptoms of, 327
therapy for, 337–339
Childhood dyslalia, 326
Childhood schizophrenia (*see* Psychotic disorders)
Chronic back pain, 16, 17
Chronic brain syndrome (*see* Brain disorders)
Chronic undifferentiated schizophrenia (*see* Psychotic disorders)
Classical psychoanalysis, 449, 450
Client-centered psychotherapy, 448, 449
Conductive hearing loss, 356–358
 causes of, 356
 atresia, 356
 cholesteatoma, 357
 external otitis, 357
 impacted cerumen, 356, 357
 otitis media, 357
 otosclerosis, 357, 358
 symptoms of, 358
 paracusis willisiana, 358
 tinnitus, 358
Conductive heating, 147, 148, 150
 heating pad, 147, 148
 hot packs, 148
 hydrocollator, 148
 Kenny wool, 148
 moist, 148
 hot water bottle, 148
 paraffin, 148, 150
Congenital amputations (*see* Congenital limb deficiencies)
Congenital limb deficiencies, 44, 45
 causes of, 44
 congenital amputations, 45
 acheiria, 45
 adactylia, 45
 amelia, 45
 apodia, 45
 phocomelia, 45
 rehabilitation goal, 45
 skeletal imperfections, 44, 45
 intercalary deficiencies, 45
 terminal deficiencies, 45
Conversion reaction (hysteria) (*see* Psycho-neurotic disorders)
Conversive heating (diathermy), 165–169
 microwave diathermy, 169
 apparatus and dosage, 169
 indications and contraindications, 169
 physiologic effects, 169
 short wave diathermy, 165–168
 apparatus, 166